# THE UNIVERSAL LAWS OF HEALING

## THE CONTRAST BETWEEN HEALERS AND PRETENDERS

C. C. Wilcher, D.C., N.D.,
F.I.A.C.A., D.N.B.H.E.

LEGENDARY PUBLISHING COMPANY
Boise, Idaho

ISBN 1-887747-28-1

Library of Congress Catalog Card Number: 99-71834

Published by:

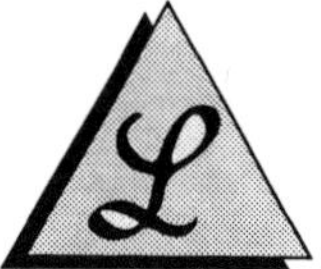

LEGENDARY PUBLISHING COMPANY

P.O. Box 7706

Boise, Idaho 83707-1706

U.S.A.

No other book has attempted to explore the world's major systems of healing in such depth, with such understanding and with as many correlations as this text does.

*The Universal Laws of Healing* documents the basic laws of each system of healing, its history, how each overlaps and complements the others, when each conflicts with the others, what is unique about each system and its relative strengths and weaknesses.

The text is actually a library of five books. The first, or Freshman, text is the introductory section written in very basic terminology. Each succeeding book — the Sophomore, Junior, Senior and Post-Doctoral texts develop the basic concepts to higher and more inter-related levels of understanding and incorporates more technical terms.

This unique book also discusses, in easily understood terminology, the quantum (energy and anti-matter) components of healing and the changes that must be implemented in standard double-blind research protocols in order to obtain valid data regarding the quantum and anti-matter components of healing.

Regardless of your education level, this insightful book will produce a paradigm shift in your understanding of healing.

## *What Others Are Saying About* THE UNIVERSAL LAWS OF HEALING:

"Dr. Wilcher receives rave reviews from our students. They expect the Sahara, and discover eclectic Eden. . . . Explores Quantum Healing in a practical fashion while keeping a sense of wonder."

Ruth Haefer, C.M.T.
Director, Idaho School of Massage Therapy

". . . Provides a firm foundation in the governing laws while setting forth a comprehensive explanation of the efficacy of Quantum Healing. . . . Should be a required teaching text as it substantiates miracles we see daily in our practices with verifiable information and sound research."

Kenneth H. Koening, D.C., D.N.B.H.E., F.I.A.C.A.
Executive Director, National Board of Homeopathic Examiners

"Quantum Healing is the medicine of the 21st Century! If you want to understand it, in a down-to-earth manner, this book is for you."
Judith Allen, R.N., M.Ed., M.B.A.

"Dr. Wilcher was one of my teachers . . . With his background, in Ayurvedic, Chiropractic, Homeopathy, Naturopathy, Oriental Medicine, etc., . . . he is able to integrate his knowledge and present eclectic insights. His book proves to be just as enlightening . . ."
L. (Ruth) Harrison, M.D., D.N.B.H.E.

". . . An incredible achievement . . . Each healing art has some of the laws but now one volume contains their collective wisdom . . . This books needs to be read by every healer . . ."

Daniel P. Towle, B.S., D.C., D.N.B.H.E.
President, Chiropractic Academy of Homeopathy

". . . A 'gold mine' for those looking for updated informative material. It is a modern, easily understood approach . . . a 'MUST HAVE' reference work."

Robert S. Hoye, C.R.Ph., F.A.C.A., D.N.B.H.E.

"Each patient must be evaluated as an individual, recognizing unique symptoms and characteristics which are the guide to proper care. This book has greatly influenced how I practice acupuncture, homeopathy and physical therapy . . ."
Simone R. Speyer, P.T., A.P., D.N.B.H.E.

". . . A one-stop source for understanding Quantum Healing. The systematic layout and progressive texts make what could be very difficult reading one of pleasure and delight . . ."

Edwin C. Floyd, M.S., D.C., D.A.C.B.N., D.N. B.H.E.
Chancellor, Quantum International University

"I am aware of the materials presented . . . and find the teaching method to be understandable on any level that the student may find him or her self."

Glen C. Mahoney, D.O., M.D., N.D., D.D.

". . . Clearly delineates the quantum components which are rapidly becoming an integral part of techniques incorporated by Social Workers, Counselors, Psychologists and Doctors in identifying the 'true' picture of the 'total' individual."

Kathy Green, M.A., L.P.C.P.

# DEDICATION

This book is dedicated to the sick and suffering of the world and to the eternal student of quantum, vitalistic, expansionistic healing who believes, recognizes and lives according to the laws of healing and the code that there, "... Is a true joy in life, the being used for a purpose recognized by yourself as a mighty one; the knowledge that you are a part of the force of nature instead of a feverish selfish little clod of ailments and grievances complaining that the world will not devote itself to making you happy."

And to those who believe as George Bernard Shaw, "I want to be thoroughly used up when I die, for the harder I work the more I live. I rejoice in life for its own sake. Life is no 'brief candle' to me. It is a sort of splendid torch which I have got hold of for the moment, and I want to make it burn as brightly as possible before handing it on to future generations."

# CONTENTS

# FOREWARD

It appears that about every one hundred years human beings take a reflective look at where we are in our progress of evolving as a race. We take this time, by innate instinct, to review our scheme of acquiring, developing and implementing the knowledge and skills we have gained. The result of this introspective period often brings an introduction, or more accurately a reintroduction, of ideas that have become more accepted due, in part, to technological advances which have occurred over the past one hundred years.

I'm not sure if the statement "**May you live in interesting times**" is a blessing or a curse. The close of each century is a time to reflect upon this. The end of each hundred-year period provides a reflective time that builds upon the previous periods, advancements and strides. After one thousand years (a millennium) mankind has had ten such periods of reflection, modification, adaptation and implication of the results of his new ways of thinking and with each hundred years, the reflective process is enhanced by more and more history. By the close of a millennium, those fortunate enough to be alive at that critical time are indeed living in **most interesting times with respect to changes in their world**.

Although every area of our existence has been impacted by this passage of time, no area has been more dynamically impacted than that of the community of health and healing. A look back on the past two centuries allows us to see these changes quite vividly.

About two hundred years ago, in the late 1790s, a German-trained physician by the name of Samuel Hahnemann introduced to the medical community a new and different approach to healing which he called "Homeopathy". This new approach to healing was centered around the vitalistic premise that all living creatures are animated by an energy which is intelligent and is found throughout the universe. Up to this time, talk of a universal intelligence was only spoken of within the realm of the church. Any talk of a universal intelligence or energy outside of the church was considered to be blasphemy, sacrilegious and even witchcraft.

In the early 1800s, Dr. Hahnemann introduced to the medical community his treatise on this new approach to health and healing. In his book, Dr. Hahnemann covers a vitalistic or energetic cause of dis-ease and introduces a vitalistic or energetic way of addressing this cause. He further documented ways in which to examine the patient as well as ways in which the patient should live in order to prevent further reoccurrence of dis-ease. The title of his book was the *Organon of Rational Medicine*. The word "Rational" created such a stir throughout the medical community that Hahnemann was forced to change the title.

About one hundred years later, Dr. D. D. Palmer introduced to the world his book outlining a further developed approach to delivering a vitalistic application to the cause of dis-ease. By this time the vitalistic banner that had been carried by the homeopathic physician was beginning to falter under the growing disagreement as to the proper application of homeopathy and the increasing number of homeopathic physicians who were abandoning the vitalistic healing approach and adopting the ease and comforts of reductionistic medical application. In his book, Dr. Palmer outlined his new healing art which he called "Chiropractic". This new health care profession took custody of the vitalistic banner that had been advocated by the homeopathic community. By the end of the World Wars, the chiropractic physician had pretty much become the major vitalistic health care professional in the United States. Up until the 1950s, when World War II and the Korean conflict ended, chiropractic was a profession grounded in vitalistic philosophy.

After the wars ended, medics and corpsmen returned to the United States and were welcomed back with the G.I. Bill. This bill allowed for the subsidy of education of veterans. It was a boon to chiropractic schools as it saved many from closing their doors. While the G.I. Bill was a very good thing in many ways for the chiropractic colleges it also played a significant role in ending the era of vitalistic chiropractic. As the G.I.s entered chiropractic colleges they brought with them the reductionistic philosophy of allopathic medicine they had learned in the military; and, as these students graduated and entered practice and the politics of the chiropractic profession, the vitalistic mission of chiropractic shifted to a mission of obtaining equality with reductionistic medicine. From the 1950s to the present, the chiropractic profession has been steadily building a reductionistic model of physical medicine which now more than ever has the doctor of chiropractic competing for patients with the physical therapist.

Today we are in the midst of a health care crisis. The reductionistic approach of allopathic medicine has pretty much failed and is increasingly being perceived as impotent in its ability to address today's health care demands. Vitalism and the vitalistic approaches to health, long dismissed by the established medical community as quackery, are now being revisited and are experiencing a great resurgence. Much of the resurgence of vitalism has been and is being fueled by the developments and deeper understanding of the insights found in quantum physics.

This book is written by one of the finest vitalistic minds of our age. As we draw to the close of another one-hundred-year and one-thousand-year period, it is very fitting that this book by Dr. Wilcher appears at this time of reflection. Dr. Wilcher's book is unlike the preceding books mentioned in this foreword.

Dr. Hahnemann's Organon was an introduction to a particular application of the vitalistic healing art which he termed "Homeopathy". Dr. Palmer's text, one hundred years later, introduced another application of the vitalistic healing art which he termed "Chiropractic". Dr. Wilcher does not strive to introduce a particular style of therapeutic application but, rather, attempts to present a comprehensive introduction to vitalistic healing in all of its applications. Rather than attempting to assist the reader to become a specific type of doctor, i.e., an acupuncturist, a homeopath, a chiropractor, etc., Dr. Wilcher attempts to assist the reader to think in the vitalistic mode. His goal is for this work to serve as textbook for the eclectic student and "Quantum Physician".

I am convinced that this book will become the classic standard of required reading for generations of quantum physicians to come. It is my hope that the following reading comforts and empowers all who are truly committed to the pursuit of vitalistic life, health and healing.

Edwin C. Floyd, M.S., D.C., D.N.B.H.E.
Chancellor/President
Quantum International University
Beverly Hills, CA, U.S.A.
October, 1996

# ACKNOWLEDGMENTS

**To my loving family, and especially my dear wife and office nurse, Pamela, for giving their father and husband the time to meditate and work and for providing suggestions for the creation of this eclectic, bio-dynamic, vitalistic textbook. Also, for their patience and proofreading. No person could have a more devoted and inspiring family with whom to meet the challenges of life. To my son Benjamin who did most of the computer generated graphics found in this textbook.**

Among the many who deserve mention for the stimulus and encouragement they gave me to write this book is Dr. Edwin Floyd, President of the Quantum International University. Few have a better understanding of the philosophy, art and science of eclectic, bio-dynamic, vitalistic healing. His suggestions in refining the concepts and wording of the universal laws taught in this text are greatly appreciated.

Suggestions, data, ideas, encouragement, reference articles and review of the text also have been received in large measure from Dr. Daniel Tole, President of The Chiropractic Academy of Homeopathy and Editor of *The Prover: The Journal Of The Academies Of Homeopathy.*

To those authors, listed in the references, who came before my time and had the courage, conviction and took the time to write text books and articles containing such golden nuggets of wisdom as the specific universal laws dealing with each of their disciplines. The laws that they taught me were the genesis of my understanding of true healing.

To my office manager, Shawn Leyba, who had the patience to endure my constant pre-occupation during the years that it took to envision, organize and write this textbook.

Nor can I forget the students and graduates of the institutions for which I have and currently do teach. Their obvious need for such a definitive volume was another prime motivational force.

Many other associates and professional friends have also had their subtle influences but space forbids mention of each and their specific contributions.

To J. A. DeCava, C.C.N., L.N.C., R. J. Hulbert, Ph.D., D. Knopp, Ph.D., and R. L. Wysong B. S., D.V.M. for their gracious permission allowing me to reproduce materials from their publications.

And above all to a kind, loving and guiding God who has inspired my mind to understand the universal laws of healing and who has allowed me to be able to teach them to others that I might leave this world little better place than I found it.

C. C. Wilcher, D.C., N.D., F.I.A.C.A., D.N.B.H.E.
Boise, Idaho
22 November, 1996

# BOOK I

# FRESHMAN TEXT

# INTRODUCTION TO THE FRESHMAN TEXT

*"Knowledge is proud that he has learned so much;*
*wisdom is humble that he knows no more."*

— Cowper

## THE NECESSARY FIRST STEP

When beginning any journey it is necessary to know our precise location.

It is also vital to have a clear understanding of exactly where we want to go. Equally important is to have confidence in the tools we choose to guide us and an ability to identify those circumstances that could cause these instruments to malfunction and lead us astray.

This is a different type of textbook. There currently is a smorgasbord of texts dealing with African, Allopathic, Ayurvedic, Chiropractic, Homeopathic, Massage, Native American and Oceanic, Naturopathic, Nutrition, Oriental, Psychology, Sufi, Quantum Healing, and other forms of healing. There is, however, a famine with regard to textbooks that organize the strengths and weaknesses of each of these disciplines into one coordinated entity. Because such an undertaking has never before been attempted on this scale, this work represents the culmination of *many* years of searching, studying, compiling of data, sifting, weeding, organizing, reflecting, discussing, unlearning, editing and deleting the 90 percent which is inadequate and maintaining and condensing the 10 percent which is the pure golden nuggets of healing knowledge.

Unfortunately, many of our so-called **educational institutions, instructors and practitioners of natural healing are in reality practicing and teaching reductionism which utilizes natural substances. They treat dis-ease A with herb B or adjustment C or acupuncture point D. Such a "cookbook" approach reveals their complete ignorance of the major distinction between sickness care and being a true healer.**

Compounding these challenges are the deficiencies of current-day medicine. Allopathic diagnosis employs techniques such as exploratory surgery, the administration of dyes followed by X-rays or chemotherapy and other dangerous drugs, all of which have a potential for harming the patient; and the more specialized these procedures become, the greater their potential risk factors. By far the greatest problem, however, is that these highly sophisticated, and extremely expensive, forms of diagnosis and treatment only consider the physical body and its pathology. **The patient's overall health status, the mental and emotional outlook, energy level, spiritual (non-corporal) composition, lifestyle, inherited strengths and weaknesses, likes and dislikes, and strange, rare and peculiar symptoms, physiology, etc., are overlooked and/or neglected** due to the pressures of academia, peer review and the medico-legal-politico-industrial complex.

These undesirable situations result in a nightmare of inadequate and/or improper treatment, medico-legal and ethical pitfalls. Not only does the patient suffer but so does the healer and society as a whole. The only viable answer is to educate ourselves to the scientific realities of both the corporal and non-corporal or quantum world. This requires a much more advanced method of thinking. We must be willing to abandon many long-cherished but inaccurate concepts regarding our universe, life, health and death. Herein lies the grand challenge. It is extremely difficult for us as individuals who envision ourselves as highly educated to realize and accept that our training has major shortcomings.

I invite you to put aside your preconceptions and come along on a wonderful and exciting journey through the pages of this book to a new and greater understanding of yourself, the sick and suffering, and the universe in which we exist.

# PRECONCEIVED IDEAS

Today, many students entering vitalistic professional training come from pre-med training. Unfortunately, this training is only oriented toward the limited, non-vitalistic, reductionistic, allopathic concept of dis-ease. While this is adequate for those wishing to become medical doctors, it is far from acceptable for those of us wishing to raise our healing consciousness beyond that most basic level. Therefore, the freshman text is designed to dramatically extend the student's education to the vast expanses of healing knowledge which was ignored and/or glossed over in most pre-medical programs.

This transition may require significant effort for some while others will find it less demanding. To a great extent, the degree of your individual struggle will reflect your total life experience, environment, cultural, spiritual belief system and intuitive understanding. Even if you have none of these vital factors currently in your favor, you can learn them. In fact, the desire to learn about the vitalistic, quantum (energy) aspect of healing supersedes all the other factors.

It is said that some are born with the gift of healing and, while this is likely true for a small percentage, the vast majority of vitalistic healers have arrived at their current understanding by old-fashioned hard work. Therefore, do not allow discouragement to lead you from your chosen path. With adequate study, reflection and role models, the reality of the laws of quantum healing will become second nature to you. In the final analysis, understanding is far more critical to your ultimate success as a vitalistic healer than your grade point average. Without a clear comprehension, you will be severely limited to that small spectrum which is encompassed within the reductionistic,  myopic concept of dis-ease, life and health. With a clear perspective, vast vistas open that will provide you an insight into the non-material aspects of the patient, your self, and the healing processes and the laws that govern the universe in which we live, move and have our being.

Best wishes as you move into a new perspective of life, health, dis-ease and your own awareness. **Your future is limitless.**

# Chapter 1
# THE NEW PERSPECTIVE

*"East is East and West is West,
And never the twain shall meet."*
— Rudyard Kipling

## FROM PARADIGM TO PARADIGM

We are accustomed to measuring our world, time, and our own being in miles, meters, feet, inches, tons, gallons and liters, A.M. or P.M., B.C. or A.D., spring or fall, historic or prehistoric, yesterday, tomorrow, minutes, hours; the feel of hot or cold, roughness or smoothness, a fragrant or carrion odor, light and darkness, happy or sad, aware or unaware; religious or atheistic, black or white. Everything seems to fit so well. Or does it?

Of all the various means we have to measure our physical reality, most of them cannot be used to measure energy and/or anti-matter. How do we measure electricity? Call the electric company and ask for two tons, or two miles or 1,000 gallons of electric energy? This cannot be done because energy does not interact in the same manner as solid state materials. The word energy comes from the Greek "energos" meaning active or quantum. Unlike the measurement of matter which provides us information in quantity, energy is measured in intensity. Therefore, it requires completely new units of measurement, ohms, watts, amps, etc. Can we measure sub-atomic components in ounces? Can we plot entities moving at faster than light speed in millimeters? Can we quantify distances within the universe in seconds? Can we understand anti-matter in grams? Can we quantify deity rough or smooth, fragrant or carrion? All require different means of measurement!

This is precisely what Einstein was referring to when he formulated his "2nd Law of Thermodynamics" which stated that we can neither create nor destroy anything, only change its form. To illustrate, it may take two men to carry in a 100-pound log but one small boy can carry out the ashes. Where did the rest of the log go? This 100-pound log has undergone a process that separated its physical parts from its energetic and anti-matter components and they can no longer be measured in length, circumference and weight. New units are required such as BTUs, lumens, gauss, joules, ohms, watts, amps, etc.

The same is true of a living being. The existence of all living beings is a combination of matter, energy and anti-matter. When addressing the physical component, we can apply all of the laws that have served us so well for so long, those of weight and mass, and so forth. The elements of the physical body conform nicely to the laws of solid state physics and molecular chemistry. However, the instant we begin **dealing with the energetic and anti- matter components of a living creature, all the laws we have utilized so successfully become inoperative. We are forced to master new laws and applications that operate in very different relationships.**

In order to successfully function in this new chaos (altered) context, we MUST progress from a linear to a non-linear mode of thinking. The one cause/one effect mentality *must* be abandoned for it is scientifically untenable within the energetic and/or anti-matter paradigm. The scientific reality of our quantum universe is that many causes can, and do, interact to produce a single effect.

If we erroneously try, as have allopathy, musculoskeletal chiropractic, reductionist naturopathy and others, to force application of solid state laws to quantum state situations, we are unable to scientifically reproduce quantum and/or anti-matter phenomena. It makes as much sense as speaking French to a person who only speaks Japanese. Yet this is precisely the error that reductionist thinking follows.

When their erroneous method fails to provide answers, they falsely assume the quantum and anti-matter components cannot exist and therefore are not scientific. This is the same rationale used for saying that it is unscientific for the small boy to be able to carry out the ashes from our 100- pound log.

Quantum healing teaches **that the solid state body without the quantum (the scientific term), innate (the Chiropractic term), vital force (the Homeopathic term), kundalini (the Ayurvedic term), num (the Kung [African] term), ch'i (the Oriental term), life force (the Naturopathic term), spirit (the Native American and Oceanic term), breath of life (the religious term) factor is nothing more than a rotting piece of meat. With the quantum factor, it is a self-repairing, self-perpetuating, living being. Therefore, it is impossible, regardless of credentials or degrees, to be a true healer without a mastery of the quantum components.**

## THE QUANTUM EXERCISE

When first encountered, this quantum shift is difficult to comprehend; like everything, it becomes easier with practice. This ability to shift is the indispensable basis for a comprehensive understanding of healing. Fortunately, there is an exercise that facilitates the development of this ability. Look at the illustration of the cube in Figure 1.1. Which side is facing you? At first, it may appear as if you are under the cube looking up at it. But if you take a second glance, you may feel as if you are on top of the cube looking down. Or it may seem as if you are looking at it from the left or the right side, or the front or even the back. As the observer, you have the choice of how you perceive the cube. But is it really a cube? Upon additional study, we realize that it is simply lines and angles on a flat surface. In reality, it is not a three-dimensional object at all.

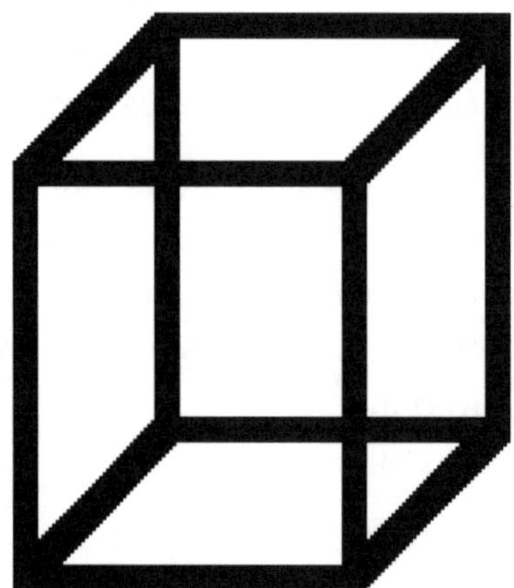

*Figure 1.1 — The Multidimensional Perspective of the Universe*

We now comprehend that there are at least seven different ways of perceiving the same object, none of which are any more correct or incorrect than the others. As the observer, you have the choice of how you will observe figure 1.1. **This does not, however, mean that the alternatives do not exist simply because you are**

**not able to observe them all simultaneously.** The living being exists in more than one plane or parallel universe at the same time. Western forms of healing view the patient only on the physical plane and totally ignore the quantum and/or anti-matter planes of the patient's health and being. As a result, western forms of healing can be only partially successful in their quest for health and healing.

Most doctors trained within the western thought (reductionist science) find it difficult to recognize the other planes upon which a living being functions. With such a limited, reductionistic, solid state philosophy in place, patients become mere machines and doctors become mere mechanics. They fail to comprehend that **every patient is a spiritual (non-corporal) being, exhibiting an energy potential, inhabiting a mechanical body that is stimulated electrically, reacts chemically but is controlled emotionally and possesses intellectual capacity.** In reality, these doctors may be trying to deal with only one-seventh of what constitutes the total being. Let us think about this from a mathematical point of view. If we deal with only one-half of what constitutes the total being, the best we can hope for is a 50 percent success rate; one-third, a 25 percent success rate; and  by the time we arrive at one-seventh, a 1.52625 percent success rate!

The enlightened healer cannot be comfortable with such statistics.  We therefore must begin to incorporate methods such as Homeopathy, Oriental Medicine and Acupuncture, Hypnosis, Sufi, Native American, African, Ayurveda, etc., as well as complementing the quantum healing arts with the advantages of the solid state forms of healing. The purpose of this text is to introduce and educate patients and practitioners of all healing arts to the multi-dimensional patient, quantum healing and vitalistic thinking.

## THE REDUCTIONIST THOUGHT

The Newtonian or western thought process revolves around the reductionistic thinking we have inherited from the ancient Greeks in which  problem solving is an elimination of possibilities until only one remains. The rationale is that what remains must be "the" cause. This is an extremely viable concept when dealing with mechanical things. In fact, it is what has made the western world excel in inventing and manufacturing.

An example of such reductionist thinking is as follows: If your automobile does not run, it could be because of problems with the fuel, electrical, or the mechanical system. We approach the problem thus: The vehicle is flooded and smells of gasoline so we assume the fuel system is functional; we turn the key and the starter motor turns over so we eliminate a potential electrical problem. This leaves something mechanical to be repaired. We have progressively reduced our problem to a single cause. This reductionistic thought process is illustrated in figure 1.2. It has, however, one inescapable deficiency which critically flaws its viability and credibility in the expansionistic universe in which we dwell. Reductionist solid state science is based upon and, therefore, bound by the material (reductionistic)laws.

Thus, according to its calculations, which are based upon this extremely limited understanding, it must conclude that all things in the universe are governed by the same restricted solid state laws. What is overlooked is that these limited solid state laws bind us to the limited solid state sphere which our reductionist educations have made us currently capable of comprehending.

**There are many things in the universe that function without the understanding of man. In other words, the universe functions in spite of limited human understanding and not because of it.**

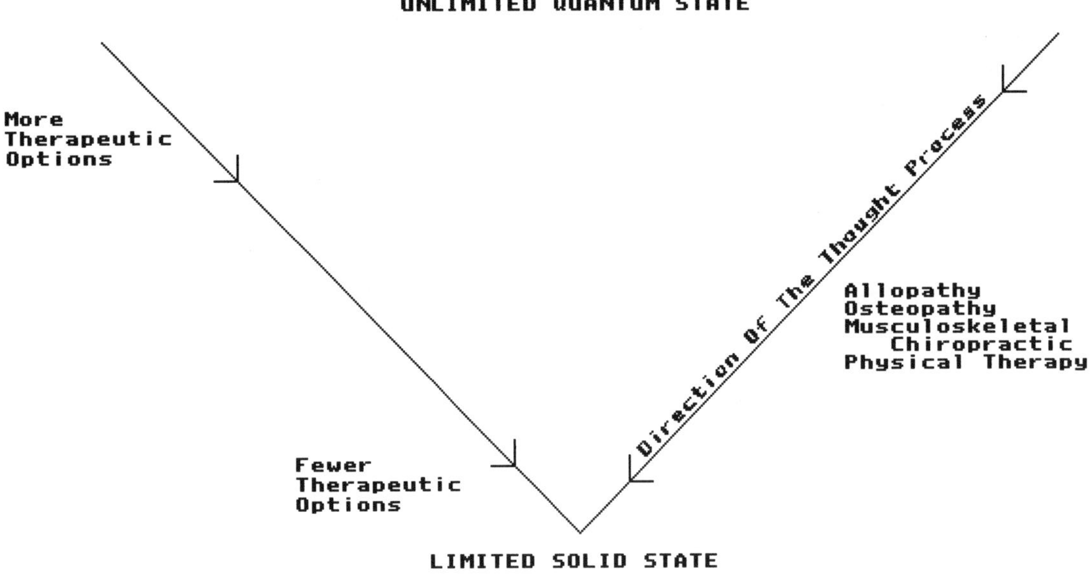



*Figure 1.2 — The Reductionistic Thought Process*

## EXPANSIONISTIC THOUGHT PROCESS

The alternate thought process is the expansionistic non-materialistic or quantum thought process and philosophy of the American Indian, the Oriental, the Ayurvedic, the African and other cultures which by Western standards have been considered to be "primitive" and "ethereal" in nature. **The problem- solving technique applied here is to expand the problem until all possible interactions are being considered and then deal with it as a unified entity - the "big picture" so to speak - to leave nothing out, to leave nothing to chance because we failed to consider all aspects on whatever plane of existence they happen to function,** as illustrated in Figure 1.3.

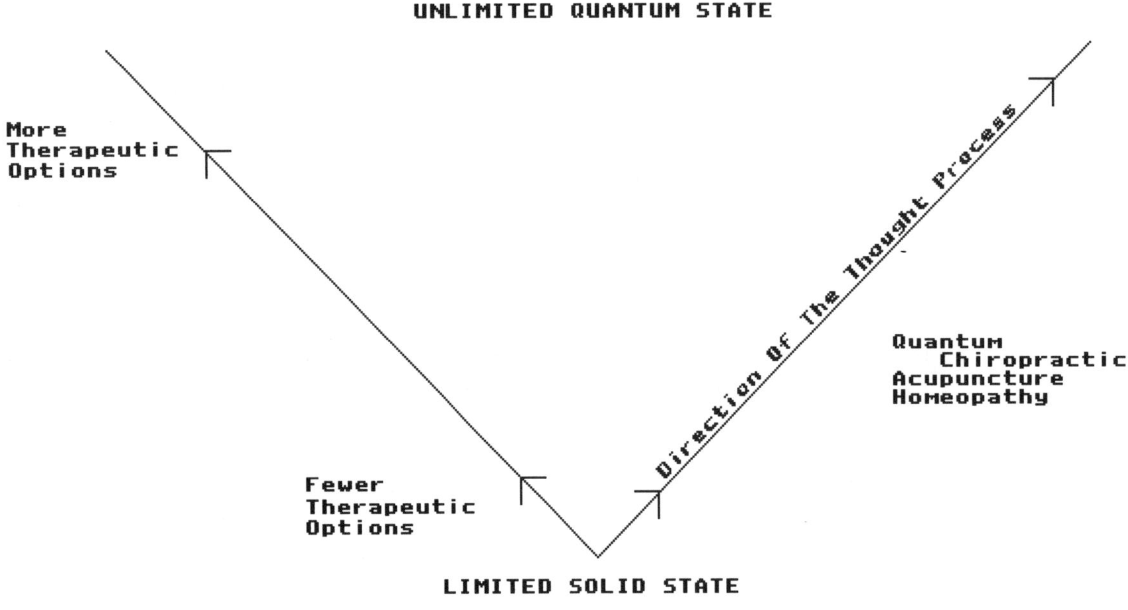



*Figure 1.3 — The Expansionistic Thought Process*

While this proves to be a cumbersome system when dealing with mechanical issues, its superiority is obvious when dealing with non-solid state factors such as the living being. For example, in Western medicine a patient is diagnosed as "Congestive Heart Failure". This gives the illusion that the problem is one of the heart only. But in reality, the heart may not even be the primary cause of the condition. The primary cause may be failure of the kidneys to eliminate fluids causing an excessive back pressure against the heart. Nor does this diagnosis acknowledge the fact that the lungs many be filling with this excess fluid much like a storm drain backing up causing the patient to drown in his own un-eliminated body fluids. But we must also consider how this physical condition is affecting the patient's energy level, his mental, emotional and spiritual functions. In the expansionistic concept, all these facets must be accounted for and dealt with simultaneously in order to have a viable answer.

## THE QUANTUM EXPERIENCE

There is an old adage, **"The only things you can count on are death, taxes and change."** The conflict between man's longing for a constant world and the reality that it is in constant change is as old as the race. The Egyptians, the Chinese and the Ayurvedics by 2,000 B.C. were discussing this principle. By 500 B.C., the Greeks debated it in attempts to explain the gods, spirit (non-corporal or anti-matter), matter and the human condition: **either all was one (constant) or all was change.**

Today, quantum mechanics and quantum physics accept the premise that the universe is in constant flux, expanding and changing moment by moment. Yet there is structure and order to this perpetual change. Each moment of flux is in direct proportion to the moment prior to it and the response is always the most desirable one. This observation leads to the conclusion that universal intelligence does not allow random change but, rather, permits order. Therefore, everything that exists in our ever-fluxing universe is required to react to these changes. This response is the universal principle known as adaptation: **For anything to continue to survive, it must adapt.**

## THE LAW OF ADAPTATION

Adaptation is a continuous process. It is never constant and unvarying as are other universal laws. Adaptation is a universal principle, the only one of its kind. It is the principle of change according to law. Universal, therefore, means covering all; unlimited; everywhere present; embracing a wide range of subjects; used for or among all; unrestricted in application; adapting to all. Adaptation being a universal law, it applies to all things including the healing arts.

## THE ENERGY PARADIGM

In the 19th and early 20th centuries, energy was regarded as the result of the motion of physical bodies (potential and/or kinetic energy). This was expressed in two supposed laws: 1) The Principle Of Conservation Of Mass, which stated that mass was indestructible, and 2) The Principle Of Conservation Of Energy, which stated that the sum total of energy in the universe was constant.

The reality of matter (mass) and energy being interchangeable was inconceivable. Of the two, matter was considered as the fundamental requirement to understand a supposedly Newtonian or mechanical model of the universe. But starting in 1905, Einstein forever shattered this overly simplistic idea by developing the concept that matter and energy are interchangeable. Thus, when matter sheds it mass and travels as light, it is energy. At greater than light speed, it is anti-matter. And, conversely, if anti-matter condenses or congeals, it becomes matter. Thus, the very foundation of all reductionistic, solid state, Newtonian "science" was proven to be inaccurate and, therefore, in desperate need of modification in order to comply with reality.

Energy is now considered to be the basic unit of all things in the universe. Nothing can exist without an energy template around which to organize itself. It is the medium that is responsible for and governs life.

We, as dense energy forms, live in a sea of energy and anti-matter which is always affecting us even if we are not consciously aware of it. It therefore makes scientific sense that quantum and anti-matter forms of healing should have even more profound effects upon our being than the solid state concepts that have been a part of traditional medicine; i.e., pharmacology, surgery, musculoskeletal massage and chiropractic, reductionist naturopathy, and others. Thus, to learn about and master the therapeutic use of these forms of healing is one of the primary goals of this text.

# THE LAW OF SUPERIOR POWER

**Nothing exists in and of itself and nothing exists by chance.** The law of superior power states there is always a source that creates, governs and allows all entities to exist. Do the laws of solid state chemistry and physics account for the beginnings of life and for its development? Living matter differs from inorganic matter in the fact that it has a far more complex structure, and in the fact that it grows and reproduces itself. A crystal structure enlarges by depositing layer upon layer but it cannot take food into itself and change it into vitalized nutrients as a living being can. This requires higher energy, num, vital, innate, life, ch'i. These laws are in effect while at the same time the lesser solid state laws continue to function.

This higher law of superior power forces us to accept the fact that there is far more to life than mere solid state chemistry and mechanics. It is what gives purpose and direction to life. It creates a tree, a bird or a man and then grows and repairs its creation according to an ideal plan. Out of common atoms, it organizes the various structures and functions. It plans, chooses, sorts, selects, directs, adapts, sees and reaches a distinct aim. See Figure 1.4.

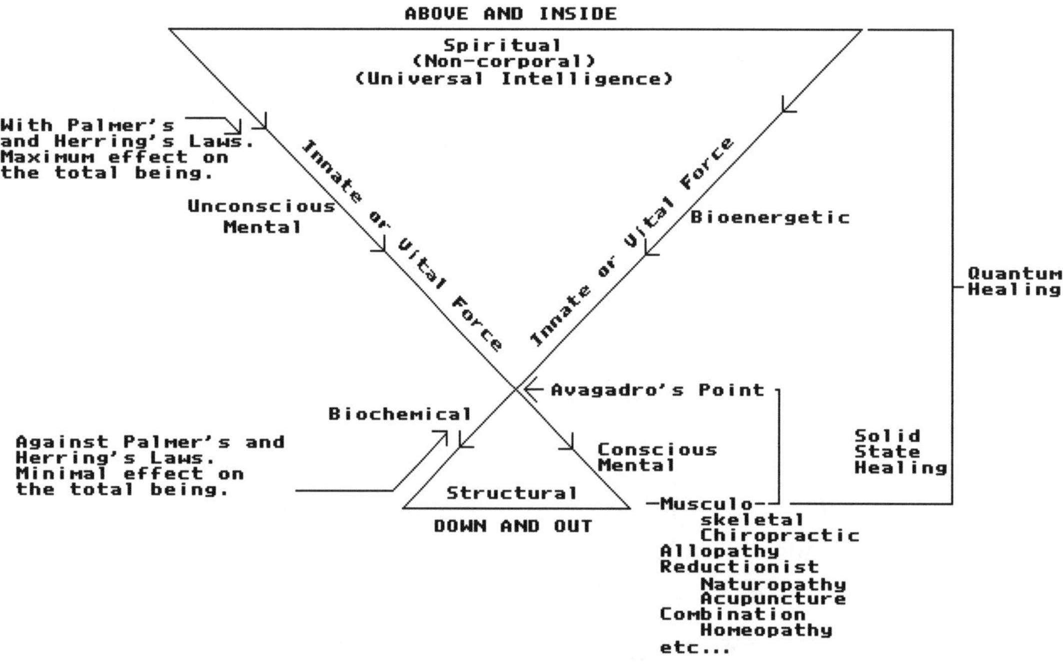


*Figure 1.4 — The Total Being*

# LAW OF LIFE = ENERGY

**There is *no* life without energy.**

It is equally true that life requires a two-way flow of energy which can take place only in a bipolar mechanism, such as a living being. Life cannot be a set polarity; the movement of energy would be only in one direction while life requires a two-directional flow. Otherwise there would be no communication between the various parts of the living organism. Energy, the life force, must meet the demands necessary for digestion following a meal or for walking, climbing stairs or hills, running, working, or to meet a hundred and one other daily survival requirements for a person to remain healthy.

The old reductionist, non-vitalistic, solid state concept teaches that life is controlled by the chemistry of the cell. This brings us to the source of cellular energy, which Dr. Alexis Carrel in his text *Man, The Unknown*, found to be the cells themselves. Otherwise, it would have been impossible for him to keep a chicken heart alive for 28 years. G. Crile, M.D., and W. Tiller, Ph.D., also documented how "the work of a cell depends on its capacity for oxidation" and that the oxidation in turn depends upon a subtle magneto-electric energy field.

This subtle magneto-electric field is the flame that keeps the chemical oxidative processes functioning in the cell. Because magneto-electricity (the electrical valances of the elements) controls chemistry and inter-molecular action, and since chemical action (oxidation) controls the production of magneto-electric energy, cells are independent entities. However, when cells form organisms there has to be a means for communication in order to coordinate the whole. Traditionally, the chiropractor has functioned on the premise that the nervous system exclusively performed this role; the oriental healer felt that the meridian (acupuncture) pathways alone performed this function; the osteopath, circulation; the allopath, chemistry. But, in the final scientific analysis, is energy independently created within a cell? **We cannot create or destroy anything, only change its form.** So what is the previous form from which cellular energy is derived?

Solar energy is trapped by and stored in vegetation and is released in living entities when the vegetation is consumed. The plants take dead, inorganic elements from the soil and transform them by biological transmutation into life-sustaining organic compounds. Yet this is not the complete answer to our inquiry. Two other phenomena require our attention.

Ultra-violet rays of the sun, for example, turn the oils of the skin into the D complex vitamins. The internal effect of the sun's rays upon body chemistry, however, isn't nearly as well understood. G. Wilson, D.C., documented that this subtle magneto-electric energy also affects the systemic acid-base balance of the living body. Additional research revealed that **a living being functions most efficiently in a mildly acid state.** Such a mild acidity has been found to decrease the resistance to neural and acupuncture meridian quantum energy flow.

It can thus be summarized that optimal life, health and vitality are a result of numerous factors. As Dr. Sakar  wrote in *Hahnemann's Organon With Commentary,* "The prevailing belief among the untrained is that any result may be explained by some single factor operating as a cause. They seem to have no comprehension of the fact that the cause of every result is made up of a combination of interacting factors, often in numbers and combinations that are absolutely bewildering to contemplate. This habit of considering only one factor when perhaps scores are involved, indicates a very primitive and untrained condition of the mind."

# THE ALL OR NOTHING LAW OF ADAPTATION

The old school Newtonians would have us believe that the living organism is nothing more than a complicated evolutionary machine and that each specialized part evolved through eons of time based upon the stimuli to which it was randomly exposed. Unfortunately, this theory does not take into consideration the fact that a living organism is a coordinate whole. **Dr. A. D. Speransky's extensive research, found in his textbook  *A Basis For The Theory Of Medicine,* repeatedly documented that a single change in any part of such a coordi-**

nated system is met by *simultaneous changes in all other parts* in order to process and accurately interpret the new data; otherwise, there is chaos and confusion rather than improvement and order. The mathematical possibility of these billions of changes (mutations) taking place simultaneously without an ordering principle is infinitely remote.

# Chapter 2
# WHAT IS HEALTH?

*"Without health, life is not life; it is only a state of
languor and suffering — an image of death."*
— Rabelais

## THE EXPERIMENT

Perform an experiment. Ask a number of your professional colleagues, **"What is health?"** You will find that no two have exactly the same answer. If we cannot agree on what health is, how can we know when the patient has achieved a state of health? How do we know that we aren't treating patients right through health and back into dis-ease again? Does this lack of agreement among practitioners mean that the patients have no diagnosable diseases? Does it mean that they have no unexplainable aches and pains? Does it mean that our patients are happy all of the time? Does this lack of agreement mean that our patients are not suicidal? Shouldn't health care providers know exactly what it is that we are striving for? Isn't health care supposed to be a consistently reproducible science? If we don't know what our goal is, or what to do to specifically achieve it, or even how to recognize it, what then do we have? It would appear that we have many theories (allopathy, chiropractic, naturopathic, oriental, ayurvedic, etc.), or guesses, and very little scientifically reproducible knowledge.

## THE MULTIPLE BEING

Before we can find answers to these questions it is necessary to review the true multi-leveled nature of our total being. As previously stated, we are basically **a spiritual (non-corporal) being, exhibiting an energy potential, inhabiting a mechanical body that is stimulated electrically, reacts chemically but is controlled emotionally and possesses intellectual capacity. Therefore, true health must cover, at the very least, all of these aspects.**

## THE ANSWER

George Vithoulkas, in his book *The Science Of Homeopathy*, provides a very workable definition of health. He states: **"Health is freedom from pain in the physical body, having attained a state of well-being: freedom from passion on the emotional level, having as a result a dynamic state of serenity and calm; and freedom from selfishness in the mental sphere, having as a result total unification with Truth."**

The first section of this definition is easily understood. **"Freedom from pain in the physical body"** is the basic underlying working principle of allopathic, dentistry, podiatry, musculoskeletal chiropractic, reductionist naturopathy, massage, physical therapy and most other western forms of medicine. Basically, if something hurts, cut it out, drug it, adjust it, ultrasound it, massage it, prescribe a herbal formula for pain relief, etc. When the pain is gone, the patient is considered to have "attained a state of well-being". Having achieved this goal of freedom from pain, any further care is unwisely considered to be "maintenance" because there is little or no knowledge of the higher levels of health discussed hereafter.

Let us now explore the second section of Vithoulkas' definition dealing with the next higher level of total health. **"Freedom from passion on the emotional level, having as a result a dynamic state of serenity and calm."** Probably the most internationally recognized example of this state of health in modern times is Mahatma Gandhi of India. Gandhi was a reserved and serene little man in a loincloth who changed the course of history. Yet, he did not do it by leading great armies, he did not do it by teaching people to hate. He did it with "serenity and calm". His dynamics brought the greatest military empire the world has ever known, the English Empire, to the conference table and won political freedom for his country. At all times, he was in complete control of himself and the situation. He did not permit passions to rule him but rather permitted himself to rule passions. One can truly say he was "healthy" at this higher and more vital level of his total being.

And lastly, **"freedom from selfishness in the mental sphere, having as a result total unification with Truth."** Children are an excellent example of this. If a parent takes a trip, what is the very first thing a child will ask of that parent upon his or her return? It's not, "How was your trip?" or, "How are you?" It's, "What did you bring *me*?" The difference between a mature adult and an immature child is the child is *me* (selfishly) oriented. The mature adult is others (service) oriented. Stratmann crystallizes this concept. To paraphrase his statement, **If we as individuals are to enjoy freedom or the ability to make choices that an adult is entitled to, then a necessary corollary of that right is that we *must* hold ourselves responsible for the results of those choices. One obvious answer to someone who says, "I am not responsible for my own actions" is, "Then you are not entitled to a full level of adult freedom, but only to that amount for which you can be held responsible."**

This brings us to "a total unification with Truth." This means becoming "one" or in harmony with universal intelligence, governing force, nature, deity or whatever other name we choose to call it. This entity serves us by governing our universe thereby making it possible for us to exist. As such, it is the source of all knowledge, laws, truth. When we live in unity with it, we also become service oriented in our lives. In other words, one of our major goals is to leave the world a better and more harmonious place than we found it. Through this process, we become healthy on this higher level of health.

# Chapter 3
# THE SCIENCE, ART AND PHILOSOPHY OF HEALING

*"When a man's science exceeds his sense,*
*he perishes by his ignorance."*
— Oriental Proverb

## PHILOSOPHY

Philosophy is the guiding rail that keeps concepts on track and moving in a coherent direction. However, if something is dynamic (moving) then there had better be some track layers out in front or it will run off the end of the rail. Thus, philosophy by definition *must* be dynamic not static. A philosophy must constantly be developing and covering new ground or it is not serviceable.

Many people confuse philosophy with theology in that they make the mistake of turning their philosophy into their religion. This is a grave error. When shortcomings are found in a pseudo-theo-philosophy, its adherents must either abandon it or defend it to the point of closing their minds to new truths. To do less would be to admit that their "god" is fallible. Therefore, they approach philosophy, art and science with tainted minds.

History documents that these pseudo-theo-philosophies have been responsible for more of the injustices perpetrated within the healing arts than all other causes combined. In 1543, Vasalius, a sixteenth century physician, a teacher of anatomy and surgery at the University of Padua in the city state of Venice, wrote of the new discoveries in human anatomy based on dissection. But the new information differed from the old views and Vasalius was denounced as an impostor and a heretic. Bitter persecution was heaped upon his head until he was forced to flee to a neighboring city state for fear of his life. Galileo, the Italian astronomer now called the "Father of Modern Science", met an even worse fate. He was thrown in prison for "Heresy" and tortured until he renounced his scientific knowledge.

William Roentgen, the discoverer of X-rays, was accused of being not only a quack but was criticized for fear his "ray" would invade the privacy of the bedroom. James Lind was considered a quack by his fellow surgeons in the British Navy for insisting that citrus fruit could cure scurvy. William Harvey, another physician, discovered what is now considered the most momentous single achievement in the history of medicine, the circulation of blood. Just because his theory was different from the current thinking, Harvey was subjected to ridicule and a storm of abuse from his peers.

Lister was declared mentally incompetent by his fellow physicians and committed to an institution because he insisted that surgeons scrub before surgery and use disinfected instruments. Semmelweis was driven to suicide by his superior because he insisted that doctors should scrub after dissection and before coming in contact with living patients. Hahnemann was ridiculed for fifty years by his peers, and forced to flee Germany for France, because of his discovery of the homeopathic principle of minimal dose which has now been scientifically proven by laws of quantum physics.

It was the founder of chiropractic, Dr. D. D. Palmer's, insistence on incorporating the quantum vitalistic concept into the chiropractic thought process that was the major factor in the irreparable schism between him and his son B.J. Palmer, D.C., Ph.C. No doubt D. D. had some books on metaphysics (quantum or energy physics); his lectures at the school he founded were along  metaphysical lines. He struggled with this new idea (chiropractic) and used metaphysical terminology in his effort to explain the new art and science of healing - material with his associates didn't quite agree. Dissension began to grow and soon it was decided that the old gentleman was a little "off balance". It was argued that Dr. Palmer was trying to infuse chiropractic with religion, metaphysics and mental therapy, and that these fields were not related to the science and art of chiropractic. The record shows that the other members of the (Palmer) school made it quite difficult for Dr. Palmer to keep control of the idea which he had established. In fact, as Dr. Palmer writes in his book *The Science, Art And Philosophy Of Chiropractic,* they actually expelled him from his own school, ostracized him from his own city  of Davenport, and persecuted him. In 1910 he wrote, "The teachings of D. D.  Palmer are not presently in P.S.C.(Palmer School of Chiropractic) today."

Philosophy is defined as "a basic theory concerning a particular subject or sphere of activity." The dictionary further defines "theory" as, "A hypothesis, a *guess,* abstract thought". Therefore, philosophy is the antithesis of science. Philosophy comes first to try to explain something that is not clearly understood but scientific knowledge eventually should replace philosophy. If science does not replace a particular philosophical concept, then there is no growth and progress and we have no hope for a more enlightened future.

Figure 3.1 represents a graphic illustration of philosophy. Note that the vertical cables of the suspension bridge attach to the mid-point of each philosophical concept and thereby make it unstable if not balanced at exactly the mid-point.

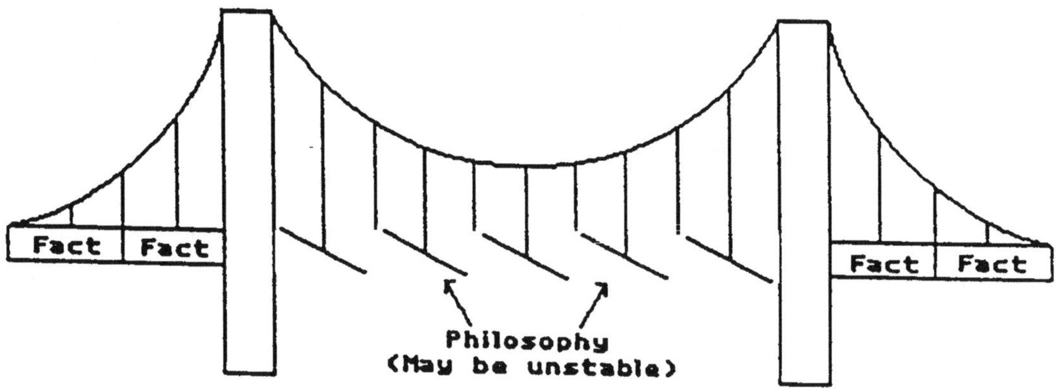


*Figure 3.1 — Philosophy*

## ART

**The general principles of any branch of learning or of any craft.**

If we ask fifty artists to paint the same picture, none of the pictures will be exactly alike. Even though they all have had the same instruction, from the same instructor, in the primary and secondary colors, perspective, composition, techniques, mediums, tone and even though they all used the same brand of brushes, pallet knives, canvas, paints, frames, etc., no two of their paintings are the same. This we call art. Thus, when we discuss the "healing arts", no two practitioners will do exactly the same thing in exactly the same way even though they graduated from the same school and in the same class.

Art is defined as "The general principles of any branch of learning or of any craft." The key words are "general principles", as opposed to specific and consistently reproducible laws of science. Another way of saying this is that "art is the mother of science." Once this transformation has begun, we leave art behind in favor of the consistently reproducible laws of science.

In figure 3.2 we see that some of the unstable philosophical elements have been replaced by scientific stable facts represented by a multiple cable suspension rendering them stable, but unstable single cable philosophical components still exist requiring that we constantly watch our positioning.

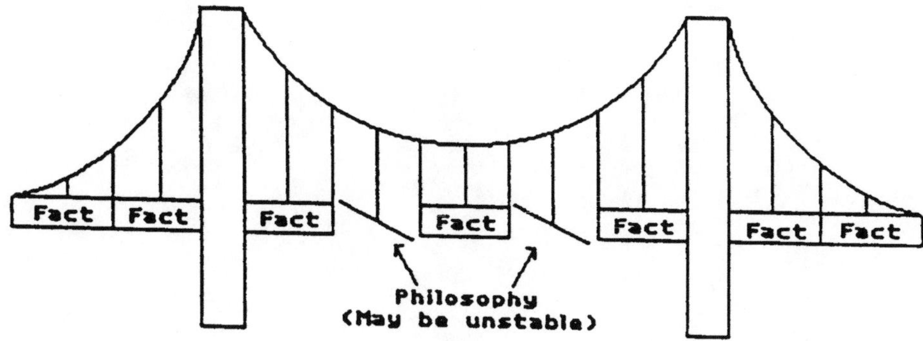


*Figure 3.2 — Art*

## SCIENCE

**"A branch of study concerned with observation and classification of facts especially with the establishment of invariable laws."**

The healing arts are not yet a complete science; in fact, the United States Government, Office Of Technology Assessment, reports that "80 to 90 percent of doctors' treatment methods are not based on scientifically proven principles and, consequently, the results are not guaranteed reproducible." Were it a science such as engineering, we would be able to consistently make every patient well. A civil engineer can build a hundred bridges, properly applying the fixed laws of engineering, and all of the bridges will stand. Science is that which works time after time. But we healers, even the best of us, do not get all of our patients well. This is because we do not yet understand all of the laws governing the living human being. Healing arts, in the strictest sense of the word, are still in the process of evolving into a science. This is why we refer to them as "arts".

In figure 3.3 we have a bridge of completely scientific facts that are capable of supporting great stress and remaining stable. **Caution must be taken not to confuse true scientific facts with so-called "facts", which are nothing more than the fad of the day and must be abandoned at some point in the future. Such were never scientific facts, only misrepresented to be so.** Relying on such false "facts" is like constructing a bridge out of fragile ornamental glass painted to look like concrete and steel rather than the true articles which have great compression and tensile strength.

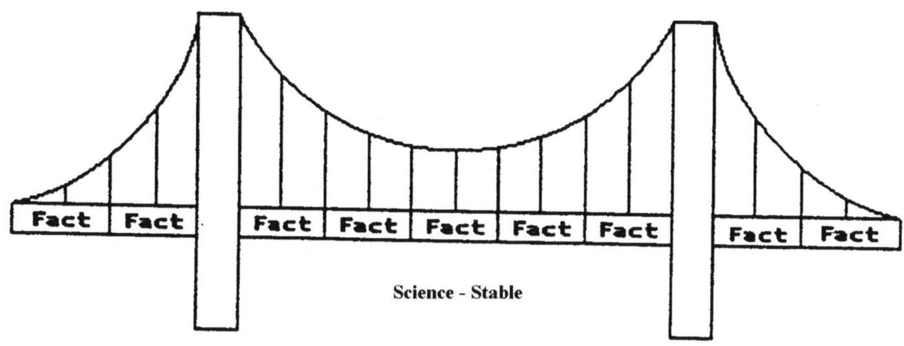


*Figure 3.3 — Science*

# Chapter 4
# THE NATURE OF TOTAL SCIENCE

*"We cannot impose our wills on nature
unless we first ascertain what her will is. Working
without regard to law brings nothing but failure;
working with law enables us to do what seemed
at first impossible."*
— Ralph Tyler Flewelling

## THE CIRCUMSCRIBED WHOLE

**Truth is a total unit and one truth, when properly understood, is never found in conflict with other truths.** When one supposed truth is in conflict with another supposed truth, one or both are incorrect or not adequately understood.

In the western materialistic, reductionistic, academic world, only things that can be proven to our five senses are considered reality. However, it must be emphasized that **a practice may be thoroughly scientific and at the same time highly irrational and even detrimental.** The scientific mind which dwells only on the physical plane and ignores the non-corporal or quantum vitalistic, expansionistic aspects of the universe can never come to an understanding of the universe and all that is within it. What these scientists ignore is *far more* than what they know and accept.

To illustrate just how limited our physical senses are between the last acoustic sensation perceived by our ears, due to 36,850 vibrations per second, and the first optical sensation perceived by our eyes, which is due to 400 trillion vibrations in the same space of time, we receive no information from our five senses. This is an enormous interval during which none of our senses provide us with data. Obviously, this does not mean that there is no information resonating within this gap. It is a well-known fact that a dog's hearing extends much further into this gap than does the hearing of a human. Therefore, we cannot accept the idea that no information is transmitted in that intermediate range. In the overall picture, our special senses miss far more data than we perceive.

Within the gap also lie radio, television and radar emissions which transmit monumental amounts of information. One hundred years ago mankind had not yet discovered these ranges but this did not mean they did not exist. Astronomers probe and learn about dead planets by means of radio waves given off by the elements of which the planet is composed. The scientific reality is that these quantum radio waves have always existed and transmitted data, even before humans developed devices to monitor them.

Another example of this point is air. We look at a distant mountain range and none of our senses tell us that there are thousands of tons of air between us and the mountains. Yet, this it is a scientific reality.

Or think about a jet plane traveling at 600 miles per hour in an easterly direction. The world is revolving at approximately 1,000 miles per hour in an east to west rotation so we are actually traveling at 1,600 miles an hour but our senses do not perceive it as such. Or even more interesting, think of the same plane traveling west; in reality, we are only making 400 miles per hour progress but our senses say 600 miles per hour. How about going north or south? If we travel 600 miles north we actually wind up 1,000 miles west of where we were originally due to the earth's rotation. Our senses don't provide us with that accurate data but only with the distorted fact that we have traveled 600 miles north.

Also, remember, that while all of the above is taking place, we are hurtling through space at tens of thousands of miles per hour as the earth orbits the sun and that the sun itself is moving through space at hundreds of thousands of miles per hour, none of which is being perceived by our senses.

## THE ERROR OF LIMITED SCIENCE

**A practice may not be "scientific" in that its procedures and action may not be explainable by our current level of scientific understanding, and yet this practice may be highly beneficial, an empirical technique, a procedure known by long experience to produce consistent and desired results. To call such a practice "unscientific" is to ignore the fact that there are laws at work. We simply have not been able to understand them yet.** This concept led Speransky to write, **"It is clear that exact knowledge of all the details is not indispensable for useful interference in the course of a pathological process. It suffices sometimes to comprehend accurately the basic condition, the 'leading link', and grasping it to manipulate the whole chain. This opens up the prospect of a scientific approach to medical practice; it is precisely this that gives rise to the need, experienced by all, for the creation of a unitary theory of medicine."**

Many biochemical processes in the living being involve exchanges of energy, but these grosser forms of energy are not what is meant when we speak of healing or subtle energy. Rather, the energy we refer to in quantum (natural) healing is more like that of a conductor of an orchestra, the choreographer of a ballet or the director of a theatrical production, each of whom envisions, integrates, directs, and coordinates the multiple parts into one cohesive and harmonious whole; that is, the subordinate biochemical and energy processes of the living being.

To further illustrate, a candle flame is the result of millions of individual atoms being heated and gaining energy to the point where each atom emits a photon. The result is visible light but it is uncoordinated or random light and the illumination fades as we recede from the candle.

Now let us take a laser whose light is an organized parallel beam capable of traveling great distances without significantly diminishing and capable of penetrating even solid objects. This laser light contains the same atoms as the candle light but its individual emissions are precisely timed and coordinated. The result is a cohesive, organized effort capable of feats the humble candle cannot do. Yet both light sources may be producing exactly the same amount of lumens.

The above example clearly illustrates that western reductionist, solid state science is in reality only a very minor fraction of total science. To make the mistake of restricting science to only what can be proven by our special senses is to pursue a "science" based upon a minuscule fraction of the data available and is in the truest sense of the word unscientific. **To be a reductionist, solid state chiropractor, naturopath, acupuncturist, nutritionist, homeopath, etc., is in reality to practice reductionist medicine with natural therapies and completely miss the mark regarding the expansionistic, quantum mechanisms of the universe in which we live and work and the true nature of healing within the living quantum being.**

Unfortunately, this is the precise trap that many of our colleagues, who think they have embraced and are practicing natural healing, have fallen into. In order to "be accepted" by reductionistic, non-vitalistic "science", they have prostituted themselves and our sciences by accepting this erroneous and severely myopic, reductionist, solid state concept of what science is. In so doing, they have stunted their own scientific growth and that of their scope of practice.

Tragically, many of these myopic, reductionistic, non-vitalistic minds have gravitated to our government licensing boards, professional organizations and educational institutions where they endeavor to restrict the minds of others. But even more undesirable, they are doing the same disservice to the minds of the next generation of our practitioners. In the end, total science, academia, the professions and above all the patients profoundly suffer from this reductionistic, non-vitalistic, pseudo-scientific mind fix.

## THE LAW OF THE UNI-SYSTEM

Traditionally, anatomy, physiology, pathology, etc., and even medical specialties have been taught and have practiced by systems; i.e., cardiology, proctology, neurology, endocrinology, massage, chiropractic, osteopathy, dentistry, podiatry, optometry, counseling and acupuncture, to name only a few. Such artificial categorization creates an erroneous comprehension which educators, practitioners, professional organizations, administrators, insurance carriers, publishers, legislators and even our legal system all unwisely continue to perpetuate to the detriment of the sick and to society in general.

In an integrated being, the nervous system cannot be segregated from the immune system, the psychological, or any other. **The scientific reality is all are members of a single inter-related, inter-dependent and inter-functional whole. What effects one effects all. As healers, we affect the entire being** not just the nervous system of chiropractic, the chemistry of allopathy and herbalism of the naturopath, the circulatory of osteopathy, the mind of psychiatry, psychology, counseling and faith healing, the energy of acupuncture, the physical of athletic trainers or even the spiritual of religion. Such concepts are relics of the bygone, overly-simplistic, under-educated, reductionist age and have no place in modern scientific health care.

## THE IGNORANCE OF ARROGANCE

Our western reductionistic culture considers itself to be the epitome of all learning as represented by the tip of the cultural and intellectual pyramid in Figure 4.1. We arrogantly believe the myth that our modern western culture has taken the best from all previous cultures and left behind all that was inferior.

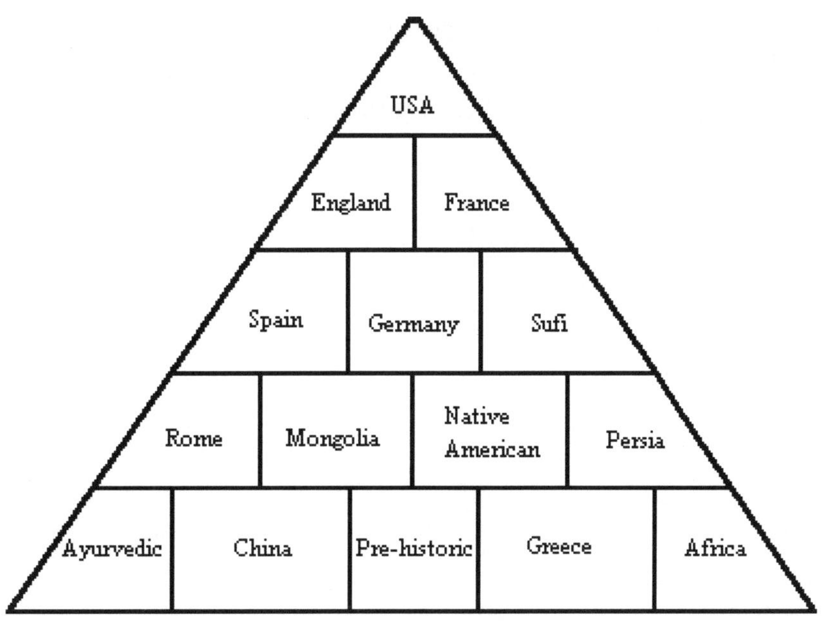


*Figure 4.1 — The Cultural And Intellectual Pyramid*

In reality, nothing could be further from the truth. For example, our modern western culture far excels the ancient Chinese culture in physical medicine such as, orthopedic, plastic, reconstructive surgeries, etc., but we lag far behind the ancient Chinese in our understanding of quantum or energy healing. See Figure 4.2. Likewise, the Romans were far superior civil engineers when it came to building structures that could endure the tests of time and use. Roman roads and aqueducts built more than 2,000 years ago are not only still standing but, even more amazing to our "throw it together as fast as you can" culture, some are still in use. For anyone familiar with modern road building techniques, it is almost incomprehensible that our modern interstate highway system, without constant repairs, could still be in use in the year 4,000 A.D. See Figure 4.2.

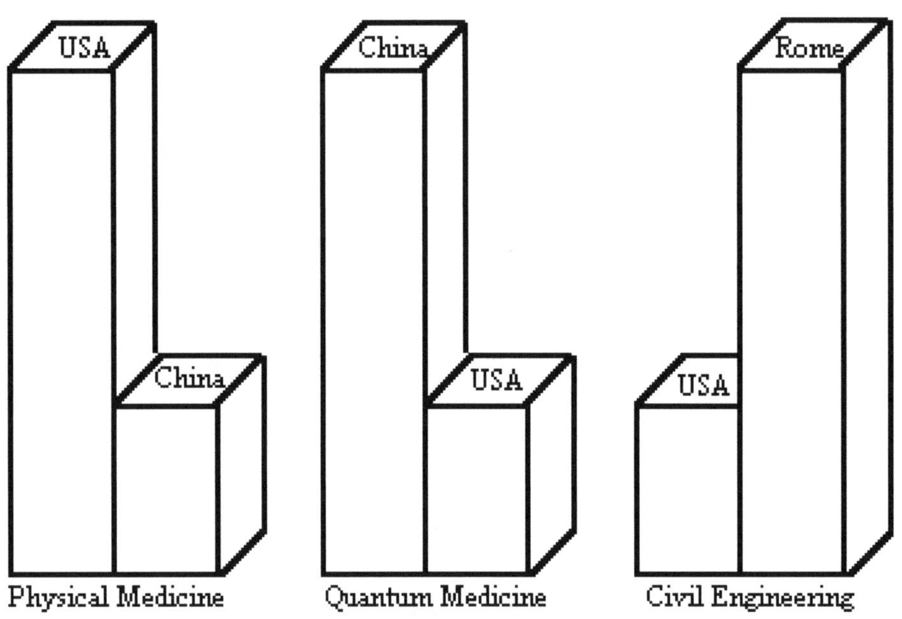


*Figure 4.2 — Cultural Variances In Skills*

So it is with every culture. Each excelled in an aspect in which our culture is weak and our culture excels in areas that the others did not. Therefore, the true goal of science is to be able to abandon our arrogance of ignorance and accept and apply truth from whatever source we find it. To do less is in reality to be uneducated and unscientific.

<h1 style="text-align:center">Chapter 5<br>THE UNIVERSAL LAWS</h1>

*"Keep one thing forever in view — the truth; and if
you do this, though it may seem to lead you away
from the opinions of men, it will assuredly conduct
you to the throne of God."*

— Horace Mann

## THE LAWS OF HEALING

Kent writes, "It is law that governs the world and not matters of opinion or hypothesis." **All things function according to universal laws.** We may not understand those laws but they function none the less. Gravity functioned long before Newton formulated his idea from observing the falling apple. **Being universal (including or covering all), these laws always function unless superseded by higher laws.** For example, the law of gravity can *temporarily* be suspended by the law of centrifugal force.

**Thus, healing becomes a study of universal laws and how they affect the living being and how higher laws can be applied by the healer to suspend or supersede lower laws and return the patient to health.** What follows in the Sophomore text is a study of these universal laws of healing and how they can be consistently applied to relieve dis-ease. (We hyphenate the word dis-ease in this text in order to constantly remind the student and practitioner of the true nature of dis-ease; that being a lack of proper function or ease within the living being.)

Many cultures have discovered these laws at different times in the  history of the world. Although they have been referred to by various names, when properly understood, the principles underlying these laws remain constant. This allows us to compare the terminology and applications of one branch of quantum medicine with the others that have discovered and utilized these laws. This is our "common ground" that becomes our grand advantage and is one of the main reasons that this textbook has been written; to allow us to communicate with each other with ease, to know when a colleague within another branch of quantum healing may be able to assist in the case management care. The fundamental goal according to B. J. Palmer, D.C., Ph.C., is **"To see HOW LITTLE we can do, at HOW FEW PLACES, HOW RARELY and HOW QUICKLY it can be done, to accomplish greatest change IN  SHORTEST SPACE OF TIME, AT LEAST COST to case, and to know WHAT to do and WHY we do it, BEFORE doing it."**

In the Junior text, we will discuss how each branch of natural healing interprets and applies these laws within its particular philosophy.

# Chapter 6
# THE HEALER'S MISSION AND REQUISITE KNOWLEDGE

*"... Unless a man or woman who administers*
*medicine to assist the human systems to overcome*
*disease understands and has that intuitive*
*knowledge, by the spirit, that such an article is*
*good for that individual at that very time,*
*they had better let him alone..."*

— Brigham Young

## THE ONLY MISSION

The physician's *only* mission is to restore the sick and suffering to complete health by the most rapid, gentle, cost-efficient and permanent means and to do so by clearly comprehensible and reproducible laws.

These laws include:

1) Knowledge of the dis-ease

2) Knowledge of the appropriate therapy

3) Knowledge of the application of the correct therapy

4) Knowledge of the obstacles to the cure and how to remove them

5) Knowledge of the existing causes in chronic dis-ease

6) Knowledge of underlying causes in chronic, constitutional and miasmatic (diathesis, doshic, phase) dis-ease

Only then does the healer truly know the patient.

**Just as importantly, the true healer is a** *preserver of health* . This role requires:

1) Knowledge of that which disturbs health

2) Knowledge of how to remove these disturbances

3) Knowledge of how to teach the patient to make intelligent decisions in the future

## LAW OF HONESTY AND CLARITY

We must be clear as to what motivates us to be a healer. Without a clear understanding as to why we are doing what we do, the personal character and discipline needed to hold true to the principles frequently is lacking. The experience has to be more than an intellectual dabbling, a quest for fame, fortune and/or social position or the founding or perpetuation of a dynasty. There must be stability of character which enables one to firmly stand by true principles regardless of the consequences.

# THE LAW OF KNOWLEDGE OF THE DIS-EASE

In accepting this dual role of knowing the laws necessary to regain health and using the laws to preserve health, the healer must not assume. **Only that which can be verified subjectively and/or objectively will give a true picture of the total patient.** Herein lies a great danger: One must not rely wholly on that which lies hidden within the patient; i.e., microbial identification, blood pressures, MRIs, EKGs, CTs, X-rays, orthopedic and  neurological tests, laboratory diagnoses, etc.

In 1931, the eminent British surgeon Edward Bach wrote, **"Disease will never be cured or eradicated by present materialistic methods, for the simple reason that dis-ease in its origin is not material." The healer realizes that we can never see the immaterial, the aberration of the vital force, which is the initiating cause of the dis-ease. It is the symptoms, the being's response to the dis-ease, that reveal how the vital force has altered the function of the being, telling the healer** *most* **reliably what must be done to restore that particular patient's health.**

Research has show that when a person becomes ill, **the first indication of declining health is an alteration in the quantum (energy) fields.** Only when all symptoms, signs and perceptions of dis-ease, on all planes of the patient's total being, have been eliminated is health restored. In this state, the energy which enervates the being reigns supreme. **Since this quantum factor is the Kundalini, Num, Vital Force, Innate Intelligence, Ch'i, Life Force, the influence of any form of care must affect it by quantum dynamics and not by molecular reactions and/or physical forces.**

**Dis-ease is not an independent entity hiding in the interior of the organism separate and distinct from the vital force that gives the being life.** There is yet to be discovered any trauma, microbe, structural dis-relationship, mental disturbance, chemical alteration, deficiency, physiological disturbance, etc., which does not, at some point, announce its presence in the living being by symptoms. **The healer can permanently remove dis-ease only by altering the quantum (energy). To do otherwise is to leave untouched the** *cause* **of the dis-ease.** It is this understanding that leads the healer to the correct choice of therapy.

# BOOK TWO

# SOPHOMORE TEXT

# INTRODUCTION TO THE SOPHOMORE TEXT

*"Dis-ease is the retribution of outraged nature."*
— Hosea Ballou

## THE PRICE OF EDUCATION

By now the burdens of obtaining your education are weighing heavy upon you and your family, if you are married. You have probably even wondered if you really want to be a healer and if there is any end to the rote memorization of anatomical features and physiological and pathological processes. Let's face reality. There are many occupations that would be less stressful. Each of us in health care have experienced exactly the same thoughts, even after being in practice for many years.

In truth, the demands of our educational curriculums, practices and personal lives are often responsible for the deterioration of our own health. What could be more counter-productive and hypocritical than forcing aspiring  healers to destroy their own health in order to make healers of them?

As you begin your study of the laws that regulate healing in the sophomore text, begin by applying their wisdom to yourself and your family. These laws will help you to survive your academic experience and, later on, will allow you to rise above the unending stress of your practice and professional life.

In other words, these laws are **a way of life**. If you fail to master and apply them for yourself and your family, you will never be capable of teaching them to your patients. Above all else, health is a teaching and learning experience. The word "doctor" actually means "learned teacher". **The laws are the missing link that every health care system abandons when it begins chasing symptoms instead of resolving the cause of dis-ease.**

If, because of time constraints, you must make a choice about the focus of your studies, choose to spend more time on these universal laws of life and health than on the more academic subjects such as pathology, etc. Without mastery of these laws, you will never know how to properly apply anatomy, physiology, and so on and assist in providing the precious gift of health. That should be the main reason that you have decided to become a healer. If you have arrived at this place and state in time for any other reason than for the sake of humanity and personal integrity, you should seriously consider another career before you become a major cause of iatrogenesis (doctor caused dis-ease) which is the result of doctors not incorporating these laws into our own beings and practices.

This discussion is not meant to discourage you but rather to encourage you in re-dedicating your life to the only proper course of health care. Our goal is care that is in **total harmony with the governing laws. Since we and the patients we serve exist within that universe,** we are bound by those laws regardless of our obedience or disobedience to them. **We can either make ourselves by applying them properly or we can ignore them and break ourselves against them. But the laws, being universal, will always remain in force.** The choice is yours.

## ALTERNATIVE AND COMPLEMENTARY

You may have noticed that we do not use the common terms "alternative medicine" and/or "complementary healing" in this text when referring to non-allopathic practices. This is because their use in that context is misleading. **Allopathy is in fact a minority practice world-wide. Therefore, in this text, allopathy is the "alternative" and/or "complementary" to the more universally practiced quantum healing.** This fact was again confirmed by a study released by Stanford University on 18 September 1998 in which a random survey of 1,000 individuals revealed that **69 percent of those surveyed used some form of "alternative medicine"** and the *Journal of the American Medical Association* in 1997 stated that there was an ". . .estimated **425 million visits to unconventional medical practitioners in 1990 exceeded visits to primary care physicians"** which numbered 388 million.

Furthermore, a 1998 article in the *American Journal of Natural Medicine* by S. Torkos, B. Sc., Phm., states that the World Health Organization estimates approximately **80 percent of the world's population relies on herbs for primary healthcare needs.** A 1993 United States poll published in the *New England Journal of Medicine* reported **34 percent of respondents had used at least one "unconventional" therapy in the past year.** A similar 1997 Canadian poll indicated that **42 percent of Canadians are using some form of "alternative" medicines or practices.**

# Chapter 7
# REQUISITE KNOWLEDGE OF THE HEALER

*"Natural forces within us
are the true healers of dis-ease."*
— Hippocrates

## LAW OF REQUISITE KNOWLEDGE

Since dis-ease is a deviation from health, expressed by symptoms, and since cure is a reversion back to health, any form of successful care must have the power to alter the way the patient thinks, feels and functions. See figure 7.1.

## ILLUSTRATION OF THE PRINCIPLE

As the patient demonstrates that he or she is returning to the self-healing mode, less and less care *must* be rendered by the healer. In both acute and chronic cases, one of the primary indications that the self-healing state is being achieved is that the *temporary* aggravations become further and further apart and less and less intense. See the right half of figure 7.1. Should this caution be ignored by the practitioner and additional care be rendered during these temporary healing crises, the healing process runs the danger of coming to an abrupt halt, or reverting to the original state, or the worst possible scenario, of actually making the dis-ease worse than it was when care began. Such a state, called iatrogenic (doctor caused) dis-ease, is totally unnecessary and is a major sign of a poorly trained practitioner.

It takes energy to run the living being and energy to heal dis-ease. When the being's energy reserves begin running out, the inborn intelligence, which controls the being, will temporarily shut down the healing process. Healing is then in a passive or coasting phase and the patient is definitely not as well as he or she was only a few days before. This is what causes the slight slump on the graph in contrast to an active healing phase which shows marked improvements. The body is resting and building up its energy reserves for the next major healing push. The innate intelligence is in complete control. If we arbitrarily continue to administer care, we deny the body its rest and make demands upon it that it is not capable of complying with. Thus, without replenishment of its energy reserves, the body is forced to function in an energy depletion mode, which causes the energy to fall below the critical level allowing the patient's health to once again begin to deteriorate.

Wisely given a few days to rest, the innate wisdom will of its own accord again re-enter the self-healing mode and there will be no iatrogenic dis-ease to complicate the case and/or embarrass the practitioner whose true and only reason for existing is to assist in protecting and building health.

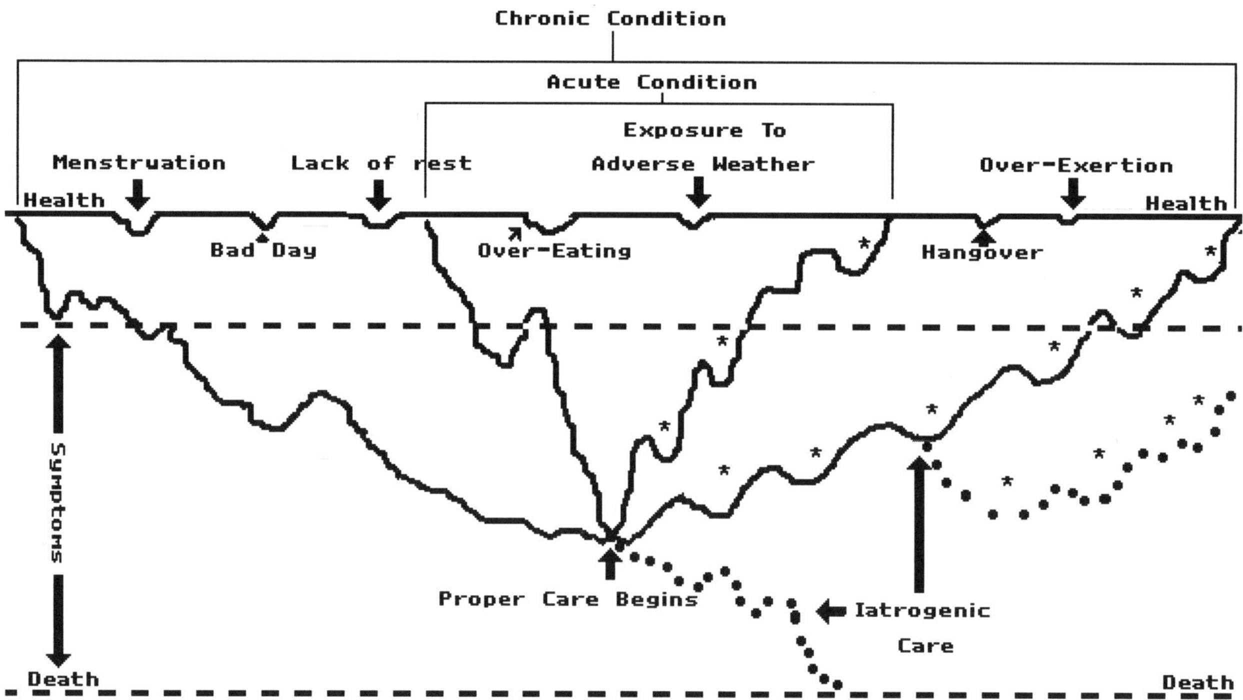



*Figure 7.1 — The Pattern Of Declining And Returning Health*

## HERING'S LAW OF THE CURE

The patient's pathology develops from outside in, from below up, and from the least vital to the most vital organs and functions. When properly cared for, the patient heals from the most vital to the least vital organs and functions, from above down, and from inside out. Old pathology may temporarily reappear in the reverse order of its original development.

## ARNDT-SCHULTZ LAW

Small doses (forces, energies) stimulate function in the living organism with little or no inhibition; larger doses (forces, energies) initially stimulate and then equally inhibit function; and very large doses (forces, energies) suddenly and dramatically stimulate for a very short time only and then dramatically and for long periods of time inhibit even to the point of death. See Figure 7.2.

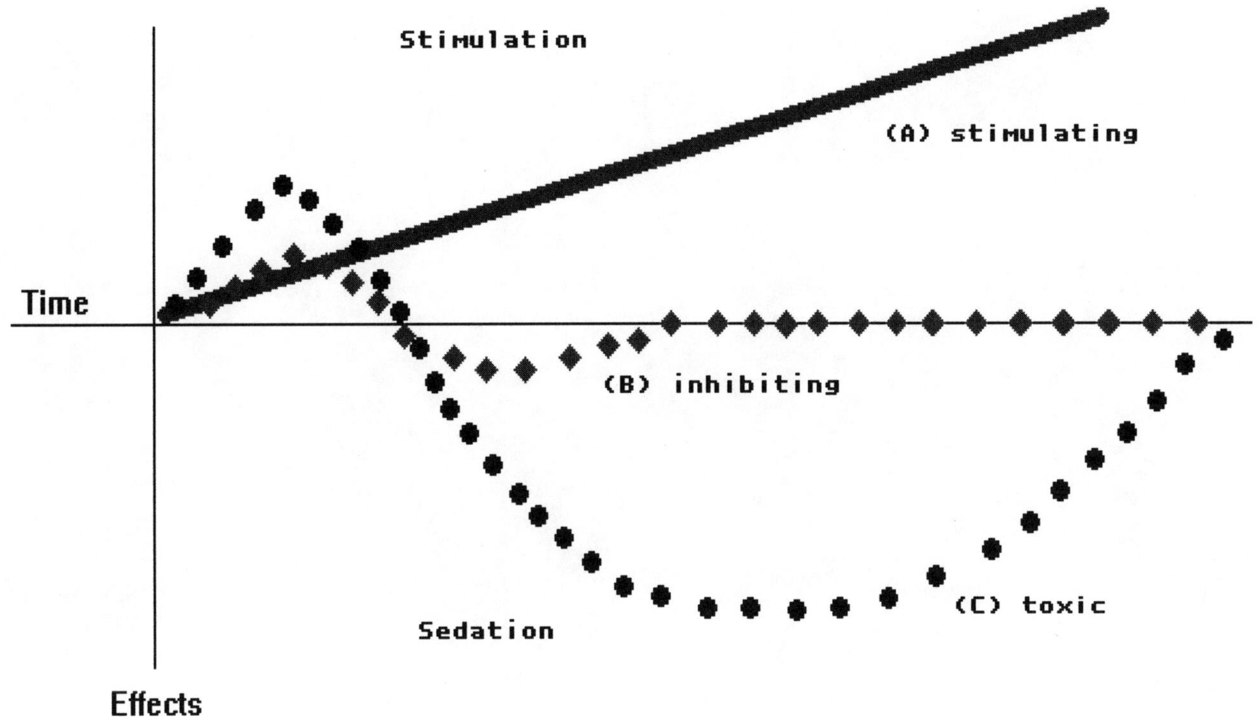


*Figure 7.2 — Arndt-Schultz Law*

## KOESTSCHAU'S LAW

There are predictable effects of a substance or force depending upon the amount administered:

A) Small amounts (homeopathic doses, mildly stimulating acupuncture techniques, light chiropractic adjusting techniques, soft massage techniques, mild psychological approaches, etc.) produce prolonged stimulation without adverse reactions. 100 percent healing in nature.

B) Corporal amounts (allopathic prescriptions, nutritional doses, medium force chiropractic adjustments, etc.) stimulate, then depress function requiring unnecessary expenditure of num, kundalini, vital, innate, ch'i, life force to return the patient to the norm. 50 percent healing, 50 percent iatrogenic in nature.

C) **Large doses (pharmacotoxic, megadose nutrients, heavy force chiropractic adjustments, heavy energy techniques, excessive stimulation of acupuncture needles, aggressive psychological confrontations, etc.) produce brief, dramatic stimulation followed by severe, long-lasting depression of function requiring excessive kundalini, num, vital, innate, ch'i, life energy to return the patient to normal. 25 percent healing, 75 percent iatrogenic in nature.** See figure 7.1 and 7.2.

## LAW OF IATROGENIC THERAPY

**Man is many times more susceptible to the adverse effects of drugs, or other inappropriate and/or excessive therapy, than to dis-ease because their dis-ease producing action(s) can be forced upon the organism.** On the other hand, in naturally occurring dis-ease, a much higher degree of susceptibility or sensitivity *must* be present in order to cause an individual to present the symptom picture. In other words, a dis-ease cannot, normally, be forced upon a healthy vibrant constitution. The body's defense mechanisms will expel it.

# Chapter 8
# LAW OF KNOWLEDGE OF CARE

*"It is the close observation of little things which is
the secret of success in business, in art, in science
and in every pursuit of life."*

— Samuel Smiles

## THE CURATIVE ABILITY

The curative ability of any therapy is in direct proportion to its capacity to *create* dis-ease in the healthy. A therapy that lacks the ability to produce dis-ease in a living organism cannot cure because it has no energy to initiate changes leading back to a state of health. The challenge, then, is to find a method that will minimize the former while maximizing the latter.

Research has proven that dis-ease symptoms, far from being eliminated and destroyed by opposing treatment, return instead with a renewed and greater facilitation after seeming for a time to have been resolved. Therefore, *none* but similar treatment can be used for the eradication of the totality of symptoms.

In accordance with universal law, a weaker dynamic dis-ease is permanently extinguished by a stronger one which is *very* similar to it. The curative virtue of any treatment thus depends on its symptoms being similar to those of the dis-ease, but stronger. Thus, The Law of Similars is recognized. A dis-ease resulting from a traumatic introduction of mechanical force responds best to a *similar* introduction of a mechanical force to re-establish health; i.e., a chiropractic adjustment. A dis-ease produced by a chemical force responds to a *similar* chemical force to eradicate it; i.e., homeopathic Croton Tiglium to cure poison ivy. An emotional dis-ease responds to a *similar* emotional release to initiate healing; a spiritual (non-corporal) dis-ease to a *similar* spiritual force to return to health. Note that in all of the above examples the word *similar* and not *identical* is used.

## LAW OF MULTIPLE INTERACTIONS OF THERAPIES

There is a *consistent* mathematical progression that dictates the potential for multiple iatrogenic interactions. See figure 8.1 In the context of this law, "multiple" means:

1) The too frequent use of a single therapy.

2) The addition of each vitamin, mineral, phytotherapeutic agent, acupuncture needle, homeopathic remedy, drug, surgery, segmental adjustment, counseling, hypnotherapy session, modality, etc., to the patient's therapeutic regiment.

1x1 = 1

1x2 = 2

1x2x3 = 6

1x2x3x4 = 24

1x2x3x4x5 = 120

1x2x3x4x5x6 = 720

1x2x3x4x5x6x7 = 5,040

1x2x3x4x5x6x7x8 = 40,320

1x2x3x4x5x6x7x8x9 = 362,880

1x2x3x4x5x6x7x8x9x10 = 3,628,800 **possible interactions**

*Figure 8.1 — The Mathematics Of Therapy Interactions*

True, certain of these interactions could be beneficial but many are also detrimental. **If the practitioner cannot** *know* **with 100 percent** *predetermined accuracy* **the precise outcome of a interaction then it** *is not science*. This is  precisely the status of so-called "medical science" today; scores of its methods and procedures rest on empiricism and even on chance, anarchy prevails, here and there corrected by separated facts, partial comparisons, speculation (guessing) and, worst of all, the profit motive. How then can the practitioner conscientiously administer care? What procedure do we discontinue? What do we continue?

# Chapter 9
# LAW OF KNOWLEDGE OF HOW TO CHOOSE AND ADMINISTER THE SUPERIOR MODE OF CARE

*"Illnesses may be identical but the persons
suffering from them are different."*
— Hsu Ta Ch'un

## LAW OF SIMILARS

The Law of Similars is in conformity with the *universal laws of healing* . **The fact that it produces consistent results is of greater importance than the mechanics of how it works.** Being a universal law may very well mean that its workings will never be fully comprehended by the finite mind of man. The great moral question, then, is, should its benefit to the sick and suffering be withheld in the name of "science"? Do we completely comprehend the atom? Do we completely understand electricity? No. Does this make the use of electrical appliances non-scientific? Of course not!

**Chronic miasmatic (diathesis, doshic, phase, hereditary) dis-eases, though weaker than many therapies, have a much longer action which dramatically disrupts the kundalini, num, vital, innate, ch'i, life force, frequently for a life-time or several life-times of affliction within the same family. These effects *cannot* be overcome and extinguished by the life force on its own without precisely administered therapy. To cure them, the healer must act on the kundalini, num, vital, innate, ch'i, life force with a very similar therapy.***

**Because the correct therapy cures dis-ease and incorrect therapies produce iatrogenic dis-ease, it is logical to assume that improper treatment, more than natural dis-eases and/or accidents, is the cause of the majority of *chronic* dis-eases affecting humanity.**

It must also be constantly remembered that the quantum and solid state dis-ease agents that the patient encounters do not have an absolute power to disrupt the organism. **We fall ill under their influence only when the organism is already sick (in a state of abnormal num, vital, innate, ch'i, life force)** but these dis-ease agents do not make everyone sick at the same time.

**Unnatural forces can be quite a different matter.** Iatrogenic, traumatic, chemical, and excessive stress dis-eases can affect all individuals at all times and in all circumstances similarly and produce predictable symptoms. This is one of the great challenges of the age. We are bombarded by designer chemicals and drugs, unnatural stresses and forces, altered food supplies, mutating microbes, excessive treatment, etc. For example, a severe force of a hyper-flexion/hyper-extension (whiplash) type injury will produce **very similar symptoms in all cases.** Highly toxic chemicals produce very similar **symptoms in all patients exposed**; for example, chemical warfare agents produce  predictable results in all exposed personnel. It is precisely because of this  consistency that governments choose to develop such weapons. Psychological warfare also produces highly predictable results among target populations.

In other words, **natural dis-ease agents have only a subordinate and conditional power to alter human health while artificial forces such as iatrogenic care have a far superior power to do so, one that is absolute and unconditional under normal circumstances.** If proper health care is to protect us from contagious dis-ease, it must possess a greater power to maintain and/or alter the kundalini, num, vital, innate, ch'i, life force than the epidemic dis-ease. (However, those dis-eases brought by un-natural forces do not have to be stronger in order to cure natural dis-eases.) **Above all un-natural dis-eases must have the greatest possible similarity to the natural dis-ease being treated.** For example, a trauma-induced structural dis-relationship will respond best to a similar, but controlled, force of a  chiropractic adjustment because the force of the adjustment is so similar to the initial cause. Chemical imbalances respond best to a similar corrective force of balancing the chemistry and psychological dis-eases to a similar psychological or counseling approach to their resolution. Further, **the corrective force must not just "dim" the kundalini, num, vital, innate, ch'i, life force's awareness of the natural dis-ease template but must completely extinguish or scramble the template, beyond access recognition, to be successful.**

# LAW OF THE MECHANICS OF DIS-EASE

1) If two dissimilar natural dis-eases (one being chronic) interact within the same patient and they are of equal virulence or **the more chronic is** *more virulent* **, the acute condition is expelled.** Thus, a patient suffering from chronic arthritis is unlikely to experience the influenza but his arthritis will remain uncured. On the other hand, if the arthritis is treated with very **virulent dissimilar treatments, a more grave and new iatrogenic disease is produced.**

2) Should the **latter acute but dissimilar dis-ease be more virulent**, it temporarily suppresses the less virulent chronic dis-ease until the acute dis-ease has run its course and then the less virulent chronic **dis-ease returns not only** *uncured* **but facilitated.**

3) A **new dis-ease, after becoming chronic, finally joins the old chronic but dissimilar dis-ease to form with it a complex dis-ease. Each occupies a region or organs for which it has a special affinity.** A patient with hepatitis can develop a case of dermatitis, **but the two dis-eases, being dissimilar**, *canno*t **cur**e **each other.** Iatrogenesis is the most frequent cause of dissimilar dis-eases.

4) **When two similar dis-eases meet in the organism, the** *more virulent acute*  **being very similar to the chronic less virulent, both are** *cured* **once the acute dis-ease has run its course. They cannot form a complex dis-ease because the acute dis-ease in attempting to invade the identical parts and/or functions affected by the chronic dis-ease process, thus they destroy each other.** Hence a chronic asthma patient who contracts pneumonia will be naturally cured of both dis-eases.

Thus nature teaches how to heal! **Such acute virulent dis-eases and forces can themselves be dangerous in natural situations. Therefore, the ideal clinical therapy is a similar dis-ease or force which is just above the threshold of the** *chronic* **less virulent dis-ease. In this way, the body easily and rapidly expels or neutralizes the curative agent as well as the dis-ease agent.** Hence the law: Only weak degrees of irritation can have a significance; strong ones invariably do damage.

The current state of "health care" is the perfect example of failure to address the above healing laws. Americans spend more on health care than does any other nation but statistically we are one of the sickest populations. This is because so-called "conventional" forms of care orient themselves to stronger and more forceful therapies in their "war" against dis-ease.

5) In "isopathy" the identical agent or force is used to try to initiate  a cure. Present immunization practices are an example of this theory; i.e., using polio virus to immunize for polio. Champions of this theory forget that the origin of immunization lies in the Law of Similars, not in the theory of identicals. Cowpox and smallpox are very similar but not the identical dis-ease. They differ in many respects, in the quicker incubation period and in

the much milder nature of cowpox, but above all in the fact that cowpox can never be contracted by man through proximity as can smallpox. **Universal law, long clinical experience and research have documented that nothing but iatrogenesis comes of trying to heal with identicals.**

## LAW OF TOTALITY OF SYMPTOMS

It has been well-stated that, **"A foot is no more the man than a single symptom is the totality of the dis-ease."** Unfortunately, the vast majority of  care rendered to patients is palliative or addresses a single symptom. This is  evidenced by the use of pharmaceuticals, phytopherapies, chiropractic adjustments, dental work, corrective lenses, massage, acupuncture and TENS units, surgeries, non-classical homeopathy, physical therapy, exercise therapy, diet, etc. Sadly, most patients subjected to this type of care are patients for life; they must keep coming back to the practitioner with condition after condition or even the same condition which is constantly recurring and progressively becoming worse. They are not truly healthy because the totality of their symptoms is not being dealt with. **Healthy people should need doctors less and less because their total being is functioning in the self healing-mode.**

## LAW OF TOO FREQUENT REPETITION OF CARE

Energy is required to heal. Too frequent care causes depletion of energy and actually is injurious. In fact, **the large majority of cases, when the original dis-ease *pattern returns* , it is temporary, and usually disappears by itself in a day or two. In those cases, we find it necessary to re-treat  because the dis-ease pattern will not disappear by itself. Where the dis-ease pattern returns without evidence of interference it is considered a normal healing pattern and will resolve itself without aid of the healer. Any attempt to give care will severely disrupt the case.**

## LAWS OF PRIMARY AND SECONDARY REACTIONS

**Every influence that affects a living organism, including therapy, must alter the kundalini, num, life, innate, ch'i, vital force to bring about modification in the state of health.** This is referred to as the primary action and is of short duration and forceful. **The action of the vital force striving to oppose this intrusion is called the secondary reaction and is long-lasting but of a much milder nature and is the curative phase.** This is in accord with the Law of Equal and Opposite Reactions. For example, an arm that has been long immersed in ice water is much paler and colder than the other (the primary reaction). Remove the arm from the water and it becomes not only warmer than the other arm but hot, red and inflamed (the secondary reaction). Excessive alertness from the use of large amounts of coffee or anti-insomnia drugs (the primary effect) eventually produces lethargy and drowsiness (the secondary effect). The person who yesterday was warmed by drinking too much wine (the primary effect) is today chilled by every draft (the secondary effect). An athlete heated by vigorous exercise (the primary effect) later feels chills if not properly clothed (the secondary effect).

This demonstrates how true health care must be rendered. Only in the most urgent of cases where there is a danger to life or limb and there is not time for the secondary reaction to take place should the true healer consider forms of care such as allopathic drugs, surgery, forceful chiropractic adjusting techniques, megadoses of nutrients and phytotherapeutic agents, aggressive needling in acupuncture, etc., that rely upon the primary action.

# LAW OF CHOICE

A therapy is not necessarily wrongly chosen just because one or more of its less important indications do not agree with the patient's symptoms, providing that the remainder of the stronger salient characteristics and strange, rare and peculiar symptoms are recognizable. These minor variants will disappear once the cure of the overall dis-ease is achieved. But a wrongly chosen therapy cannot normalize a disrupted vital force.

A palliative therapy produces a condition completely different from pathological dis-ease and therefore leaves the dis-ease intact. Since all palliative therapy must be given in large doses, an opposing secondary reaction MUST follow. Thus an anti-pyretic (the primary short-term effect) will cause the fever to increase (the secondary long-term effect). The dis-ease symptoms become facilitated after the palliative effect has worn off. When each therapy has completed its action it is necessary to re-evaluate the case in order to select the next appropriate therapy.

# LAW OF THE DOCTRINES

1) Dis-ease is a survival adaptation, it is the best response of the being's num, kundalini, life, innate, ch'i, vital force, to the present conditions.

2) An understanding of the totality of symptoms is necessary in order to be able to cure rather than palliate the patient.

3) Palliative treatment in chronic conditions always facilitates the dis-ease process.

4) Care is successful only to the extent that it can re-tune the kundalini, num, vital, innate, ch'i, life force.

5) Natural dis-eases cannot be cured by therapies that oppose the short- term primary response.

6) True healing takes place only during the secondary long-term response.

# Chapter 10
# LAW OF THREEFOLD KNOWLEDGE OF THE HEALER

*"I have entered through the door of nature.*
*Her light and not the lamp of an apothecary's shop*
*has illuminated my way."*

— Paracelsus

## THE NATURE OF DIS-EASE

Dis-eases are groups of symptoms that, when eliminated, allow the organism to return to health by means of the body's own num, kundalini, vital, innate, ch'i, life healing force. Thus, cure comes down to:

1) How the healer ascertains what he/she needs to know about the dis-ease;

2) How the healer investigates the therapeutic power of the care; and,

3) How the healer can use the therapeutic power most effectively.

## LAWS OF THE CURE

Acute dis-ease is rapid progressive disruption of the kundalini, num, vital, innate, ch'i, vital force. Chronic dis-ease is slow but progressive disruption in which the automatic healing power, normally intended to preserve the health, can only offer imperfect, inappropriate, and/or ineffective resistance and cannot extinguish the dis-ease process in and of its own accord, so the organism must allow the dis-ease to progress until the offending miasma (diathesis, dosha, phase) finally destroys the organism.

There are acute dis-eases affecting **single individuals, dis-eases brought on by harmful influences** to which the person may have been exposed such as excesses or privations of diet, trauma, hypo and hyperthermia, fatigue, mechanical strains, psychic stress, poisons, etc. **Most of these dis-eases have as a root a dormant miasmic (diathesis, dosha, phase) weakness** which can be quickly inactivated by the kundalini, num, vital, innate, ch'i, life force.

The **sporadic** acute dis-eases affect a **limited number** of individuals at a time. Dis-eases brought on by adverse weather conditions are an example.

**E**pidemic dis-eases affect **many** individuals and tend to become **contagious** in congested quarters. Because these dis-eases have a similar genesis, they manifest similar symptoms. Left untreated, they result either in death or recovery within a limited period of time. Common causes of epidemics are natural disasters, wars, famine, lack of hygiene, etc.

Lastly are the **acute miasmas (diathesis, doshas, phases)** that occur in their own particular forms. Some are contracted only once in a lifetime, such as smallpox, measles, whooping cough, scarlatina, mumps, etc., while others occur frequently and in fairly similar ways, like influenza.

Among chronic dis-eases we must include all those widespread and voluminous illnesses of iatrogenesis, chemicals, allergies, megadosage, mechanical, thermal and mental stress, etc. All of these relentlessly disrupt and weaken the num, kundalini, ch'i, life, vital force, each in its own characteristic way and to such an extent that it requires an alteration in the organism's function in order to maintain life. **Sensory functions must be exaggerated or inhibited or even destroyed in order to allow the organism to survive as long as possible. This results in the most incurable miasmatic (diathesis, dosha, phase) dis-eases on all levels of the being. No doctor is capable of repairing this damage. It must be removed by the num, kundalini, vital, innate, ch'i, life force itself. In the past, we were taught that the damage could arrive at a point where it was so extensive that it was not possible for it to be healed.** In such a case, it was said that the dis-ease had gone beyond the "limitations of matter" and that there was so much damage that the kundalini, num, life, vital, innate, ch'i could not successfully repair the body. This is to a significant degree inaccurate. **We now know that what, in many cases, were called "Limitations of Matter" are reversible if the practitioner's skill level is adequate.** This condition is more accurately termed **"The Limitations of Knowledge"**.

Dis-eases produced by self-inflicted, prolonged exposure to **avoidable** noxious influences should not be categorized as chronic because they will go away on their own with improvements in living habits if no miasma is present. Such indiscretions include:

1) habitual indulgence in harmful drugs, food and drink;

2) habitual excesses of passions that undermine health;

3) prolonged deprivation of components necessary to life;

4) residing in unhealthy locales;

5) lack of exercise and/or fresh air;

6) physical and/or mental over-exertion;

7) continuing emotional and spiritual stress.

Many **Chronic** dis-eases arise from an **unavoidable miasma (diathesis, dosha, phase)** and, without proper care, continue to increase in spite of a robust constitution, a well-ordered lifestyle or a high energy level. Psoriasis, gonorrhea, and/or syphilis tendencies, which can be hereditary and/or acquired, either in the individual or in the familial history, are the root causes of most of these chronic miasmatic (diathesis, dosha, phase) dis-eases. By far the most widespread is psora which is the underlying common denominator of multitudinous, and otherwise seemingly unrelated, dis-eases such as neurasthenia, hysteria hypochondria, fatigue, depression, epilepsy, bone softening dis-eases, scoliosis and kyphosis, neoplasms, fungal and yeast infections, jaundice, cyanosis, dropsy, amenorrhea, gout, hemorrhoids, hemorrhagic dis-eases, asthma, impotence and infertility, migraines, deafness, cataracts, renal calculi, paralysis, sensory deficits, and pains, hematomas, mental deficiencies, twitches and tremors to name only a few.

When first encountered, the miasmatic (diathesis, dosha, phase) basis of chronic disease seems overwhelming and unbelievable. With the realization that these dis-eases have had hundreds of generations and billions of human organisms through which to mutate, it becomes understandable. Envision the great number of variable internal and external influences experienced by the human family; i.e., climate, diet, cultural and religious restrictions, co-habitation with indigenous animals, insects, microbes, etc., exposure to phytological agents, mineral content and chemical pollution of drinking water, industrial, agricultural, and electromagnetic pollution, stress, deficiencies, contagious disease, immunization, nuclear pollution, air pollution, iatrogenic factors, poor hygiene, malnutrition, moral abuse, excessive passions, education or lack of it, individual constitutional make-up, neglect, personal habits, genetic weaknesses and strengths, mental ability, mental stability, endogenous (origination from within) toxicity, levels of individual hormone production, balance of acupuncture meridians, presence or absence of spinal subluxations, surgical removal of body parts, sexually transmitted dis-ease, occupational related dis-ease, trauma, congenital defects, and on and on.

For the true healer, diagnosis is a moot issue. **Statistically, it would be an extreme scientific rarity that would produce two individuals with exactly the same background leading to exactly the same dis-ease. A second point that becomes obvious is that no cure of such a chronic and diverse dis-ease can be achieved unless the healer is willing to piece together the perceived symptoms and peculiarities of the individual case. In such chronic cases, it may require much time and many searching question to learn the following:**

## INFORMATION NEEDED BY THE PRACTITIONER

1) Patient's case history;

2) Relatives' and/or associates' descriptions of the symptomatology; along with anything **strange, rare or peculiar** they have observed;

3) What the healer observes, hears, palpates, or perceives with any of his/her other senses;

4) Of least importance are the results of laboratory tests and physical examinations, X-rays, etc. The reason for this is that there are literally hundreds of thousands, if not millions, of chemical, neurological, psychological and other reactions that take place in the living being. Laboratories have also been known to change their "normal" ranges from time to time. If test values were not correct in the first place how could they be of diagnostic value?

## HOW TO OBTAIN NEEDED INFORMATION

1) Record of the data revealed in the verbatim descriptions of the patient and observers.

2) Whenever possible, remain silent and let the patient, relatives and/or friends finish without interrupting as long as they do not digress unduly.

3) If the patient, relatives and/or friends speak too fast, only ask them to slow down so that you may record the significant data.

4) Leave blank spaces in your notes so that you can record additional data if the patient, relatives and/or friends revert to a former subject.

5) When the speakers have finished, the practitioner should ask additional clarifying questions that must be answered by additional comments rather than simple yes or no statements. In particular, the healer is interested in the modalities, times, descriptions of sensations, mental/emotional responses, etc.

Unfortunately, no individual or group of practitioners, regardless of the extent of their training or their IQs, are capable of considering all of the potential data generated by the above outlined method. **The reality is that the more data we amass the more likely we are to make oversights.** (L. Timberlake states in *Born To Win* that the knowledge available at the time of Christ doubled by the year 1750 or in 1,717 years, it doubled again by the year 1900 or in 150 years,  and again in 1950 or 50 years, and again in 1960 or 10 years, again in 1965 or five years, again in 1968 or 2  years, and by 1990 knowledge was doubling every 3.5 months.) **Such a system of amassing cumbersome amounts of data can become unmanageable and therefore unreliable. The alternative is to simplify, to understand the resulting symptomatic deviation from health, on all levels of the** *total* **being. This allows us to properly care for cases that involve principles that are not yet scientifically understood, as well as those we fully comprehend. The above principles provide the totality of the case rather than bits and pieces.**

As J. T. Kent, M.D. said, "We may never ascertain causes but we may observe results." Kent, however, cautions against complete abandonment of the amassing of vast amounts of knowledge in these words, "There is more to be learned about diagnosis and prognosis by studying the complex of symptoms than by any form of physical examination, but . . . all methods of examination should be used, as they confirm each other, and often where one is defective the other is strong and helpful."

## TAKING THE CASE

**When asked questions that can be answered, Yes or No, the patient is being led by the practitioner's preconceived idea of the case.** This results in incorrect care. If, on the other hand, volunteered information has provided no strange, rare or peculiar data, the practitioner should ask general questions such as: What about your bowels? What about sleep? What foods do you enjoy or dislike? Only when the patient is finished and the picture is fairly complete should the healer ask more precise questions to determine the best indicated therapy; i.e., how frequent are your bowel movements? In what position do you sleep? What causes the pain to increase? How thirsty are you? After this process is completed, the practitioner then records what has been observed during the consultation. Was the patient nervous, hesitant in answering questions, let the spouse answer for him. What was his voice like, color of skin, body odor? Does he sit erect or slouch, etc?

The symptoms exhibited by a patient during or just after a course of care do not give an accurate picture of the dis-ease. **Only the symptoms suffered before any treatment was rendered are the true dis-ease symptoms.** The rest are iatrogenic symptoms. If you are unable to determine accurately the pre-care symptoms, have the patient discontinue the previously prescribed care for several days and the old dis-ease symptoms will clarify. If the dis-ease is a rapidly progressing one and there is no time to allow clarification of its original symptoms, the healer must put together as complete a picture as possible by subtracting all known iatrogenic symptoms from the patient's present complaints.

**If the dis-ease has been brought on by a stressful event, the patient usually will spontaneously mention it.** If, however, the origin of the dis-ease is from an embarrassing situation, i.e. venereal dis-ease, not following the physician's instructions, etc., it may be necessary to investigate its source without friends or relatives present.

In chronic cases, the practitioner should also carefully evaluate daily activities, habits, diet, domestic situations, menstrual history and so on. **Remember that chronic patients can become so accustomed to living with their symptoms that they come to ignore them. Frequently, these seemingly insignificant symptoms prove to be the strange, rare and peculiar data that strongly confirm the proper choice of care.**

## THE ACTUAL NATURE OF THE CURE

**No amount of reductionist solid state research will ever document the mechanism by which a therapy cures.** This is because a **therapy does not cure. The energy (innate, life force, Ch'i, etc.) that inhabits and runs the being is what cures.** This is proven by administering the correct remedy, adjustment, acupuncture treatment, herb, drug, surgery, massage, mental therapy, etc., to a cadaver. Nothing happens.

However, a properly chosen therapy **does provide a particular energy template which along with the vital life force, (innate, Ch'i, etc.)** does allow the being to again access the quantum self-healing mode.

## LAW OF THE OPEN PATIENT

In some cases, hypochondriacs or the extremely sensitive and co-dependent patients may exaggerate their symptoms and the healer must down-play their significance. **With these patients, the symptoms, they present on different visits frequently fail to confirm each other and may even conflict and so are considered of little value. Placebos should be considered to prevent too frequent and potentially iatrogenic care being rendered. The mentally ill who fabricate their dis-eases are a different matter and great attention should be paid to them.**

## LAW OF THE CLOSED PATIENT

There are others who seem to be very closed and do not seem to want the practitioner prying into their affairs, even though they have come for help. **These patients keep back vital data, intellectualize symptoms away or minimize the importance of symptoms. The value of the information provided by these patients must be** *enhanced* by the astute practitioner.

Because of these different types of patients, the healer must have great tact and be constantly evaluating the input from the patient, friends and relatives, including physical symptoms and laboratory test results. Evaluating an acute case is a much easier task because the details of the symptoms are still fresh in the patient's mind and do not require as much **probing** by the practitioner.

## LAW OF EPIDEMICS

**The healer cannot assume that all cases occurring during an epidemic are the identical disease, even though many symptoms are similar.** When confronted by the life-threatening nature of the epidemic, however, the astute healer can  begin to see trends developing. In such cases, she/he is free to **concentrate on the exceptions.** As more cases are seen, the characteristics of the dis-ease become precisely qualified. (This does not imply a more wordy description but rather a better understanding of the dis-ease.) This, then, allows the healer to determine if the previous care is **the most appropriate for a particular case.** See Chapter 32 and 33 for a more in-depth discussion of the immunization theory and iatrogenic antibiotic effects.

## LAW OF CHRONIC MIASMAS (DIATHESIS, DOSHAS, PHASES)

The same understanding can be applied to chronic miasmatic dis-ease. Thus, the total symptom picture of a miasma can be established only from **many individual cases.**

# Chapter 11
## HOW TO ACQUIRE KNOWLEDGE OF THE THERAPIES

*"If it were possible to restore the sick to health in*
*several ways, we should choose the least difficult."*
— Hippocrates

## LAW OF THE SECOND VISIT

Writing down the pertinent data on the first visit allows the healer to systematically evaluate the tools of his/her trade for their effectiveness in each case and at each visit; the second visit then is much simplified. Symptoms cured are eliminated, **those still present are left intact or decreased or enhanced in value and any new ones are added.**

This educational process must not stop with the symptoms in one case. **It is extremely rare that any one patient will exhibit all of the symptoms for which that therapy is effective.** Therefore, healers would not learn how to successfully use this therapy in the case of patients who exhibit different symptoms. For this reason, it is essential to also know how the therapy affects the healthy. The effects it produces in the healthy are the *identical* symptoms that will respond when the therapy is correctly administered to the sick.

The most successful means of investigation is to search the literature for adverse results from the potential care. For example, if an improperly administered chiropractic adjustment can cause cephalgia (a headache) it is a strong indication that this type of therapy can also be an effective therapy for the same dis-ease. When acupuncture administered to a healthy individual causes mental irritability, it can be administered to an irritated patient to cure irritability. A phytotherapy agent(herb)that causes burning of the stomach in the healthy, if properly administered will cure the same condition in the ill. This is the **Law of Similars; each therapy in improper amounts and/or applications can produce those specific, fixed, consistently reliable dis-ease symptoms which it is capable of healing in small properly administered amounts and/or forces.**

**Only narcotics seem to be an exception to this rule. In their primary action, they take away sensation, sensitivity, or irritability; in moderate experimental doses on the healthy there is a noticeable increase in sensitivity and irritability during the secondary action.** Therefore, their action is less predictable.

In the primary action of some therapies there can be a few symptoms that are opposed to the majority. They should not be considered contra-indications but variables or **alternating actions** within the primary action. It must be remembered that, in testing therapies, some symptoms are produced in the majority of patients, others less frequently, and a very few in a very limited number of cases only. This last category is termed **idiosyncrasies or hypersensitivities** and means a peculiar disposition in otherwise healthy persons to become ill from certain things that do not appear to have an effect upon the vast majority. In hypersensitivity, two things are required; 1 the inherent power of the therapy to act, and 2 the ability of the num, kundalini, vital, innate, ch'i, life force to respond to it. Therefore, hypersensitivity is the ability of an individual constitution to react to small units whereas the general population requires much larger amounts or forces to experience similar effects. Today these types of cases may also be referred to as "Environmental Illness".

# LAW OF INDIVIDUALITY

**Every therapy exhibits specific effects in the human that do not occur from any other therapy in exactly the same pattern. There can be no surrogates.** For a practitioner to utilize therapies without first proving them is analogous to a madman in an artist's workshop grabbing tools unfamiliar to him to "work" on the art around him. Such irresponsibility can only ruin the masterpiece. So it is with health care. Therapies upon which life depends must be distinguished from each other so that quick, permanent and harmless restoration of the health and well-being of the total individual can be achieved.

# Chapter 12
# LAWS OF MOST SUITABLE MODE OF EMPLOYING CARE

*"Nature knows no trifling; she is always sincere,*
*always serious, always stern, she is always in*
*the right, and the errors and mistakes*
*are invariably ours."*

— Goethe

## LAW OF TOTALITY

Let us now consider the **most effective employment of the primary and secondary reaction of therapies for the cure of dis-ease.** Clearly, the therapy with a documented symptom picture that **most nearly** corresponds to the totality of the patient's symptoms will produce the most dramatic and permanent cure. However, the true healer must constantly guard against the reductionist mistake of considering the dis-ease to be the result of something within or without the living being. Research has repeatedly documented that the **num, kundalini, vital, innate, ch'i, life force must first be altered before foreign influences can have an effect upon the physical being. In other words, barring trauma, the quantum component must be dis-eased** *before* **the solid state can be affected by an entity within or without the living being.**

## WILDER'S LAW

**The most critical factor is the varying sensitivity of the individual organism (patient) to a given dose or force; the same dose may be "small" for one individual, "medium" for another, and "large" for the third person, thus yielding different effects in each.** See Figure 7.2 Arndt-Schultz Law. **The critical issue is to accurately adjust the dose and/or force to the individual's need at that particular time.**

## LAW OF MICROBES

Pasteur put forth the misguided hypothesis that micro-organisms caused dis-ease because he could isolate them from all sick individuals. But under close scientific scrutiny, his theory cannot support itself. If we were to visit garbage dumps and record all data observed, we would likely document that all sites were infested by rats. According to Pasteur's pseudo-scientific thinking, because we could isolate rats at every site, the cause of garbage dumps is rats! Far more scientific is the concept that rats are found in garbage dumps because dumps provide an ideal environment for them. There is a constant food supply, shelter and  the inability of enemies to attack them. Alter any one of these necessary factors and the rats will not be able to survive. So it is with dis-ease; the defense mechanisms have to deteriorate **prior to** the establishment of pathogenic microbes. Scientifically speaking, then, **exogenous agents, such as microbes, are the result and not the cause of dis-ease.**

# LAW OF ACUTE VS. CHRONIC DIS-EASE

The cure of chronic dis-ease, especially those that are complicated dis-eases, can require **much time.** Iatrogenic dis-ease in particular falls into this category.

One or more minor symptoms should not be considered a full-fledged dis-ease requiring major intervention. Experience demonstrates that slight adjustments of diet, life style, etc., or even if given a little time, the life force may resolve these dispositions on its own. If, however, the patient complains of a few intense symptoms and the healer finds several other, minor, symptoms that complete a dis-ease picture, then an intervention may be warranted.

The worse the acute dis-ease, the more numerous and striking the symptoms. The larger the volume of useful symptoms, the more surely the most appropriate therapy can be determined. The more general and unqualified the symptoms, the less value they are in achieving the cure. **The more strange, rare and peculiar the symptoms are, the quicker and easier they reveal to the practitioner the correct therapy. To illustrate, "headaches" provide nothing of significance but the report of headaches that "start in the neck and radiate to the eyes accompanied by dizziness and nausea" is a rich source of data leading to the *one* correct therapeutic approach that produces few or no iatrogenic side effects.**

This is true because the numerous remaining symptoms that be treated by this one therapy can remain entirely inactivated. No trace of them can be perceived because the therapy being administered, **at just above threshold,** is  too weak to affect the healthy parts. Thus, **symptoms not already an intrinsic part of the aggravated picture are not affected during the retracing process. Extremely sensitive patients may experience, when the therapy exceeds threshold, some very slight new symptoms; but recovery proceeds in spite of these minor irritations and these aggravations soon pass away** if not perpetuated by errors in living, excess passions, iatrogenic influences, etc.

**Minor aggravations within the first hours or, on rarer occasions, within the first few days are an excellent indication that the *acute* dis-ease will be cured. The closer to threshold the therapy is in *acute* dis-ease, the shorter and milder is the primary aggravation (retracing). Conversely, the more over-threshold the therapy is, the greater the primary aggravation.**

**With *very* chronic dis-ease and a properly chosen threshold therapy, it is much less likely that the patient will exhibit a significant aggravation. Experience has documented that this is especially so when indicated subsequent therapy is slightly modified. When this procedure is utilized, aggravations of the original symptoms appear only temporarily when the cure is near completion.**

# LAW OF EXCEPTION

**Because there are very likely laws and therapies that we healers have not yet discovered, it is not always possible to achieve the perfectly matched threshold therapy.** In such cases, a cure without aggravation is not possible but if the therapy selected is close to the threshold, the aggravation will be very mild.

**When, however, there are strange, rare and peculiar symptoms associated with a particular therapy, even though there are many lesser or common symptoms, cure will follow without marked aggravation (retracing). If none of the symptoms are rare, strange or peculiar but are, instead, very general symptoms such as nausea, weakness, headaches, etc., then the healer must not expect a favor-**

able outcome. Such situations, should be *rare* for the properly trained healer. If aggravations from improperly selected therapy do take place, the healer must not allow the patient to suffer through them. The case must be re-evaluated for a more precise therapy.

If the symptom complex of the dis-ease is not sufficiently covered by any one therapy but one therapy is compatible with one group of symptoms and another therapy compatible with a second group of symptoms, it is not advisable to administer both. If the better of the two therapies fails to cure and has produced additional or altered symptoms, it would not be advisable simply to give the second choice. Nor is it advisable to give both therapies simultaneously. Experience has documented that a closer similimum therapy must be found to be successful in producing a cure. Here, as in all cases where there are changes in the symptom picture, a re-evaluation is necessary.

In *chronic* dis-ease, usually arising from the psoric miasma (Pittic dosha, fire phase) it may be necessary to use several therapies in succession to bring about the cure. Each of these therapies must be chosen based upon an update of the symptoms *after* the num, kundalini, vital, innate, ch'i, life force has *completed* its action initiated by the previous therapy.

The same rules also apply in rare defective chronic internal dis-eases when the patient does not exhibit enough symptoms to clearly indicate a precise therapy. The choice of therapy often requires an intuitive judgement on the part of the practitioner. With these rare cases, the first therapy usually proves to be only partially effective and frequently may produce adverse side effects, requiring urgent relief because of their intensity, which may inter-mix with the original symptoms. Even more important, the correctly selected therapy will bring out additional symptoms of the dis-ease process itself. These new dis-ease related symptoms facilitate the choice of a more precise therapy.

In defective chronic local (external) dis-eases, the new symptoms appear externally but the protocol is similar to defective chronic internal dis-eases. The great error in caring for this class of dis-ease is treating them as isolated local dis-eases which causes them to become even more chronic. What may appear to be a currently developed local condition is most frequently a local manifestation of chronic systemic dis-ease. It may become necessary to help the afflicted part by chemical, mechanical or surgical means to remove impediments to the num, kundalini, vital, innate, ch'i, life force but it must be remembered that such "local" conditions affect the entire organism and that systemic evaluation is necessary. Such a position is confirmed by the administration of a constitutional or miasmatic (diathesis, dosha, phase) therapy which produces changes to what was thought to be an isolated "local" condition.

## LAW OF TOTAL DIS-EASE

A local condition is never anything but a *part* of the total dis-ease. Local treatments of surgery, ointments, liniments, salves, poultices, adjustments, modalities, etc., can appear to cure but may drive the condition deeper into the constitution of the patient creating a chronic disturbance which the num, kundalini, vital, innate, ch'i, life force cannot overcome. To use "local" therapies simultaneously with constitutional or miasmatic therapies, or to use a local application of the constitutional or miasmatic therapy has the serious disadvantage that the "local" dis-ease *appears* to be cured before the constitutional or miasmatic, doshic, phase dis-ease is fully resolved. The result is a false impression of cure when in reality the dis-ease has only been temporarily palliated and will return with a greater severity due to facilitation. Additionally, if the correct constitutional or miasmatic, doshic, phase therapy has not yet been determined, palliation of the "local" symptoms eliminates vital data making the practitioner's work much more difficult. See Figure 12.1.

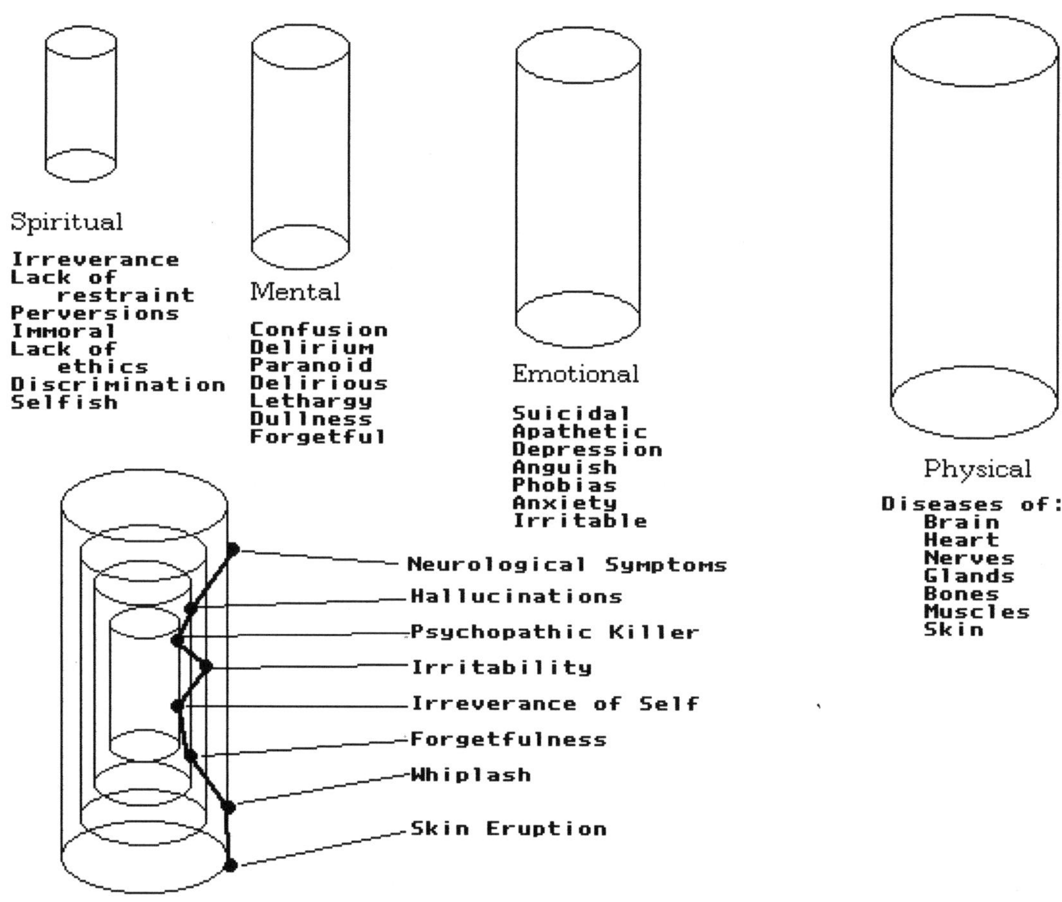


*Figure 12.1 — The Total Being/Total Dis-ease Graph*

## LAW OF MIASMAS (DIATHESIS, DOSHAS, PHASES)

**It must be understood that a miasma (diathesis, doshic, phase) occupies the entire organism. It creates "local" as well as systemic symptomatology and because a "local" therapy cannot remove the holographic totality, such palliative care facilitates the miasma.** Therefore, in **any** case with a personal or familial history of any of the miasmas (diathesis, dosha, phase), that is what **must** be addressed in order to truly heal the patient. Miasmatic (diathesis, dosha, phase) weaknesses are the most frequent underlying cause of chronic dis-eases. It is also necessary to inquire as to previous palliative care of "local" dis-ease which will have facilitated the chronic dis-ease.

This miasmatic (diathesis, doshic, phase) influence can be compared to an iceberg. The local symptoms are the minor and least dangerous portion that can be seen above the waterline while the miasmatic (diathesis, dosha, phase) influences are like the submerged, unseen, and most dangerous portion of the iceberg. The total iceberg (miasmatic, diathesis, dosha, phase) must be dealt with in order to truly make the organism safe (healthy). See Figure 12.2.

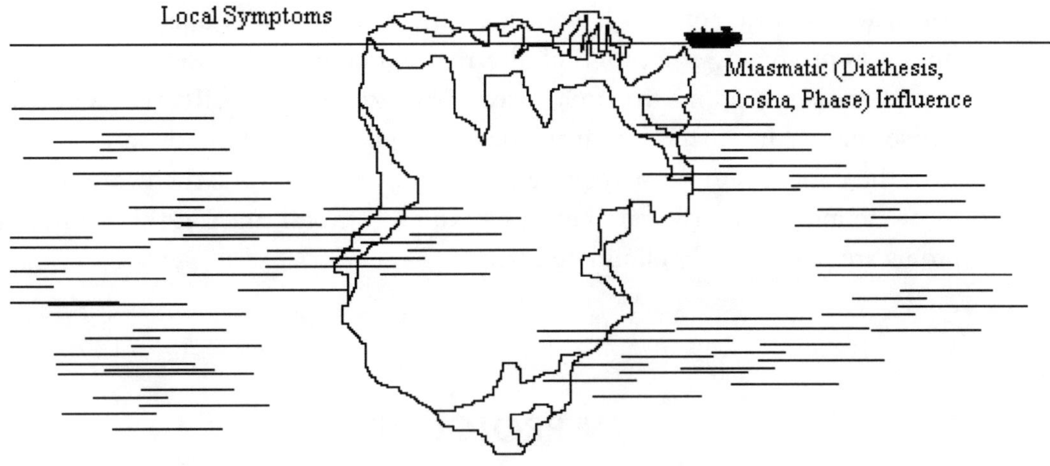


*Figure 12.2 — The Miasmatic (Diathesis, Dosha, Phase) Iceberg*

## LAW OF SPIRITUAL, MENTAL AND EMOTIONAL DIS-EASE

**To psora belong all defective dis-eases, dis-eases in which all the other symptoms are hidden behind a single dominant one.** This makes the higher (spiritual, mental, and emotional) levels of the patient's total being the critical factors in choosing the correct care. In fact, so much so that we arrive at the **Law of Spirit, Mind and Emotion: There is no dis-ease or therapy which does not markedly alter the spiritual, mental and emotional state of the patient in its own destructive manner. Therefore, one can never cure according to nature without considering the spiritual, mental and emotional states of the patient.**

**These defective dis-eases are cured in exactly the same way as all other dis-ease is cured, by choosing that therapy which in the healthy produces the symptoms to be cured. This is especially true when there is a history of a life-threatening physical dis-ease being palliatively treated and the patient is deteriorating into mental illness. This aspect of masking must be investigated thoroughly in taking the case history.** This may mean carefully reviewing not only the narrative of the patient but also that of his relatives and/or associates.

**If, on the other hand, spiritual, mental and/or emotional dis-eases suddenly present themselves in an otherwise calm, well-adjusted individual with no significant physical symptoms, the non-miasmatic, non-diathesis, non-doshic, non-phase should be cared for immediately with non-miasmatic, non-doshic, non-phase, non-diathesis care. Once the presenting symptoms are no longer a part of the patient's symptom picture, then and only then should miasmatic care be rendered. Care must be taken not to over-treat because this will facilitate the miasmic, diathic, doshic, phase and change it from an acute to chronic case. Without this proper psoric, diathic, doshic, phase care, the condition will recur and more severely than it occurred in the first attack.**

When dealing with such spiritual, mental and emotional cases, the practitioner and staff must always behave as if they believe the patient to be in full possession of his/her faculties. For only then will the patient divulge the true inner feelings that are critical to a total understanding of the case.

# LAW OF INTERMITTENT AND ALTERNATING DIS-EASE

Chronic psoric (and occasionally syphilitic) dis-eases in which the same symptoms occur, in the midst of apparent well-being, at **definite intervals** or which alternate with other dis-ease, one being asymptomatic while the other is active, i.e., in fevers producing symptoms of alternating hot and cold sweats, the critical issue is to accurately determine the non-crisis symptoms. **In such cases, care proves most effective when administered immediately after an episode.** To administer care at the beginning of an attack tends to weaken the patient and aggravate the attack. If the intervals are close together, such as in grave fevers, then care is best given just as the symptoms are subsiding. In most cases, the care must be rendered several times at this point in the attack before the cycling symptoms are permanently eliminated.

# LAW OF PROTOCOL

**As long as there is improvement, no additional care should be rendered.** Each subsequent application of care must be **altered slightly** so that the program used by the num, kundalini, vital, innate, ch'i, life force cannot be facilitated. When this law is observed, **in chronic cases, the same type of care can be rendered daily for weeks or even months if necessary without aggravation and with increasing benefit. If new symptoms develop near the end of care, or if the remaining dis-ease symptoms worsen near the end of therapy, then the frequency of care must be reduced or stopped for several days.** Any care that brings about new symptoms will not resolve the original problem. If aggravations are *dramatic,* a counteracting therapy *must* be instituted immediately because **the aggravating therapy was not appropriate; it never means that the therapy was below threshold.** A more precise therapy *must* be chosen.

**If, with a properly chosen therapy, the symptoms continue to exist, there is something in the patient's life style, work environment, diet, previous treatment, etc., that must be dealt with in order to successfully resolve the case.** This is especially critical in the case of chronically ill patients.

**Excessive and/or excessively forceful care, especially if repeated frequently, is iatrogenic to the patient.** Because of facilitation, it may not be possible to counteract the engram produced by long-term improper care. For this reason, all therapy ideally must be administered at **just above threshold.** Care should be continued, with slight modifications each visit, until such time as the original symptoms begin to return. This indicates complete cure is imminent and that the num, kundalini, vital, innate, ch'i, life force has no further need for care to be administered. To confirm this, the patient should go without care for a period of time. If the symptoms again disappear, he/she is cured. If the symptoms are still manifested, further care is indicated but at reduced force, frequency, volume, potency, use of a different technique, etc.

**In** *all cases* **, improvement of the psychic and energy levels is the most reliable, early, indication that the health problem will be successfully resolved by the administered therapy. Greater sense of ease, composure, mental freedom, higher spirits and the normal demeanor of the individual** are early indications of cure. Aggravations, on the other hand, are announced by a deterioration of the same factors.

# FAVORITE THERAPIES

The healer must guard against the overuse of "favorite" therapies, administering only those therapies that are truly indicated.

# LAW OF CONTRADICTIONS

When dealing with extremely chronic patients, the symptomatic picture can reverse itself from that normally described in the textbooks; i.e., instead of being mentally restless (hyperactive) or irritable, patients become lethargic or depressed; instead of chronic constipation, the patients will frequently complain of diarrhea; rather than ravenous, their appetites may become anorexic; instead of excessive body heat, they complain of coldness. Complaints such as these mean that the patient has entered the "Exhaustion Phase" where the physical and quantum (vital, num, kundalini, life, ch'i force) components required for healing are failing. At this point, the practitioner must understand that the patient's progress can be very slow. Even correctly chosen therapies are frequently capable of stimulating the healing process only with difficulty.

# BOOK THREE

# JUNIOR TEXT

# INTRODUCTION TO THE JUNIOR TEXT

*". . .Physician heal thyself. . ."*

— Jesus Christ

## INTRODUCTION AND CORRELATION

The Junior text is meant to be an introduction and correlation of the various quantum healing arts and is not to be considered an extensive treatise on them. Nor is it to be considered a complete listing; there are literally hundreds of variants within quantum healing. Rather, what we are presenting is an overview of the most widely used forms. It should not be interpreted that the forms listed are more acceptable, more reliable, more scientific, etc., than those forms of quantum healing not listed here.

A general tendency is to pay particular attention to the aspect of natural healing in which you are most educated and gloss over the other specialties. This is a most grave error for you will never gain a perspective of how your particular discipline correlates with the others. You will lack an understanding of when and how another aspect of quantum healing, and even at times allopathic (complementary, alternative) medicine, can result in a synergistic enhancement of benefit and better serve the patient. This is the grand and arrogant mistake made by allopathy, the illusion that all knowledge and healing skill resides within their particular concept of healing. If we as quantum healers make the same mistake, how are we any different than they are?

Our goal is to become the best healers that the world has ever known. In order to achieve this lofty status we must be willing to leave our bigotries, prejudices and discriminations behind. That is the price demanded. The grand question is are we, as individuals and as a group, developed to the point that we can meet the challenge and live with the results? If not, then we must take stock of what changes need to be made and have the courage to follow through with them. If so, then we must constantly guard against self-inflated egos that will most definitely cause us to lose that which we struggled so hard to achieve.

Thus, in the final analysis, we not only strive to obtain proper healing knowledge but also struggle with the universal weaknesses of our race. Few individuals in history have achieved our target goals but those who have become glowing beacons for the rest of us. The price is high but the reward is great.

B. J. Palmer, D.C., Ph.C., once said, **"When our work becomes a standard for the whole world, it also becomes a target for the shafts of the envious. If our work is mediocre, we are left serenely alone. If we achieve a masterpiece, it will set a million tongues a-wagging. Whatsoever you think, write, or build, no one will strive to surpass or to slander, unless your work be stamped with the seal of superiority."**

How superior do you truly want to become?

# Chapter 13
# WESTERN MEDICINE

*"The successful physician is a doctor who can
manage to keep the patient calm until nature
has time to heal him."*

— Hugh Allen

## THE GENERAL TERM

"Western Medicine" is a general term used to classify multiple types of medical practice which, generally speaking, have as a common bond the reductionistic, non-vitalistic, mechanistic concept of health and dis-ease. This type of medical thinking has its origins in the atomistic theory of science which developed about 200 years ago. Fortunately, more and more of these practitioners are beginning to see the need for dramatically modifying their practices in order to incorporate modern quantum healing principles.

## HISTORY

Almost from the beginning, man has been susceptible individually or collectively to dis-eases from physical and/or moral causes. Man started with the simple task of treating dis-eases. As the civilization of man increased in complexity, the need for complex medical aid increased in equal proportion. Since the death of Hippocrates, western man has occupied himself with addressing the ever-increasing multiplicity of dis-ease.

With the new pre-occupation with dis-ease came varying dis-similar ideas. This led to what is now referred to as systems of medicine, each of which was at variance with the others and many being very contradictory even within themselves. Some of the ideas brought forth were in concert with the order of nature while others most definitely were not. Some, such as "blood letting", were merely theoretical webs woven loosely together by cunning minds.

Independent of all of these, there arose a system of healing utilizing a mixture of unknown (in that they produce side-effects not anticipated when prescribed) substances targeted towards some material (solid state) objective completely at variance with the natural order of life. This system has became known as allopathy. Its practitioners are referred to as Medical Doctors (M.D.s).

The allopath has been primarily trained to believe that the cause of dis-ease is material (micro-organisms, mal-functioning chemistry, traumatic injury, etc.) Today, it is increasingly obvious that this philosophy has not proven successful as more and more causes of dis-ease are proving to be non-material (quantum, energetic) in nature. A second complication is that the solid state drugs prescribed for energy disturbances are not consistently predictable in their reactions.

## ALLOPATHY

Allopathy is based upon the antiquated premise that the living being is **not** an innate self-healing entity but, rather, requires the superior education and invasive knowledge of the practitioner in order to be healed. Passive patient participation is the required norm. Treatment centers around the hypothesis that dis-ease is the result of exogenous etiologies, with which  the practitioner is at war. This philosophy requires the practitioner to control, destroy and/or exorcize, by means of drugs and/or surgery, those external dis-ease-producing demons and the tissues which they inhabit. **Little or no consideration is given to the living being's innate defense mechanisms that can assist the being to strengthen and repair itself.**

This misguided reductionistic, non-vitalistic philosophy tends to produce, at best, disrespect and, at worst, arrogance toward the living being and its auto-healing abilities. Heroic measures are therefore routinely resorted to in the mistaken belief that another heroic intervention can be easily employed when iatrogenic dis-ease results. Such an approach, while very theatrical, unfortunately, quickly produces a hypnotic dullness of the mental faculties of the practitioner and prevents practitioners intoxicated with their own self-importance from comprehending the scientifically untenable position of their philosophy.

Such mental paralysis has, for over 100 years, even prevented these practitioners from comprehending the dying words from their high priest Louis Pasteur who said with great regret, **"Bernard was correct, the bacterium is nothing, the soil is everything."** Meaning, of course, if the body's resistance is adequate, a microbe cannot produce dis-ease symptoms. Claude Bernard, the "Father of Experimental Physiology", agreed with Pasteur when he said that not everyone exposed to cold would come down with pneumonia, only an occasional exposure turns into pneumonia. Bernard's deduction was that unless individuals are predisposed, even powerful causes will have no effect on them. He wrote that this issue is the pivot of all experimental physiology and the true cause of almost all dis-ease.  Unfortunately, in their obsession with micro-organisms, allopathic researchers have ignored and continue to ignore these words of wisdom to pursue the illusion that microbes cause illness.

This lack of basic understanding of the nature of a living organism has led them, in spite of their dismal results in chronic dis-ease, to continue to develop increasingly stronger and more toxic drugs, which are themselves now the leading causes of iatrogenic dis-ease and a major public health hazard. In fact, so much so that M. Lappe in *When Antibiotics Fail* states that from excessive exposure to antibiotics we are creating new microbes through mutation faster than we are developing drugs to counter them.

But this is certainly not the first warning on the subject. Fleming, the researcher who developed penicillin, cautioned against the over-use of antibiotics in these words, "There may be a time down the road when **80 percent to 90 percent of infections will be resistant to all known antibiotics."** The scientific reality is that antibiotics have been frequently used indiscriminately for fifty years and we are now down that very road that Fleming feared. Even the prestigious *New England Journal Of Medicine* echoed this fear, albeit in somewhat cloaked terms, stating that infections have to be treated with "less ecologically disturbing techniques." See Figures 13.1, 13.2, 13.3.

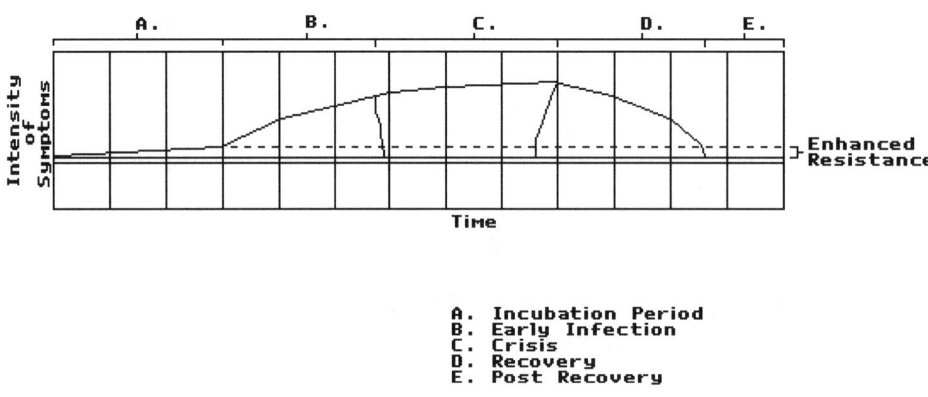


*Figure 13.1 — Infection And Recovery By Natural Means*

This graph illustrates a healthy immune system's response to a localized, moderately severe infection. **Note the lengthy recovery period leading to an enhanced natural health (immunity) base line thus indicating that the individual's immune system has successfully counter-acted the infection. Furthermore, it has retained a "memory" of this encounter and has become stronger and better able to successfully deal with any future episodes of the same nature.**

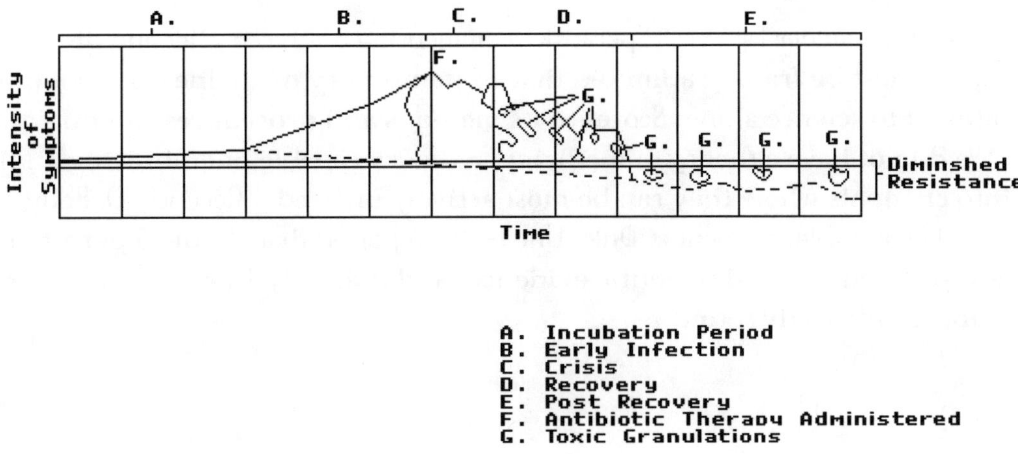



*Figure 13.2 — Infection And Recovery By Means Of Synthetic Antibiotics*

The acute infection pattern with antibiotic intervention provides **a faster recovery time but ongoing iatrogenic problems arise with "Toxic Granulations" released by the microbes, plus the natural base line of resistance is lowered. The antibiotic did the immune system's work for it and the innate defense mechanisms were never triggered; therefore, the individual's body has no retained memory of the encounter and the immune system is actually weaker than before. Another complication is that unless all the microbes were eliminated, the remaining ones will mutate and develop a resistance to the antibiotic with the result that recurring future infections are more likely.**

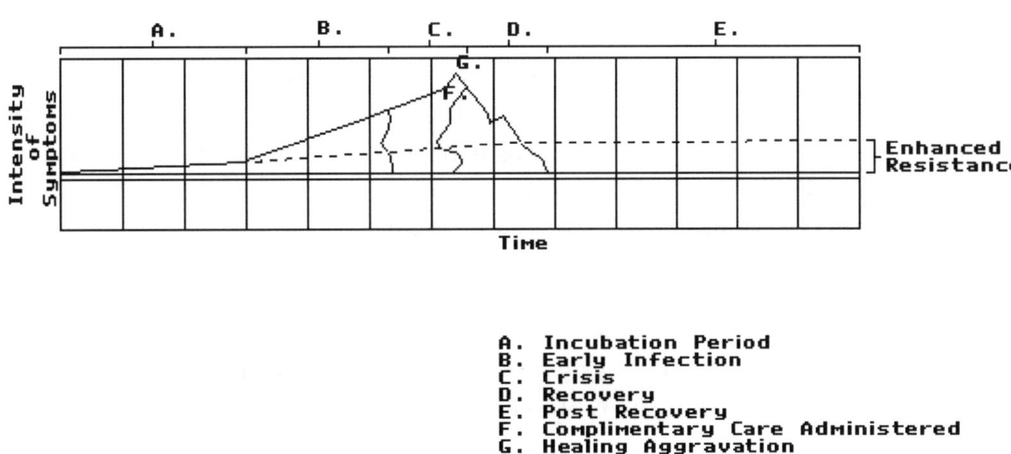



*Figure 13.3 — Infection And Recovery By Means Of Quantum Care*

This figure represents an acute infection in which **the immune system has been enhanced by means of quantum procedures. Note the comparison of the time frames for the illness and recovery, the lack of downstream complications, and the substantially higher natural health base line (resistance).** *Proper* **quantum care helped the immune system first fight off the infection and then retain the immune response memory. The end result is an immune system that is enhanced in its ability to deal with future challenges.**

# FURTHER SUPPORT

Jonas Salk, M.D., of polio fame, also came to this same conclusion years after developing the "Salk Polio Immunization". In 1976, he stated that there are two distinct ways of attempting to heal. First, one can **try** to control the individual symptoms; **the second stimulates the patient's own immuno-defense system and thus allows the body to heal itself.**

The famous Russian researcher Dr. A. D. Speransky commenting on the conflict and disorder of allopathic concepts wrote, ". . . **It must be frankly admitted that contemporary medicine does not owe its success in the sphere of treatment to science alone. Scores of its methods and procedures rest on empiricism and even on chance. We do not have a theory of medicine, a theory capable of embracing all the data and directing them into channels where they can be most actively utilized.**" Recently D. Eddy, M.D., Ph.D., professor of Health Policy and Management at Duke University reported that **about 15 percent of all medical interventions are supported by solid scientific evidence, and that only 1 percent of all the articles in medical journals are scientifically sound.**

# STRENGTHS AND WEAKNESSES

Allopathy's strength lies in acute heroic intervention. If an individual has been in a serious accident and is hemorrhaging or is having a heart attack or suffering from anaphylactic shock, he or she needs to be rushed to the hospital emergency room. Its weakness is in health maintenance and treatment of chronic, constitutional and miasmatic dis-ease. In what case has the allopathic treatment cured diabetes, arthritis, hyperactivity, epilepsy, enuresis, depression, colitis, etc.? Insulin never cures diabetes; Ritalin never cures hyperactivity but only drugs the patients to the point where they are so lethargic they can no longer cause mischief.

# THE GRAND DIFFERENCE

Allopathic medicine and its branches share an obsession with identification of the infectious agent supposedly causing the dis-ease rather than the strengthening and support of the patient's defense mechanisms. This can be traced back to the "germ theory" of Pasteur which states that different dis-eases are caused by different organisms. The majority of Pasteur's professional life was consumed by his search to find these "pathogenic organisms". While his work has greatly advanced the symptomatic treatment of such dis-eases, it has only dealt with the very limited scope of the virility of the infectious organism.

Contemporaries of Pasteur, Bernard and Virchow did not follow the same road. They elected to primarily research the internal deranged environment of the host or, as Bernard termed it, the "milieu interieur" as the dominant factor in the genesis of dis-ease. They taught that **the physician's primary responsibility is to make the internal environment of the individual inhospitable to the pathogenic organism and no dis-ease can develop.**

Speransky's entire volume of research *The Basis For The Theory Of Medicine* proves Bernard and Virchow to be correct. Dr. Murray also discusses the work of another Russian, Metchikoff, the discoverer of the white blood cell. "He and his associates consumed cultures containing millions of cholera bacteria. Yet none of them developed cholera. The reason: Their immune systems were not compromised."

In their later years, Pasteur and Bernard engaged in lively scientific debate. As previously stated, on his death bed Pasteur finally acknowledged his monumental error by stating, "**Bernard was correct. The pathogen is nothing. The terrain (environment) is everything.**" Unfortunately, for over a century, Pasteur's revelation has had little or no impact upon allopathy. It still chooses to pursue the narrow road of the abnormal (pathology) instead of the broad scientific expanses of what is required to keep the patient normal (healthy).

This is the grand distinction between allopathy and other forms of healing. All forms of quantum healing share the principle of strengthening the individual's defense systems while allopathy tends to ignore the state of the body's defenses, believing that drugs and surgery have the inherent ability to "control" dis-ease.

## DENTISTRY

Dentistry is considered a limited licensed specialty and is restricted to conditions of the oral cavity. Allopathic thinking and modes of treatment dominate and, therefore, dentistry's strengths and weaknesses generally reflect those of allopathy.

## DIETETICS

Dietetic is a subservient branch of allopathy. Practitioners are not considered competent to practice without physician supervision. The great irony, however, is that very few allopathic practitioners have studied nutrition.

Amounts of nutrients needed are based upon Minimal Daily Requirements/ Recommendations with little or no consideration for individual constitutional variants such as absorption ability, miasmatic (diathic, doshic, phase) influences, bio-availability, racemic molecules or increased metabolic requirements. Growth of foods in nutrient-depleted soil is generally regarded as insignificant. Chemical residues from pesticides, fungicides, herbicides, etc., are for all practical purposes ignored. Synthetic foods are generally regarded as equal in nutritional value with natural foods because complete vitamin and mineral complements and synergy are generally disregarded. Nutrients are considered as non-related factors in non-metabolic dis-eases.

## LABORATORY DIAGNOSIS

A laboratory diagnosis is a reductionist procedure held in common by all subdivisions of allopathy. The goal is to isolate abnormal factors and exogenous agents in the belief that all dis-ease can be identified and resolved by the reductionist equation.

## NURSING

Nurses are subservient paraprofessional assistants to the physician. Practitioners are not considered competent to practice without supervision. Thought and practice are rigidly controlled along the allopathic model.

## OPTOMETRY

Optometry is a limited licensed specialty which is denied the use of drugs and surgery. The optometrist's main activity has traditionally been the prescription of corrective lenses for the eyes. More progressive practitioners are exploring the possibility of more natural and permanent means of correcting visual abnormalities.

# OSTEOPATHY

Osteopathy was once a distinct philosophy of manipulative healing based upon the premise that all dis-ease was caused by a deficiency of blood supply to the involved tissue. Today, it has been assimilated and is indistinguishable from allopathy. Most practitioners are now un-educated in and therefore incapable of non-iatrogenic manipulative therapy. Osteopathy, therefore, currently reflects the same philosophy, strengths and weaknesses of allopathy.

# PHYSICAL THERAPY/PHYSIATRY

Physical therapy and physiatry are the allopathic attempt to duplicate the services of masseuses and the previous generations of chiropractors and osteopaths. Lacking expansionistic, vitalistic perspective and training, therapists fall back on standard allopathic procedures and tend to incorporate their same strengths and weaknesses.

# PODIATRY

A podiatrist is a limited licensed practitioner specializing in the pedal foundation. Philosophy, practices and procedures are generally in line with reductionist allopathic standards.

# PSYCHOLOGY

A psychologist is a limited licensed mental health practitioner who is denied the use of drugs and surgery. Practitioners tend to polarize between the reductionistic allopathic orientation and the vitalistic expansionistic concept of health care. Limitations and advantages reflect these respective polarizations.

# SURGERY

Surgery is the practice of removing non-functional, damaged and/or supposedly extraneous body parts. Its strength is in the elimination of parts that have become deleterious to health and are beyond the limitations of matter (knowledge of the practitioner to heal). Its major weakness is that the organism, in many instances, can no longer function maximally and/or properly with missing or mutilated parts.

# VETERINARY

Veterinary, the allopathic practice upon animals, generally contains the same strengths and weaknesses as its parent allopathy.

# Chapter 14
# QUANTUM MEDICINE

*"Whatever elements nature does not introduce into
vegetables, the natural food of all animal life,
directly of herbivorous, indirectly of carnivorous
animals - are to be regarded with suspicion. The
disgrace of medicine has been a colossal system of
self-deception, in obedience to which mines have
been emptied of their cankering minerals, the
vegetable kingdom robbed of its noxious growths,
the entrails of animals taxed for their impurities,
poison bags of reptiles drained of their venom, and
all the inconceivable abominations thus obtained
thrust down the throat of human beings suffering
from some fault of organization or nourishment
of vital functions."*

— Oliver Wendell Holmes

## THE FORMS OF MEDICINE

Those forms of medicine that have allopathic principles as a common root exhibit certain unifying characteristics and it is for this reason that they can interrelate with such ease. They share basic philosophy, protocols, procedures, and understanding of each other's arena of practice, etc.

The same is not true of quantum medicine. True, there is a root philosophy but unfortunately few schools are currently teaching these common bonds. In fact, many, such as chiropractic, naturopathy and oriental medicine, have incorporated the territorial attitude of allopathy and do all in their power to prevent others from "infringing on their scope of practice". Nor do practitioners receive formal training in related disciplines. For example, the doctor of chiropractic receives no formal training to acquaint him with methods used by the oriental medical doctor, the native healer, the ayurvedic practitioner or the massage therapist. Therefore, quantum medicine cannot as easily refer patients back and forth as allopathic practitioners do. This shortcoming, obviously, deprives the patient of the best possible care.

Reality dictates that **there is no single healing principle which is all- encompassing.** Each succeeds where others have failed. Each complements the others. Each overlaps others. A topic discussed under one heading may very well apply to another discipline also. This does not mean that the discipline under which it is discussed has a monopoly on that knowledge or concept. This is the grand eclectic lesson that all quantum practitioners must master and is the main topic of this section. We must each learn to understand and appreciate how the various quantum healing arts interrelate. To do less is to make the same arrogant mistake that is the major stumbling block of the allopathic profession, the self-defeating attitude that, "We know it all."

# Chapter 15
# AFRICAN MEDICINE

*"The village raises the child."*
— African Proverb

## THE SCOPE

The practice of African medicine occurs over a large geographic area from the Sahara and Kalahari deserts to the tropical rain forests, from the vast grasslands to the summit of Mount Kilimanjaro. Within this vast territory, with its great diversity of climate, many phytotherapeutic agents grow and their uses have been mastered by the local populations.

African medicine also encompasses a huge time span, extending from the crude medicines of early man to the refinements developed by ancient Egyptian civilization and the black empires of central Africa and the Islamic or Sufi influences of north Africa. The latter is found under the separate heading of Sufi healing in this text.

African medicine inseparably connects healing, culture, society and spirituality while in the western mind there are clear-cut, but artificial, separations between healing, culture, society and religion. **In order to comprehend African healing, such artificial categorizations must be abandoned.** Once we begin to appreciate the vitalistic, expansionistic concepts of African health care, we can perceive the great wisdom encompassed within the indigenous African mode of healing.

## HISTORICAL PERSPECTIVE

The western academic study of African healing has barely begun. The main reason for this delay appears to be the western cultural and academic reluctance to accept anything of value coming from the indigenous inhabitants of the "Dark Continent". It is imperative that such prejudices be set aside and that attention immediately be given to African healing for, like so much other indigenous knowledge, it is rapidly being lost forever.

A second problem is that very few authors seem to have the ability to accurately express what is taking place in native African healing in terms of traditional culture. Even the references at the end of Book III, some of the best available, are in many instances noticeably lacking in this perspective. Therefore, much study, reflection and correlation with vitalistic, expansionistic principles is necessary in order to segregate the scientific realities of African medicine from preconceived prejudices.

One fact is absolutely certain and well documented however. David Living stone, the great Scottish missionary and explorer, was deeply impressed by the **comparatively few dis-eases present among the indigenous peoples** he met during his exploration of Africa in 1869. He further wrote that the dis-eases most prevalent were those promoted by sudden and extreme changes of temperature and weather. These became rare as the people adapted standards of better personal protection from the elements - and **not because of changes made by western medicine.**

## LAW OF NUM

Among the people of the Kalahari desert, healers commonly discuss the "Num" (vital or life force, innate, kundalini, ch'i). Similar concepts, are also known, but by other names, among other African tribes.

## THE TSWANA HEALER

Among the Tswana, the Ngakas (healers) are not distinguished from other citizens. Their ability to treat dis-ease does not isolate them as a separate class in society as are physicians in western society. When not engaged in healing, the Ngaka leads exactly the same life style as every other member of the community producing his own food and following a necessary trade. The amount of time spent in healing depends entirely upon the chronicity and extent of the dis-ease. Simple dis-eases are dealt with by family members, relatives and neighbors. Only when they are not successful in their care is the Ngaka normally consulted. Therefore, **the degree of respect and authority accorded a particular Ngaka in the community is proportional to his professional success** and not by the extent of his training as in custom in western cultures.

A Ngaka does undergo extensive and involved training under the supervision of an older practitioner. This training is called "teaching to dig" as most medicines are obtained from plants that must be dug up. Because of the extent of training that can last for years, apprentices usually become members of the Ngaka's family and community. By attending consultations with the patient and the Ngaka, the apprentice hears much confidential information as well as family and personal "secrets" of the community. He thus learns the virtues, vices and personal strengths and weaknesses of each member of the community which aid in prescribing correct remedies and giving wise council and advice. (One might compare this to the homeopathic case-taking process, the determination of the phase within Oriental medicine or arriving at the proper dosha in Ayurvedic medicine.)

How well these "secrets" are guarded further enhances the professional prestige of the Ngaka. It is frequently necessary for an apprentice to obtain approval from the chief and elders before beginning his training. In short, **the Ngaka is not only the community's healer but also the keeper of social order and values.**

Another skill associated with the Ngaka is the ability to throw bones (*go thela bola*) as a way to diagnose. In Tswana tradition, *go laola* (the ability to interpret the bones) is believed to be a gift from Modimo (God, or Universal Intelligence). Although, in western minds, the bones are commonly associated with diagnosis, they are not generally used by the Ngaka for this purpose but rather for religious and ceremonial purposes. The correctness of the thrower's interpretation of the bones appears, in western minds, to be attributed more to the Ngaka's extensive knowledge of his community's members, their personality traits and their "secrets".

## LAW OF A TOTAL HEALING ENVIRONMENT

Inherent within native African medicine also is the concept that an individual is not in a state of health, as a total person, when he/she is not abiding by the familial-social-religious standards of the community. Therefore, restoration to health is not merely a practitioner-patient relationship but a normalizing of familial-social-religious relationships as well. All individuals associated with the dis-eased person are thus required to be involved in the cure. **To heal in totality requires dealing with the physical, social and spiritual realm of the patient.**

## THE MAGIC QUESTION

While there is no doubt that there is an element of magic in African healing, it would be a tragic mistake to dismiss all of what is practiced as unscientific and, in so doing, miss much that can be consistently (scientifically) applied to aid the sick and suffering of the world.

## THE LESSON

The proverb appearing as the heading to this chapter is an excellent example of the social awareness of African cultures in general. No individual, other than by his or her own choosing or as a severe punishment for a crime, is left without an extensive support system in any aspect of life. **This cultural belonging, caring and nurturing is the basis of all African healing and one of its greatest strengths.** It is a lesson that could well be incorporated into the sterile non-social, non-religious, non-cultural, reductionist, non-vitalistic, doctor-patient only practice of western medicine.

## LIMITATIONS

There is obviously much more that needs to be studied and written regarding African healing. It remains one of my goals to further expand upon it and other deserving topics in future editions of this text. Much of the data discussed in the chapter on Native American And Oceanic healing may also apply to African healing.

# Chapter 16
# AYURVEDIC MEDICINE

*"The Science of Life shall never attain finality.
Therefore, humility and restless industry should
characterize your every endeavor and your
approach to knowledge. . . . The entire world
consists of teachers for the wise and enemies for
the fools. Therefore, knowledge conducive to
health, longevity, fame and excellence, coming even
from an unfamiliar source, should be received,
assimilated and utilized with earnestness."*

— Charaka Samhita

## HISTORY

In the ancient (circa 2,000 B.C.) Sanskrit language of India, "ayur" means life or healthy life and "veda" means science; thus, Ayurvedic Medicine literally is the science of life and health. Truth relating to health must be accepted and utilized with conviction even if it comes from unfamiliar or opposing sources.

The Charaka-Samhita (Annals Of Charaka)record that Asoka (273-232 B.C.), an Indian ruler who was totally distraught by the unrelenting internal wars and power struggles of his time, turned to Buddhism and its non-violent doctrines and established the first public hospitals. Interestingly, Mobile Surgical Army Hospitals (MASH) units appear to have been the norm as early as 1,000 B.C. In such MASH units, blood transfusions appear to have been nearly as commonplace as complex herbal pharmaceutical formulas.

## LAW OF BALANCE (PRAYOJANA)

The main objective of ayurvedic practice is health, the restoration and maintenance of metabolic and mental equilibrium and balances of the five senses (smell, taste, sight, touch, and hearing) with the organs of action (mouth, hands, and feet) and the organs of speech, excretion and reproduction.

## LAW OF DIS-EASE (DUKKHA SAMYOGA)

Dis-ease is defined as imbalance of physical comfort, pain or suffering, as well as mental anguish including the pangs of jealousy, fear, anger, avarice, hate, passions, **all that is unpleasant to the body and mind.** Dis-ease is fourfold:

1. AGANTUKA - or "adventurous dis-ease" resulting from external factors such as cuts, bites, stings, accidental injuries, etc. Generally speaking, such conditions are cared for surgically; i.e., by removing the stinger, suturing the incision, setting the bones.

2. SHARIRAKA - or "physical dis-ease" consisting of internal, nutritional, metabolic imbalances, growth defects, inflammations, infections, and degeneration. (Infectious dis-ease, in Ayurveda, is considered physical, as no infection can take place in the presence of immunity, an internal trait.) Generally, treatment is by means of medication, diet, herbs, gemstones, drugs, glandulars, vitamins, and minerals.

3. MANASIKA - or "mental dis-ease" differs from mental dis-ease in western medicine. In Ayurvedic medicine, dis-eases that can have both mental and physical symptoms are not considered mental. The Ayurvedic concept is represented by states of anger, wrath, pride, vanity, greed, avarice, treachery, falsehood, undisciplined desires, hate, fear, cruelty, distress, sorrow, anxiety, unhappiness and laziness. In Ayurvedic medicine, these conditions are generally cared for by psychological means.

4. SVABHAVIKA - refers to "natural dis-eases" of birth, death, old age, natural hunger, thirst, and sleepiness where the care rendered is generally spiritual guidance.

## LAWS OF PHARMACODYNAMICS

Ayurvedic pharmacology is an elaborate and sophisticated science.

It is designed and administered in such manner as to eliminate adverse reactions while enhancing desirable effects. These goals are clearly stated by Charaka in the following statements:

1. **"By proper processing, even poisons can be converted into an excellent medicine."**

2. **"By proper processing, even small amounts of medicine(s) produce potent effects."**

After determining the action required, the healer formulates substances into what would be considered in the west a polypharmacopoeia to produce the desired synergism, antagonism, and/or modification but in ayurvedic medicine the components are considered to have formed a single new substance with unique properties.

## LAW OF PRESCRIBING

**There is nothing that is not therapeutic IF PROPERLY UNDERSTOOD AND PROPERLY ADMINISTERED.** Substances, drugs, surgeries, diet and therapies can be prescribed in Ayurvedic medicine according to multiple philosophies which cover the concepts of allopathy, homeopathy and naturopathy. According to Ayurveda, they are alternate approaches to a common objective and philosophy. These alternatives can be classified under the following headings:

1) Contrary to the cause of the dis-ease;

2) Contrary to the symptoms of the dis-ease;

3) Contrary to both the cause and the symptoms of the dis-ease;

4) Similar to the cause of dis-ease;

5) Similar to the symptoms of the dis-ease;

6) Similar to both the cause and symptoms of the dis-ease.

## LAW OF NEW KNOWLEDGE

In order for a new principle to be scientifically valid it has to **be supported by three distinct and different sources of previously proven knowledge:**

1) Pratyaksha - direct sense perception

2) Anumana - logical thought

3) Aptopadesha - complies with the previously proven truths.

## THE LAW OF THREE CONSTITUTIONS

Within Ayurveda there are three basic constitutional types or doshas (the concept referred to as the miasmatic influences in homeopathy, the five phase principle of oriental medicine, the diathesis of chiropractic). **These are Vattic, Pittic and Kephaic and there is nothing that can be conceived that does not fall under one of these grand types.** However, no true mono-doshic types exist because life is not possible in the absence of even one Dosha  type. (This is similar to the bi-phase concept of yin and yang in oriental medicine or the pure miasmatic type in homeopathy.) It is the general predominance of the functions of a particular dosha pattern in an individual that determines his or her "type". **No psychic, physiological, physical or spiritual phenomenon can exist without the tri-doshic influence on living matter; however, one dosha (constitutional, diathic, phase type) will always be dominant over the other two.** It is the identification of the dominant type that holds the key to successful Ayurvedic health care for it directs the practitioner to which therapies will be ineffective, which will aggravate, and which will be beneficial. Constitutional types (in western medicine, ectomorphic, mesomorphic or endomorphic types) or doshas differ in health, the type of dis-eases experienced by each, their reactions to drugs, surgery, herbs, adjustments, nutrients, psychoanalysis, diet, acupuncture treatment, spiritual counseling, and physical therapy, as well as response to seasons, climates, and emotions. Thus, **in western medicine the emphasis is on what type of dis-ease the patient is suffering from while in Ayurveda, the vital factor is to determine the constitutional type or dosha of the patient suffering from the dis-ease.** (This is similar to Oriental Medicine in which yin type patients respond better to herbs, because of drug side-effects, while the yang type patient generally responds without side-effects to drugs.)

## THE AUTOMOBILE EXAMPLE

Dr. S. Sharma gives an excellent and comprehensive example of the Ayurvedic thought process in his book *The System Of Ayurveda.* He illustrates it in the following manner: it is only when the automobile springs into action that the comparison between it and the unit of life is feasible. The state of motion is possible only because there is a body of the car. In the absence of the body there can be no motion. But the body and motion cannot exist together without producing or losing energy. In the case of the moving automobile, the energy is produced in the form of heat. To control the heat thus produced, the machine has to be provided with an anti-heat factor, a lubricating and cooling system, to save it from disintegration through uncontrolled heat.

In this extremely simple and crude example, if we compare the motion with Vattic, the heat with Pittic and the lubricants with Kephaic of the human body, we have a base to explain tri-doshic equilibrium. In the analogy of the moving car, the existence of the single factor of motion is inconceivable; pure motion without a body can have no base to exist. For example, if a car moved at the speed of light, it would cease to exist as a physical car. According to the laws of modern quantum physics, it would become a streak of light. The heat, too, has to act within its laws. When it falls below a certain (critical) level, the car freezes up and refuses to move. But, conversely, the car cannot overheat. If the automobile turned uni-doshic, for example, just to heat, it would be automatically burnt and destroyed; without heat and motion there will be no moving body but a lifeless mass of inanimate matter.

Even the lubrication has to remain within certain limits (laws); otherwise, the oil will clog the plugs, parts of the engine, etc. There is plenty of latitude for the equilibrium to fluctuate within the normal limits, but the fluctuation must not exceed the permissible limits (laws). Even in the case of the car, an imbalance indicating disturbance beyond the maximum  permissible limits (laws) will stop the efficient functioning of the car.

An Ayurvedic physician maintaining correct data from both modern and the Ayurvedic (traditional) angles will be in a good position to accurately evaluate the patient. In Ayurveda, there is very little danger of injurious medicinal, surgical, nutritional, adjusting, diet, modality, or other deleterious side-effects. The drawback lies in the pure observational and intuitive approach which, however well-developed, is subject in certain cases to diagnostic mistakes. For example, a cerebral tumor, undetected by the physician in the absence of modern diagnostic facilities, can be mistaken for migraine. This can be prevented by the judicious collaboration technique offering modern diagnostic facilities, primarily allopathic facilities.

Of course, our analogy of the car has major limitations. The automobile, unlike man, is incapable of auto-repair. It cannot adjust itself to changed conditions. Every car of similar brand behaves identically. It has none of the complexity characterizing human nature and functions. There are no male and female cars, nor is one car attracted by another car, creating a number of psycho-somatic complexes. They do not laugh or cry. They do not tell lies. They do not want to destroy each other nor do they display a vast number of other non-material aspects and emotions).

## THE LAW OF THE VATTIC TYPE

Vattic individuals are usually slender, restless, fast moving, and have dry skin and hair. When out of harmony they are subject to digestive and nervous dis-eases.

This category of dis-ease includes every concept associated with **motion**. Motor, sensory, central and autonomic nerve system dysfunctions such as subluxation, dislocation, dilatation, constriction, tremor. The five senses, anal and penal perception, circulation, elimination, micturation, defecation, perspiration, expectoration, sneezing. Sighing, yawning, lachrymation, ejaculation, enthusiasm. Conception, fetal development and delivery. It controls and inspires mental activity and harmonious organ action, digestion and secretions. It dries abnormal secretions and regulates breathing.

This type of dis-ease is ameliorated (made better) by consuming heavy, hot, greasy food such as eggs, kidney beans, wheat, cream, butter, yogurt; by sweets, sour, salt; by rest, reserved sexual activity, sleep; regular balanced, light, in-season meals; relevant brief conversations; in the spring time and from 6 to 10 A.M. and 6 to 10 P.M.

This type is aggravated (made worse) by excesses of light, cooling, drying,  bitter, pungent, astringents, over-exertion, excessive sexual indulgence, swimming, falling, injury, suppression of bowel movements, urination, passing of gas, sneezing, yawning, tears, eructation, coughing, hunger, thirst, sexual urges, lack of sleep, passion, fear, sorrow, anxiety, fasting, starvation, poor nutrition, irregular meals, poorly balanced diet, excessive eating (before the previous meal is fully digested) irrelevant talking, shouting, chatter, emaciation, senility, wetness, by emesis, purgatives, hemorrhage anf from 2 to 6 P.M. and from 2 to 6 A.M.

## THE LAW OF THE PITTIC TYPE

Pittic individuals are generally of medium build, intelligent, and well organized. When out of balance they frequently suffer from heartburn, skin condition, cramps and fevers.

This type of dis-ease deals with all concepts having to do with **heat**. Indigestion, disturbances in clarity of vision or absence of vision; hyper- and hypo-temperatures; unnatural coloration of the skin; cowardice, anger, lack of intellectual brilliance, low ideals; unhealthy changes in the blood, especially hemoglobin-related problems; non- or mal-absorption of substances applied on the skin.

It is ameliorated by sweets, bitter and astringent foods, cooling foods, serenity, nutrition, fats, milk, night, physical contact with opposite sex (not arousal, only pleasure), food and drink, winter and spring, from 6 to 10 A.M. and from 6 to 10 P.M., by eating, childhood and old age, diarrhea, sweating and urination.

It is aggravated by pungent, sour and salty foods and drink, heating foods, anger, fasting, sunshine, day, excessive sexual intercourse, suppression of thirst and hunger, alcohol, autumn and summer, from 10 A.M. to 2 P.M. and 10 P.M. to 2 A.M., during digestion, youth, constipation, and decreased perspiration.

## THE LAW OF THE KAPHAIC

Kaphaic persons are most commonly big boned, with oily skin and crave sweets. When experiencing imbalances they exhibit lethargy, sluggishness and/or depression.

This type of dis-ease deals with all aspects of **lubrication**. Dryness, abnormal looseness, softness, instability and porousness, sliminess, viscosity, firmness, coldness, whiteness, heaviness, sweetness, unctuousness (greasiness), oiliness. Unsteady character, frailty, laziness, revengeful, discontented, intolerance, greedy. Sensations of lightness, leanness, emaciation, impotence, sexual debility. Physical weakness, anorexia, torpor (lack of response to normal stimuli), stiffness, heaviness of limbs, sweetish taste, salivation, mucous expectoration, large stools, indigestion, pericardial heaviness, increased stomach acid secretion, post-nasal discharge, atherosclerosis, goiter, obesity, sub-normal temperature, uticaria (hives), pallor, whitish urine and feces.

It is ameliorated by pungent, bitter and astringent foods and drinks, Non-greasy substances, dry and/or light foods, staying awake at night, physical exercise, rainy weather, from 2 to 6 P.M. and 2 to 6 A.M., when digestion has been completed, old age, heat, sexual intercourse, emesis (vomiting), sternutation (sneezing), thirst, walking and running.

It is aggravated by sweat, sour and salty food and drink, fats, liquids, heavy foods, napping, lack of exercise, spring, from 6 to 10 A.M. and 6 to 10 P.M., by eating, childhood, cold, continence, greasy hair, excessive fluid consumption and rest.

Some symptoms appear under more than one dosha but their physiopathology may not be the same. For example, sweating is both Vattic and Pittic but the sweating is due to heat in its Pittic form and to fear in its Vattic form.

## SURGERY

Ayurvedic medicine has at least a 4,000-year history of sophisticated surgery and even blood transfusion. Much of the ayurvedic surgical knowledge was derived from the ancient Indian Aryans' tradition of protracted warfare and the necessity of dealing with severe wounds. But the high degree of Aryan civilization also allowed time for the study of surgery which greatly added to the basic skills of an army surgeon. In fact, between 1,000 and 600 B.C., even plastic surgery was a highly developed art within the Aryan culture of India. By 1,000 B. C., Charaka describes in detail the hundreds of surgical instruments and many procedures used in ancient Indian surgeries.

## CHAKRAS

The chakra can be defined as, "A vortex or window allowing energy to enter or leave the living being." This is also an excellent description of an acupuncture point used in oriental medicine. (See Chapter 25.)  B. Brennan, M.S., in her textbook *Hands Of Light: A Guide To Healing Through The Human Energy Field* states that as human beings mature, each chakra develops and  represents the psychological patterns evolving in the individual's life. As the individual experiences certain life circumstances, his chakras may become blocked with stagnated energy, spin irregularly or backward or counter-clockwise which depletes innate energy and, in the case of dis-ease, may become severely distorted or torn. When the chakras are functioning normally, each will be 'open' to incoming energy, spinning clockwise to metabolize the particular energy needed from the universal field.

Generally speaking, care rendered to chakras consists of bringing energy into, removing energy from and/ or stabilizing energy within the patient. Figures 16.1 and 16.2 illustrate the locations of the major chakras in relation to acupuncture points in oriental medicine.

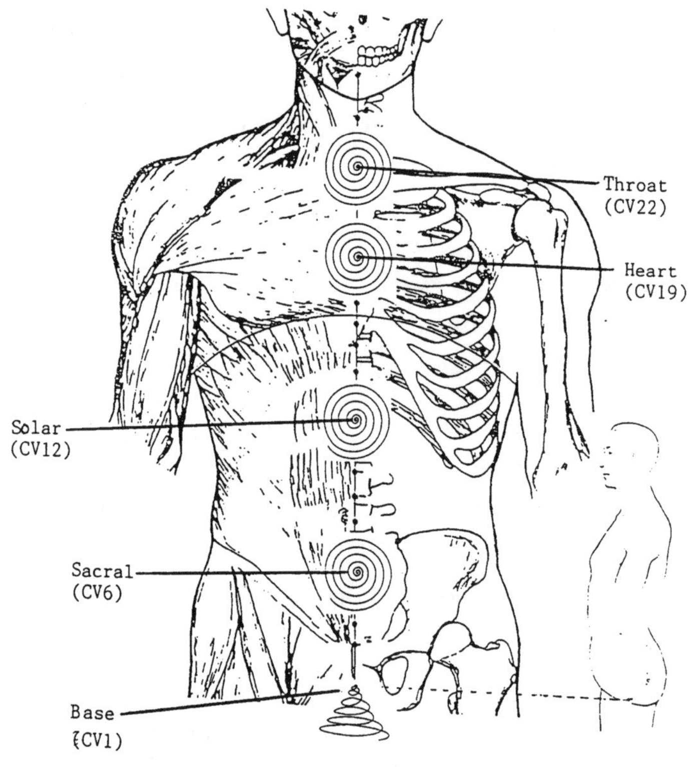


*Figure 16.1 — Major chakras in relation to acupuncture points, Anterior View*

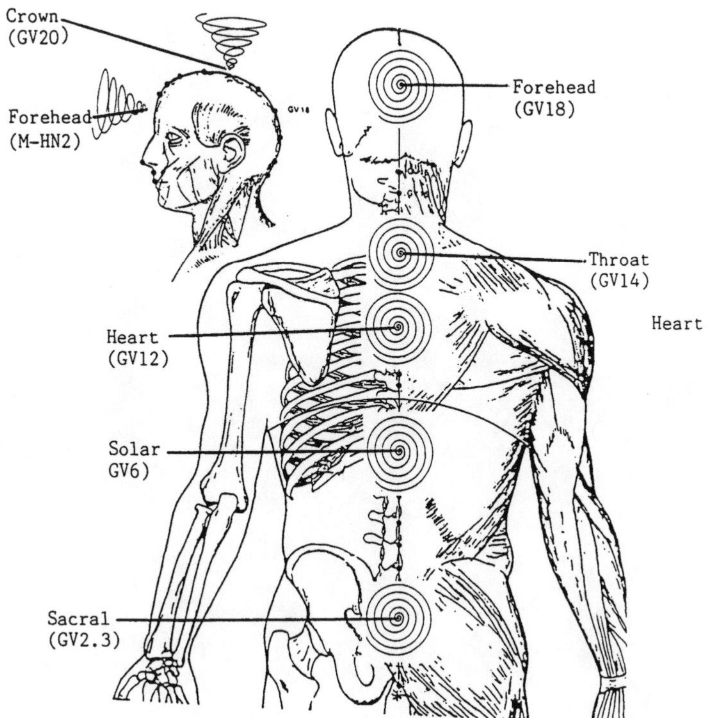


*Figure 16.2 — Major chakras in relation to acupuncture points, Posterior view*

## MAJOR CHAKRAS AND AREAS OF BODY/MIND CONTROL

The base chakra controls the adrenal glands, the spinal column, the kidneys, physical functions, and the will to live.

The sacral chakra regulates the reproductive organs, feelings of sexual love, and the ability to give and receive.

The solar plexus chakra controls the pancreas, stomach, liver, gall bladder and sympathetic nervous system, thought conception, spiritual wisdom and understanding, and the ability to heal one's self.

The heart chakra governs the thymus gland, heart, circulation, blood, parasympathetic vagus nerve, brotherly love and will power.

The throat chakra rules the thyroid, bronchial and vocal apparatus, lungs, alimentary canal, touch, smell, taste, assimilation of thoughts, sense of self and belonging.

The head chakra relates to the pituitary gland, lower brain and parasympathetic functions, the left eye, ears, nose, nervous system, spiritual and emotional level, and the ability to visualize, understand and execute abstract concepts.

The crown chakra regulates the pineal gland, reasoning, right eye, and integration of self with the universal intelligence (God).

# Chapter 17
# CHIROPRACTIC

*"Too much or too little is dis-ease."*
— D. D. Palmer, D.C.

## CHIROPRACTIC, THE UNKNOWN ENTITY

What is chiropractic? That is a question that chiropractors themselves have fought over for a hundred years. Some see it as a very restricted, spinal adjusting concept while others comprehend it in a very broad naturopathic perspective.

## HISTORY

The origins of adjusting the osseous structures of the body have been with us since antiquity. One of the first recorded references appears in the Chinese Kong Fou, a book written about 2,700 B.C. Greek papyruses dating from 1,500 B.C. give instructions on the adjusting of the lower extremities and on low back conditions. Cultures as diverse as the Japanese, Indian, Egyptian, Babylonian, Syrian, Hindu, Tibetan, Native American, Polynesian and European all share this common mode of therapy in their history.

Hippocrates, the Father of Medicine in the western world, wrote a book about 200 B.C. entitled, *Manipulation And Importance To Good Health And On Setting Joints By Leverage* in which he stated, **"Get knowledge of the spine, for this is the requisite for many dis-eases."** It is a recorded fact that Galen healed the paralysis of the right hand of Eudemus, the Roman scholar, by adjusting his neck. Like Hippocrates, Galen comprehended that the mechanical adjustment of the spine had a profound impact upon the nervous system when he said, **"Look well to the nervous system as a key to maximum health."**

As with so much of mankind's knowledge, the skill and therapeutic understanding of adjusting seems to have been lost during the Dark Ages. It was not until the 1890s that D. D. Palmer again began to understand the relationship between the spine and the nervous system and incorporated the adjusting principle into an organized therapeutic science called chiropractic.

# LAW OF UNIVERSAL INTELLIGENCE

There is an intelligence that creates energy (kundalini, quantum, innate, vital, life force, ch'i) in a purposeful manner and it expresses itself through this energy in *all* things, giving to them their characteristic life, properties and actions and thereby defining and maintaining their existence. Without this intelligence there can be *no* energy or matter.

# LAW OF LIFE

The union of intelligence (anti-matter) and matter by means of the quantum (energy, force) is the **Law Of Life**. In order to experience 100 percent life (health) there must be 100 percent intelligence, 100 percent energy, 100 percent matter and 100 percent anti-matter. **Total life and health are total energy.**

# LAW OF TIME

There is *no* process that does not require time.

# LAW OF LAWS

Universal Intelligence functions by means of well-defined spiritual (non-corporal or anti-matter), quantum, and physical laws. All adaptations within the framework of these laws are for the *positive benefit* of the being.

# LAW OF CAUSE AND EFFECT

Dis-ease is an interference with the expression of universal intelligence by aberrant energy flow resulting in abnormal function of matter.

# LAW OF ENTROPY

**Life and health are expressions of negative entropy or increasing degrees of order, organization and growth.** Positive entropy is the decrease or loss of order, organization and growth.

# LAW OF INBORN INTELLIGENCE

*All* things exhibit an inborn governing intelligence (num, kundalini, innate, vital force, ch'i, life force) the mission of which is, to the maximum degree possible and without injuring or destroying it, maintain and regulate the being by adapting it within the parameters of universal laws and forces.

## LAW OF MEANS OF FUNCTION

Num, kundalini, innate, ch'i, life, vital force operates by way of the quanto-psycho-neuro-immuno-endo-mechano-trophic (QPNIMT) system which can and does malfunction causing dis-ease. (Due to a lack of understanding of the Law of Coordination, the QPNIMT mechanism has been abandoned and, as a profession, chiropractic has progressively restricted itself to only the neuro-mechanical subluxation as the cause of abnormal function and disease.)

## LAW OF COORDINATION

The principle of harmonious action of *all* the parts and functions of an organism is known as the Law Of Coordination. Were the spinal subluxation the *only* cause of dis-ease, individuals who have never received a chiropractic adjustment could not get well. This would mean that only 3 to 4 percent of the world's population who have received chiropractic adjustments could be well. Obviously, this is not scientifically supported and can only lead to one conclusion. **There are other means of affecting mal-functioning organisms in addition to the mechanical chiropractic adjustment. One thing must be kept in perspective, however. When the cause of dis-ease is neuromechanical, a chiropractic adjustment is the most effective and cost-efficient means of caring for that particular patient.**

## LAW OF SUBLUXATION (DIS-EASE)

**A subluxation is a condition of a bone that has lost its normal juxtaposition with one or more adjacent bones to an extent less than a luxation but sufficient to produce aberrant QPNIMT phenom-enon. A subluxation can be the *cause* or the *effect* (symptom) of QPNIMT dysfunction. If the sublux-ation is repeatedly recreated following an adjustment, it is a symptom and not the cause of dis-ease.**

## LAW OF CORD INTERFERENCE

**A subluxation (dis-ease) does not have to occur exclusively at the  intervertebral foramina. Edema and/or space-occupying lesions (i.e., a bulging disc) within the spinal canal can cause pressure, tension and inflammation of a spinal track.** Such situations can result in dis-ease far removed from the subluxation site.

## LAW OF JOINT INTERFERENCE

*Any* joint can exhibit a structural disrelationship which can produce pressure, tension and/or inflammation on adjacent nerves resulting in the criterion of a subluxation (dis-ease).

# LAW OF FREQUENCY OF ADJUSTMENTS

R. Stephenson, D.C., Ph.C., indicates in *The Chiropractic Text Book*, that **adjusting at too many locations or adjusting too often makes a patient very weak and if carried to excess is chiatrogenic. The patient often gets well faster after the care-giving is stopped. For this reason, after one or a series of adjustments, the patient should be allowed to rest entirely from care for a while.** This is what D. D. Palmer meant when he said, **"Too much or too little** *is* **dis-ease."**

# LAW OF MAJOR AND MINOR

This law is one of cause and effect. **When an adverse condition is present for a** *sufficient period of time* **it begins to affect other parts, functions and/or capacities. Directing care to these secondary (minor) conditions (compensations) will not resolve the primary condition (subluxation), but resolution of the** *major* **condition (subluxation),** *which is most critical to the total health of the patient,* **will almost always resolve the entire malfunctioning complex. In the** *rare* **instances when this does not take place, the remaining** *dominant* **condition (subluxation) then becomes the** *new major* **. This is the chiropractic concept of caring for** *the* **cause and not symptoms. Secondary conditions are symptoms of the major.** Unfortunately, this makes the majority of so-called "chiropractic adjusting" the treatment of symptoms which is the practice of non-vitalistic, reductionistic medicine.

# LAW OF ADJUSTING

If the patient is feeling better but is getting weaker, he/she is over-adjusted and there is no hope of cure until adjustments are dramatically curtailed.

**If the patient is feeling worse but getting stronger, he/she is retracing; all is well and no additional care is currently needed. If the patient's symptoms are improving and he/she is getting stronger, everything has been done correctly. No additional care is currently needed.**

This law can be summed up in the old chiropractic (universal law) adage **"The less you adjust or render any form of care, the oftener you can. The more you adjust or render any form of care, the less you can."**

# LAW OF KINESIOLOGY

Current kinesiological protocols are based upon the premise that alteration or re-administration of the therapy is indicated when the strength of the muscle being tested changes. This hypothesis, however, leaves a great deal to be desired. **A far more rational approach, based upon the universal laws of healing, is to refrain from any alteration and/or additional administration of** *all* **forms of care as long as change, the alteration of muscular strength, is continuing. This is because the previously administered therapy is still working. As long as changes continue, the body remains in the self-healing mode. Only when changes cease, as documented by repeated muscle tests producing the identical test results, should the prudent practitioner consider administering additional care.** Such lack of continuing changes indicates that the self-healing process has ceased.

## LAW OF MACHINES

The same considerations discussed in the previous paragraph also hold true for electronic machines that are used by some to test for remedies.

## LAW OF FACILITATION

That which the patient's being persists in doing becomes easier, not because the nature of the task has changed but rather because the individual's ability to do it more efficiently has increased. When speaking neurologically, this principle is referred to as the "Law of Facilitation". However, it is a universal law of life and not merely a neurological principle. **The longer a dis-ease process exists, the harder it is generally to eradicate or alter it to the point where it is no longer capable of triggering the totality of the symptom picture.** See Figures 17.1 - 17.4

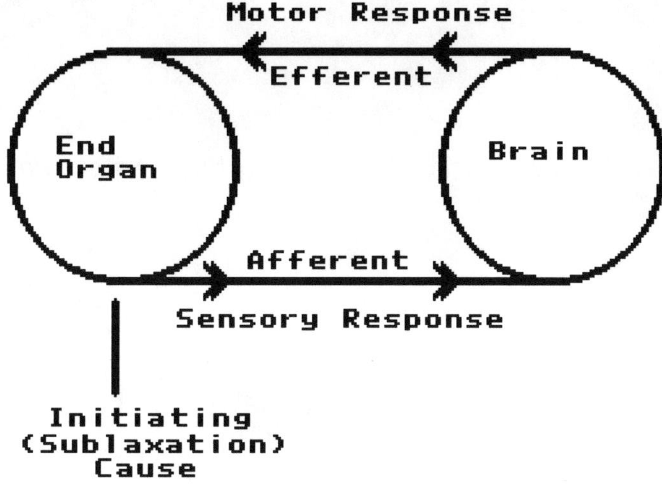


*Figure 17.1 — Simplistic Safety Pin Cycle*

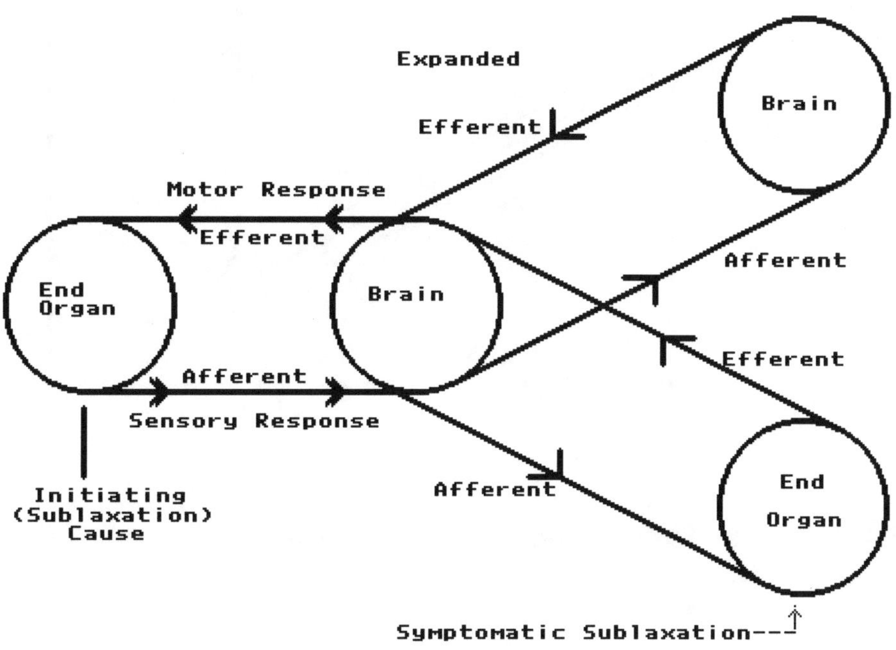


*Figure 17.2 — Expanded Response of Basic Safety Pin Cycle*

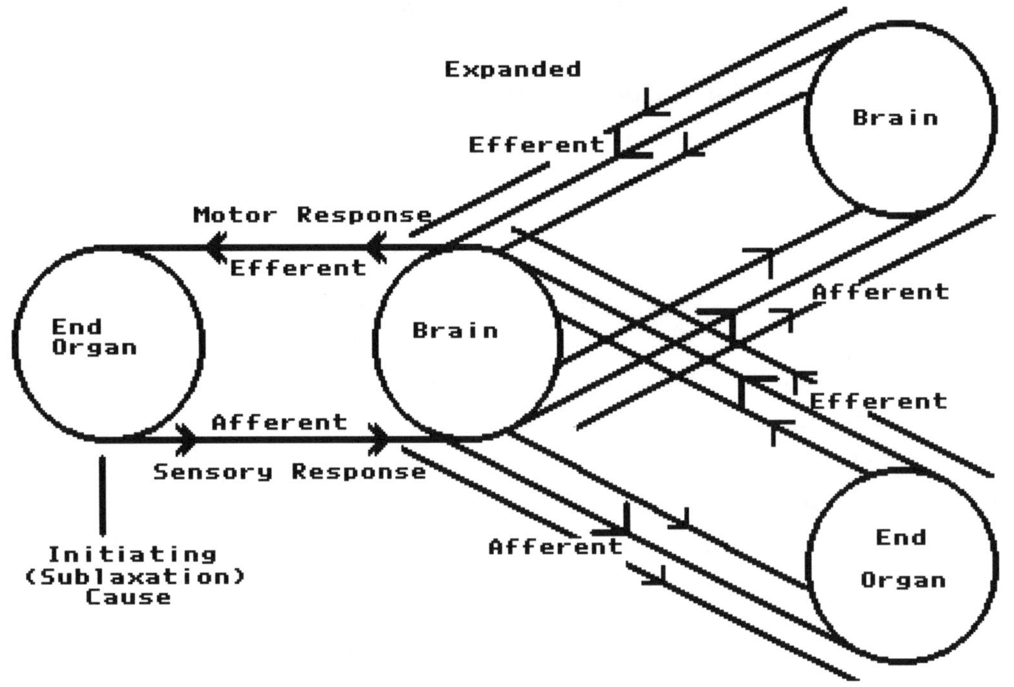


*Figure 17.3 — Facilitated Response of Basic Safety Pin Cycle*

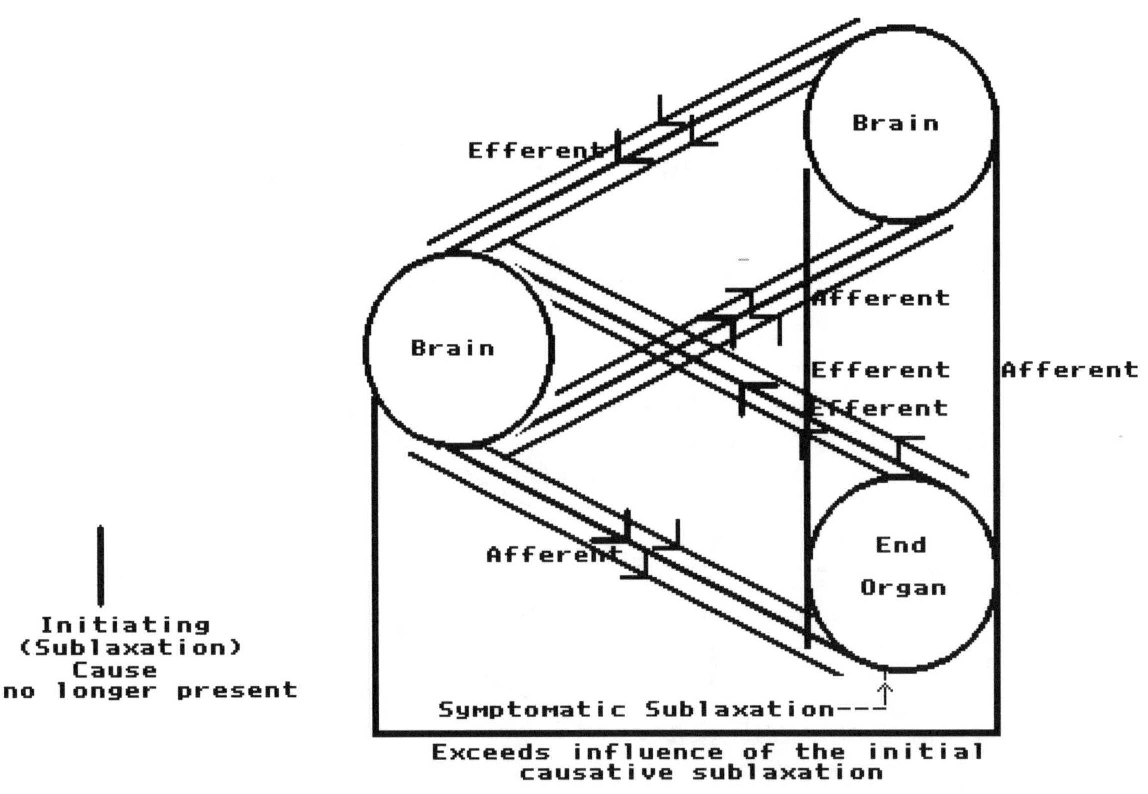


*Figure 17.4 — Chronic Subluxation Syndrome of The Facilitated Safety Pin Cycle*

## LAW OF SYMPATHETIC VS. PARASYMPATHETIC

**Tissues and their functions are, generally speaking, neurologically regulated by an interplay of sympathetic stimulation and parasympathetic inhibition. Therefore, to adjust both the sympathetic (the thoraco-lumbar) and parasympathetic (cranio-cervico-pelvic) during the same visit is *unscientific and counterproductive* . The body cannot do two diametrically opposed things to the same tissue at the same time.**

## LAW OF PROGNOSIS

1) Older patients, as a rule, respond more slowly.

2) The more knowledge and ability the practitioner has at his command, as a rule, the better the prognosis.

3) Chronic cases, as a rule, require more healing time (not the same as treatment time) than acute cases. Constitutional cases routinely require even longer periods of healing and miasmatic (diathic, doshic, phase) cases may take the longest time.

4) The rule of patient compliance has a profound impact on the outcome of the case. If they comply, the outlook is good; if they do not comply, the outlook is poor.

## SHORTCOMINGS OF THE MECHANICAL SUBLUXATION (DIS-EASE) THEORY

Plato once said, "The great error of our day in the treatment of the human body is that the physicians separate the soul from the body." B. Sakar writes in *Hahnemann's Organon With Commentary*, "The prevailing belief among the untrained is that any result may be explained by some single factor operating as a cause. They seem to have no concept of the fact that the cause of every result is made up of a combination of interacting factors, often in numbers and combinations that are absolutely bewildering to contemplate. This habit of considering only one factor, when perhaps scores are involved, indicates a very primitive and untrained condition of mind." Hippocrates, the father of medicine (460-377 B.C.) stated, "The physician of the future will treat the whole man - body, mind and soul." D. D. Palmer, D.C., wrote, "Chiropractic is a name given to the principle of restoring the body, mind and the soul to normal."

Thus we learn that no true doctor of chiropractic can concentrate only on the neuromusculoskeletal; to do so is to ignore the reality of chiropractic. The living being is an integrated whole. It is clinically, scientifically and philosophically impossible to treat only a portion of the living being. To try to segregate the living being's systems and functions is the folly of non-vitalistic, reductionistic medicine

## MODIFICATION OF ALL OR NONE LAW NEEDED

The All or None Law states that all nerve impulses are identical and therefore the varied physiological responses are mediated by the cells of origin and the end organs (i.e. muscle, special senses, glands, etc.) stimulated. Some current research, however, casts strong doubts on such a concept. Insulin injections are normally followed by a drop in blood sugar levels *if* the nervous system is functioning normally, but the injections initiate no changes at all in blood sugar levels if the nervous system is anesthetized and thereby unresponsive. Potassium cyanide in lethal doses will cause convulsions and sudden death through the neuropathy initiated in a responsive nervous system but an anesthetized animal given the same dose shows no symptoms at all. The poison is excreted in the saliva and the animal arouses from the anesthesia quite unharmed. Likewise, the majority of clinical symptoms, such as fevers, changes in the blood counts and even antibody production, are all part of an interrelationship of the hormonal and nervous systems.

Further, extra-neural control of the nervous system has been substantiated by the work of Sperry who found that after slipping off the torso skin of a young frog with a loosened belt-like strip rotated to place the belly side on the back and the back side on the belly, tickling belly skin now on the back caused the frog to scratch the belly and tickling the back skin now over the belly caused it to scratch the back. The eye was cut loose and rotated 180 degrees upside down and the nerves again allowed to re-grow. The frog would strike downward to reach a fly in the air and upward to reach a fly on the floor. Next, the eye was cut and rotated back to its normal position. Upon recovery the frog again would strike but now in the old normal direction. Weiss did similar work and found that when the gastrocnemius muscle was transplanted from the hind leg of a young frog into his front leg, the frog could walk and hop; but when the nerve to the hind leg was stimulated electrically, the transplanted gastrocnemius muscle jumped along with the other rear muscles. These experiments clearly demonstrate that there are other factors at work in conjunction with the nervous system.

## SIGNS OF HEALTHY LIFE

1) **Assimilation** - the intelligent ability of an organism to take into itself, selectively, trophic materials and make them a part of itself.

2) **Excretion**- the selective ability of an organism to give off waste deemed not useful in its functions.

3) **Adaptability** - the selective ability that an organism possesses of responding through sensory, motor, calorific and/or secretory means to forces to which it is exposed.

4) **Growth** - the ability to expand according to an intelligent plan, to mature in function, to repair, dependent upon the power to assimilate.

5) **Reproduction** - the ability of an entity to perpetuate its own kind.

## LAW OF RETRACING

Retracing is the course of restoration from dis-ease back to health. *Every* case retraces for if there is a departure from health, there *must be* a return if care is properly rendered. When a case retraces, it passes back through the successive steps, in reverse order, that it passed through in becoming dis-eased.

## LAW OF POISONS

1) Any substance that is no longer usable in body metabolism is a poison.

2) Any substance, even food and drink, that is in excess of what the organism can use is a poison.

3) Any substance not manufactured by the cells or glands of the body is a poison; i.e., drugs.

4) Any glandular product in the wrong place or at the wrong time in the body is a poison.

5) Any foreign substance, be it liquid, solid or gaseous, even if chemically inactive, can be a poison.

6) Any excretory substance is a poison.

7) Anything that excessively stimulates or inhibits is a poison,

8) Too much or too little water acts as a poison.

9) Excess exercise produces large volumes of waste substances which are poisons and must be removed from the body.

10) Strong emotions affect the chemistry of the body producing inappropriate secretions which are poisons.

## LAW OF MICROBES

It is unscientific to believe that microbes are the cause of dis-ease. Microbes are opportunists. They can only survive where conditions are ideal for them. The body's QPNIMT system normally is able to control and eliminate them. *Only* when the QPNIMT system fails can microbes survive in significant numbers to produce dis-ease symptoms. They do so by excretions from their bodies that are highly toxic to particular tissues. In small numbers, the body can neutralize these toxins with no symptomatic effects. In large numbers, the body is no longer capable of neutralizing such large amounts and it then presents the symptoms of the dis-ease.

## LAW OF INHERITANCE OF DIS-EASE

Diathesis (miasmas, dosha, phase) is not a dis-ease; it is a type or form of family characteristics that can be inherited just the same as one can "inherit" the shape of nose belonging to his father or grandfather. If an individual has a diathesis (miasma, dosha, phase) for tuberculosis, that does not mean that he has tuberculosis or that he is obligated to have it. The term is used to indicate that such a person has a body with a predisposition to that type of dis-ease. True, one's parents may have tuberculosis. The offspring of these parents with a family resemblance will have the same kind of tissues with a likeness in strength and resistance and the same type of spine, subject to the same subluxations (dis-eases). *If* subjected to the same environmental conditions that his parents were forced to suffer, such as living or working in unsanitary quarters, he will have the same adaptive battles to fight that they did. He is likely to be overcome in the same way they were. If, however, he manages to improve his environment, he is no more likely to have tuberculosis than anyone else.

## UPDATE: THE NEURAL COMPONENT

The chiropractic profession currently envisions a static subluxation with accompanying static dis-ease. Dr. Peterson's work documents the subluxation (dis-ease) complex to be dynamic in nature. He states, "It now seems likely that the . . . **subluxation, rather than being the static cause of dis-ease, can play a dual role. It may both initiate and/or reflect neural dysfunction, manifesting itself both as a cause and a symptom of a more profound disturbance deep within the nervous system.**" (emphasis added.)

Chiropractic made a quantum leap in realizing that **interference as we now understand it is neither a blockage nor an abnormal stimulation of the normal impulse.** Rather, as Peterson believes, **it appears that which is corrected is a build-up of neurological dysfunction which, once set in motion through various factors, is capable of existing without further abnormal irritation.** Having once reached this state of development, abnormal function becomes a reflection of established abnormal neural control. In its superficial or acute aspect, it is observed as a zone of reflex aberration, a change in mode or design of appropriate response to normal stimuli. In its totality or chronic state, it may represent a completely new nervous system, programmed on modified premises, responding in abnormal function, unable to integrate normal defense mechanisms, and even ultimately initiating its own pathology.

Peterson further indicates that **it is now understood that it is only necessary for the subluxation to be present momentarily, from a historical standpoint, to initiate a type of injury to the neural elements whose latency of repair of such injury is extended in time beyond the more spontaneous recovery of the musculo-skeletal strain of the articulation.** Petersen continues his concept by postulating that regardless of the manner in which it was set into motion (trauma, toxicity or auto-suggestion), the segmental neuropathy once established becomes self-supporting in the sense that the initiating factor (subluxation) need not remain as part of the abnormality for the process to continue to exist and expand itself. Continuous neurological facilitation is imposed onto these associated networks until a new conditioned reflex of the total complex is impressed as a new behavior pattern upon the central nervous system.

**In chronic cases we must begin to think of the brain neurons as efferent to the pathological irritation of the spinal subluxation (dis-ease) site. As more and more brain neurons are drawn into the pool of central nervous system tissues affected by the subluxation, their total (neural and non-neural) influence on the patient's health begins to far exceed the initial influence of the causative subluxation (dis-ease). At this point, the spinal subluxation has lost control of the QPNIMT mechanism! These Frankenstein-like holographic engrams have ceased to obey their creator!**

# LAW OF HOLOGRAPHIC BRAIN FUNCTION

The chronic subluxation syndrome (CSC) cannot be clearly comprehended without mastery of the holographic principle of brain function. A hologram is a very interesting multi-dimensional scientific phenomenon.

For example, the 3-dimensional holographic picture is much like dropping two pebbles into the water of a still pond simultaneously. Each pebble produces expanding concentric wave circles. When the expanding circles interface with each other one of two phenomenon takes place. They will, depending upon their interfacing positions, either cancel each other's effect or becoming a single enhanced wave. A similar effect occurs with light. This takes place when two lights strike an object from different angles. They produce multiple shadows of differing degrees of darkness called an interference patterns.

Between 1948 and the early 1960s, Nobel prize winning, Professor D. Gabor demonstrated that such interference patterns could be photographically recorded producing a 3-dimensional image.

Holograms, however, exhibit an even more interesting scientific phenomenon. A holographic photography can be ripped into several pieces and all but one of the pieces destroyed. The remaining fragment is then holographically reproduced and the **entire picture is once again present.** This is contrary to solid state physics which states, "The parts are never greater than the whole." Einstein, however, reminded us that all laws learned in solid state physics must be modified when we move into quantum physics. **In quantum physics, the sum of the parts is always greater then the whole.** To illustrate this principle, we could dissect a cadaver into fifty parts and suture them back together. The parts equal the whole in the solid state concept but when the vital, innate, ch'i, life force enters into these parts their sum is greater than the physical whole. **Life, the quantum factor, is greater than the physical whole.**

A similar phenomenon is at work within the brain in the CSC. In the CSC, the causative subluxation (dis-ease) may be repeatedly corrected; or the causative subluxation (dis-ease) may no longer even exist, but the brain's holographic engramming nevertheless is capable of recreating the entire QPNIMT complex to include a symptomatic subluxation. **Thus, the more we adjust the symptomatic subluxation (dis-ease), which is now only a part of the total QPNIMT complex, the more we reinforce the body's ability to recreate the entire holographic complex.** See Figures 17.4 and 17.5

This is called facilitation, a basic law of neurology. **The effect produced in nerve tissue by the passage of an impulse causes the resistance of the nerve to diminish so that a second application of the stimulus evokes the reaction more easily.** This process may reach the point where the body facilitates so efficiently that it is impossible, for all practical purposes, to alter the course and progress of the dis-ease process. At this point, we have created a chiropractically induced dis-ease entity.

Research conducted at Harvard University shows that brain programming is essentially stored on a global or holographic level, not in discrete, little pockets from which it is then retrieved. It must also be recognized that, over time, there is a great deal of reorganization in the brain and its memories. As the memories age, they generally become independent of the medial temporal lobe structures such as the hippocampus. This reorganization also includes some connections. At the same time, new associations are being made and things are being forgotten on the conscious level. Evidence also indicates that, at least in learning complex tasks, information may be stored simultaneously in several parts of the neural circuitry. This phenomenon is called "parallel processing" in computer jargon.

Care must be taken, however, not to confuse dynamic holographic engramming with the antiquated static neurobiology "engram" or "mystery molecule" that was supposedly similar to a computer's silicon memory chip. After forty years of intense research no such memory molecule has ever been identified or its existence even scientifically supported.

## THE QUESTION AND ANSWER

**This presents a monumental dilemma! If the causative subluxation (dis-ease) no longer exists but the patient is still sick, what then do chiropractors adjust?** Dr. D. D. Palmer, the genius who conceived modern chiropractic, answers in *The Art, Science and Philosophy of Chiropractic*, "The determining causes of dis-ease are traumatism (mechanical), poisons (toxins), and auto-suggestion (psychological)." Realizing that the definition of "adjust" is to settle; to free; to bring to a satisfactory state; to bring into proper relationship; to bring into harmony or balance, Dr. Palmer taught that chiropractic care that adjusts the mental and toxic imbalances is just as much within the chiropractic scope of practice as adjusting the structural imbalance.

## TRAUMATIC (MECHANICAL) VECTOR

Literally thousands of articles have been written that deal with the musculoskeletal aspect of the subluxation (dis-ease). We will therefore not address the subject other than to quote A. Homewood, D.C., N.D., **"Irritation of a mechanical, chemical or mental nature alone or in any percentage of combination, may be sufficient to overcome the normal resistance of the body, causing structural distortion, or subluxation, which interferes with normal transmission of nerve force; somatic and visceral structures show disturbances of function, with symptoms and tissue changes of dis-ease."**

# LAW OF HYGIENE

Hygiene is the restoration of natural and healthful environmental conditions which have been made abnormal by the necessities of a particular lifestyle. In instances where it in not possible to restore natural conditions, compensations must be made. The student must not think that having a natural lifestyle is reversion to primeval conditions. The goal is to provide the being with properly balanced diets, fresh, clean air, adequate light and exercise, sanitary surroundings, personal hygiene, a calming, relaxing environment, opportunities for personal enlightenment and development, etc. This does not mean, for example, that cooking of food is unnatural, but it does mean that over-cooking of foods decreases their nutritive value. The health benefits of natural living can be had without adopting a Tarzan-like lifestyle; in fact, civilized life can produce a much richer and more fulfilling experience than that mythical figure could ever have hoped for, if the excesses and deficiencies can be compensated for.

# TOXIC (POISON) VECTOR

V. Logan, D.C., writes, "A sick body is a dirty body, inside if not outside." A. E. Homewood, D.C., N.D., in *The Neurodynamic of the Vertebral Subluxation* concurs, "**Toxicity may be considered as a failure of** the body to rid itself of end-products of metabolism." F. M. Pottenger, M.D., in *Symptoms of Visceral Disease* agrees, "**Toxemia causes an increase in the normal excitability of nerve cells, lowering the threshold of response, thus making the individual more receptive to harmful stimuli. The entire nervous system is influenced by toxemia, but that particular group of nerves which shows the greatest degree of peripheral stimulation, as indicated by disturbed organic function, belongs to the sympathetic system.**" With an increased irritability the response to stimuli becomes more pronounced, the hyper tonicity of muscles increased and the likelihood of subluxation more certain.

D. D. Palmer, adds, "**Any substance which, when introduced into the animal economy, acts in a noxious manner on the vital properties, on the . . . organ, or on the system at large, is a poison.**" He continues, "**We are not opposed to agencies which neutralize the poisons and remove the accumulated waste materials and thus give nature the opportunity to assist itself and aid the entire system to harmonize itself in every part and organ in the body.**"

Logic dictates that the removal of these toxins will decrease the irritability of the nervous system, decrease the hyper tonicity or increase the hypotonic state of muscles as appropriate and thereby decrease the likelihood of subluxation (dis-ease). Stephenson writes, "**Poisons impair the condition of tissues so that they limit Innate's expression. . . . Poisons produce a shock as any other penetrating force, causing subluxations (dis-ease).**"

# PSYCHOLOGICAL (AUTO-SUGGESTION) VECTOR

D. D. palmer writes, "**In auto-suggestion which is also known as psychological suggestion . . . the will and judgment are more or less suppressed and auto-traumatic action is directed to any organ or portion of the body, thereby modifying bodily functions, exciting or relieving morbid conditions by mental processes independently of external influences. This condition is due to an underlying psychical impressionability exhibited in paralysis, contraction of muscles, impairment of vision, sensory and functional disturbances, more or less of the nervous system.**"

Palmer acknowledged that other non-neural factors could also be involved. He said, ". . . .Thots produce disease - malice, revenge, remorse, grief, worry, spite. . ." Joy, a Ph.D., adds that according to "the generous statistics of psychologists, we are about 20 percent aware and 80 percent unaware of our actions and motivations. I would suggest, more realistically, that we are less than 0.0001 percent awake and more than 99.999 percent unconscious." Neither 80 percent nor 99-plus percent is comforting to the practitioner who senses how important the emotional state is to the patient's health.

V. Strang, D.C., in *Essential Principles of Chiropractic* writes, "The supreme health care concept that all individuals should understand is this: the conscious and unconscious mind cannot be disturbed without dire physical consequences. If the emotions are continually in shambles, there will eventually be a serious psychological consequence. A most trying task for a chiropractor is to attempt to correct the spine of a genuinely distraught individual. The subluxations are apt to return again and again. The nervous energy that accompanies conscious and unconscious mental conflict wracks both smooth and striated muscles, not only initiating psychological dysfunction, but perpetuating it through the resultant subluxation." See figure 17.5.

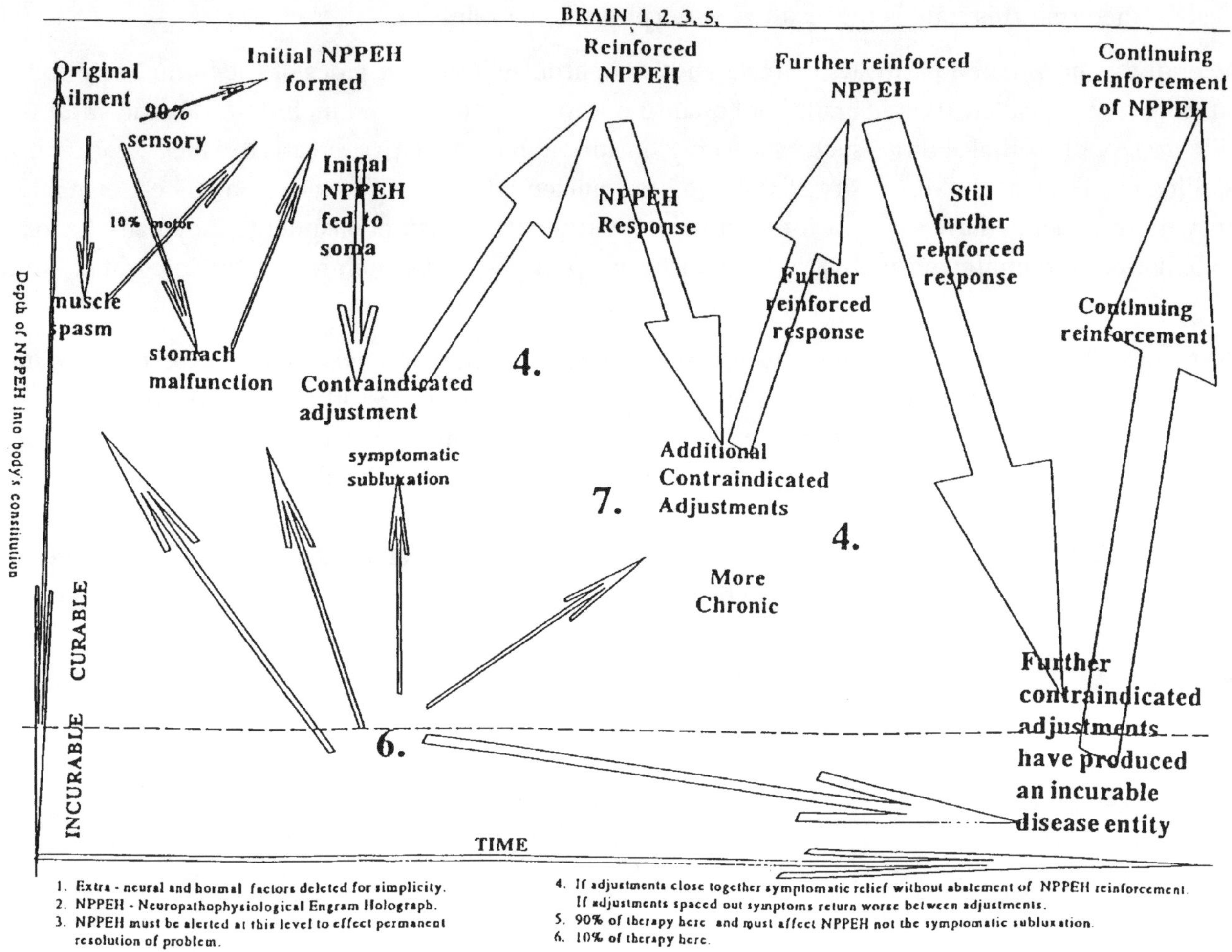


*Figure 17.5 — The Chiatrogenic Subluxation*

Cranes in *Managing Your Mind* finishes Strung's thought, "Tension is caused by a bombardment of desires, wishes, fears, anxieties, that is by attitudes, that stimulates, the hypothalamus. . . The over activity of the hypothalamus, in turn, causes an excessive number of impulses to be sent down the sympathetic and parasympathetic nervous system. When these extra impulses reach the heart, the heart beats faster when they reach the blood vessels, the blood vessels become spastic and the blood pressure is raised; when they reach the intestines, the intestines contract and cause spastic colitis or diarrhea, constipation." Thus we learn that **the physical dysfunctions are symptoms of mental/emotional tensions and will not resolve until the mental/emotional program is resolved.**

Brisance's research discussed in *Minding The Body, Mending The Mind* confirms this virtual reality (VR) principle, **The body cannot tell the difference between events that are actual threats to survival and events that are present in thoughts alone.**

# HIGHER LEVELS OF ORGANIZATION

Prigogine's Nobel Prize-winning research on how complex systems, such as the human nervous system, evolve to higher levels of function establishes the fact that very specific signals stimulate the creation of new neural connections between the left and right hemispheres of the brain. EEGs documented that most research subjects experienced a deep, trance-like meditative state of the type achieved only by experienced yogi masters. It was established that this state is the result of endorphins being released.

Secondly, as new neural pathways connect and "synchronize", the two sides of the brain begin to function in what is now being called "whole brain" or "quantum leap" function which includes dramatic improvements in a wide variety of mental abilities such as learning, intuition, mental clarity, creativity, focus, concentration and intelligence. Levy at the University of Chicago has commented on this phenomenon, "Great men and women of history did not merely have superior intellectual capacities within each hemisphere. They had phenomenonal levels of emotional commitment, motivation, attentional capacity - all of which reflect the integrated brain in action."

Every time the nervous system reorganizes itself at a new and higher level, the being experiences himself or herself and the world in a totally new way. The threshold of stress, regardless of the type of stress, goes up and many of the uncomfortable, dysfunctional feelings, behaviors and limitations we all experience from time to time begin to fall away. For most people, this means dramatic, deep changes in mental and emotional health and release and elimination of self-defeating behavior, childhood traumas and self-imposed limitation. Release of unresolved anger, fears and depression also are common along with an increased ability to feel positive about oneself as the ability to express oneself and to become self-aware increases.

# Chapter 18
# ADDITIONAL VECTORS

*"If what we say proves right, then none can break it
down, therefore, discussion will help it. If it proves
wrong, then discussion will bring out errors and it
should be corrected."*

— B. J. Palmer, D.C., Ph.C.

## THE REST OF THE STORY

In view of the universal requirement for continuous adaptation, it is extremely likely that numerous other vectors are also involved in the CSC. What, then, are some of these additional vectors the doctor must address which applied under a favorable set of circumstances can dramatically augment the chiropractic adjustment (or any other form of care)?

## BIOMAGNETIC VECTOR

D. D. Palmer writes, **"Some persons seem to be surcharged with magnetism, are magnetic. They are always giving off their life-force, they affect not only persons, but animals and plants as well; while others seem to be shut up like clams and some are even absorbent - living upon (the energy) of those with whom they are associated. (Emphasis added.)** House plants thrive under the care of some persons, and wither and die by the hand of others whose very presence seems to be poisonous. Persons of a highly sensitive organization are affected pleasantly or otherwise by those whom they meet. Those who are delicate in health may be made to feel stronger or weaker by a call from a neighbor. Some persons seem to tire while others enliven; one person exhausts the invalid while another refreshes. These facts have been recognized for many centuries; they have survived all sorts of opposition, ridicule and argument."

In 1530, the greatest scientific mind of the age, Paracelsus, a Swiss physician and alchemist, indicated that the vital force is not enclosed inside an individual but radiates within and around him or her like a luminous sphere which can be made to act at a distance. Today every electrical engineer knows that accompanying an electric field there is a magnetic field (quantum or energy vector). When a nerve conducts a pulse along its axon, magnetic fields accompany it. One might say we have magnetic personalities!

In 1964, Josephson, Nobel Laureate and physicist at the University of Cambridge, developed magnetic detectors many thousands of times more sensitive than ever before and Williamson, Kaufman and Brenner of New York University, in 1975, successfully detected the magnetic field produced by a human head while a person was thinking! It is the ability of a magnetic field to pass through and out of the living body that makes it so useful for sensing what takes place inside the body. These realities are the basis of Magnetic Resonance Imaging (MRI) technology.

J. Gerber adds, SQIDs (pronounced squids - Superconducting Quantum Interference Devices) as magnetic measuring tools have detected weak but significant increases in the magnetic field emanations of a healer's hands during the healing process. Zimmerman at the University of Colorado, School of Medicine, again using SQIDs, documented that **the intensity of the magnetic fields emitted by healer's hands was several hundred times larger** than that of non-healer's hands. One might then say that the kundalini, vital, innate, ch'i, life force seems to be associated with negative entropic characteristics. **(Negative entropy meaning: The energy utilized by cells or organisms to produce increasing degrees of growth, order, organization and communication.) When a body dies and the life force vacates the physical form, the remaining unoccupied shell returns, via earthly microorganisms (positive entropy), to its raw constituents in characteristic positive entropic fashion. The ethereal (energy or quantum) body, a self-organizing holographic energy template, demonstrates negative entropic properties.**

C. W. Smith and S. Best studying the biological effects of healers, documented in their book *Electromagnetic Man: Health And Hazards In The Electrical Environment* that magnets "could only produce a non-specific increase in the activity of enzymes. On the other hand, the energy fields of healers could cause variable changes in different enzymes. The direction of change was always consistent with greater health of the cell and organism." This is the one major weakness of magnetic therapy as practiced today. There is no known configuration of bio-static magnets that can duplicate the bio-dynamic negatively entropic fields of a genuine healer's hands.

See Chapter 35 for additional data relating to the DC currents that work in conjunction with the neurological impulse but are not identical to it.

# LAW OF ENTRAINMENT

D. Black, Ph.D., who holds a doctorate in physics, has also shown that the living nervous system does not function by "Reflex Neurological Arcs" (Safety Pin Cycle see Figures 17.1 - 17.5) but rather by "oscillators". He states, "The reflex arc is neatly scientific, perfectly within the atomist tradition, and contrary to vitalism. **No energy or 'force' exists within (the arc). If no outside force strikes the reflex arc, nothing happens . . . And when an outside force does strike the reflex arc, it reacts in an entirely predictable way. The body's actions are determined by what strikes it from outside.**" (Emphasis added.)

Black indicates that the basic units of the nervous system are oscillators that swing back and forth, or pulses in wave-like cycles. The heart, for example, is an oscillator. Every cell is an oscillator. Even atoms are oscillators, which is why we have atomic clocks. We have oscillators that operate in seconds, minutes, hours, days, months (as women well know), and even years.

The important point about oscillators is that they don't stand still, at least not until we die. **An oscillator has its own built-in source of energy. It is a vital force that resides within the (living) body.** But the difference between neurological reflex arcs and oscillators is even more profound. **Oscillators "entrain"**, meaning their energies interact with each other, and this interaction is a major factor in keeping the body in harmony. As the energy of one oscillator interacts with another, the combined energies cancel disturbances and lock (entrain) together or synchronize.

Entrainment obviously follows laws, the most critical of which is: to entrain, **oscillators must be free from outside interference. Such interference would be spread from one oscillator to another.** This is yet another of the non-neural components of the vertebral subluxation. **Every tissue of the living being can be affected by oscillating entrained responses, even when the neural stimulation is not great enough to reach the neurological threshold and cause structural mal-positioning.**

The Law of Entrainment also provides another vehicle explaining how homeopathic remedies can act as energy templates causing an alteration in the physical health and energy of the living being. One must look at entrainment as an algebraic equation a + (the remedy energy or frequency) and a - (the dis-ease energy or frequency) cancel each other out and return the being to a state of health.

## BELL'S LAW

The world renowned physicist J. S. Bell in 1964 published a mathematical formula called Bell's Theorem, also termed the "Chaos Principle", which establishes the fact that **on the sub-atomic (or energy and anti-matter) level, data and effects within one unit are transmitted to every other unit at "super luminal speed" (faster than light speed).** Thus Bell's work also establishes that **these sub-atomic energy and anti-matter fields do not comply with the laws that govern energy transmission in the solid state mode because they are not dissipated by time or distance.**

Therefore, in conformance with Bell's calculations, **all entities must instantaneously communicate with every other unit by non-neural means.** R. Sheldrake in *The New Science Of Life* terms this communication process "morphogenic", morpho "form" and genesis "coming into existence". This means that not only do living organisms communicate within themselves and with every other living organisms but also that **so-called "inanimate objects" communicate with other inanimate objects and with living entities. Thus, our environment has a profound role to play in our health and dis-ease.**

## ORBITALLY RE-ARRANGED MONO-ATOMIC ELEMENTS

In chronic and degenerative dis-ease, the DNA codes within cells assume aberrant patterns termed "Junk DNA". **Permanent restoration of health cannot be accomplished until the DNA norm is restored.** Hudson has been reported to have achieved this with oral administration of orbitally re-arranged, mono-atomic, non-metallic gold which resonates at a single frequency. In other words, it functions as a superconductor producing a "Misner Field" composed of one magnetic field rotating clockwise and another counter-clockwise. This results in no north/south pole orientation, no voltage potential and, therefore, no electrical current flow. Nevertheless, the elements within cells resonate with each other producing "High Spin Nuclei" capable of transmitting information from one cell to another, even at a distance, with no net loss of energy. This produces an energy field up to 1,000 times more intense than found in conventionally generated fields because, having no particles, it allows *any* amount of energy to exist within a given space/time frame. This causes material objects to appear to lose weight, but not mass, and even levitate due to their intense magnetic fields repelling gravity.

## TILLER-EINSTEIN MODEL

According to the Tiller-Einstein Positive/Negative Space/Time Model, matter and energy are interchangeable and must be primarily electrical or magnetic in nature. W. Tiller, Ph.D., indicates that positive space/time (+S/T) is the realm of electromagnetic emissions (EM). On the other hand is negative space/time (-S/T) energy and anti-matter, which is distinguished by its primary magnetic nature and which is described as magnetoelectric (ME) emissions. Because it moves faster than light, ME radiation does not interact with conventional EM detectors. Besides its magnetic nature, -S/T energy and/or anti-matter has another unique characteristic, the tendency toward negative entropy. That is, the energies of the ethereal (energy or quantum and antimatter) bodies have qualities that move solid state (cellular) systems toward states of higher order and organization (health). To clearly understand this principle, it is necessary to modify Einstein's basic formula as noted in Figure 18.1.

$$E = \sqrt{\frac{mc^2}{(1-v^2/v^2)}}$$

E=Energy    c=Speed of Light

M=Mass      v=Velocity

*Figure 18.1*

This comprehension of the multi-dimensional (physical, energy and anti-matter) nature of the universe allows otherwise unsolvable problems to be answered. The accompanying diagram gives a visual expression of the relationship between velocity and matter in our multi-dimensional universe. As matter accelerates until it approaches the speed of light, its kinetic energy increases exponentially. In the past it was considered physically impossible to accelerate matter beyond the speed of light as the ascending curve approaches the speed of light (C) but never intersects with it and continues off into infinity. See figure 18.2.

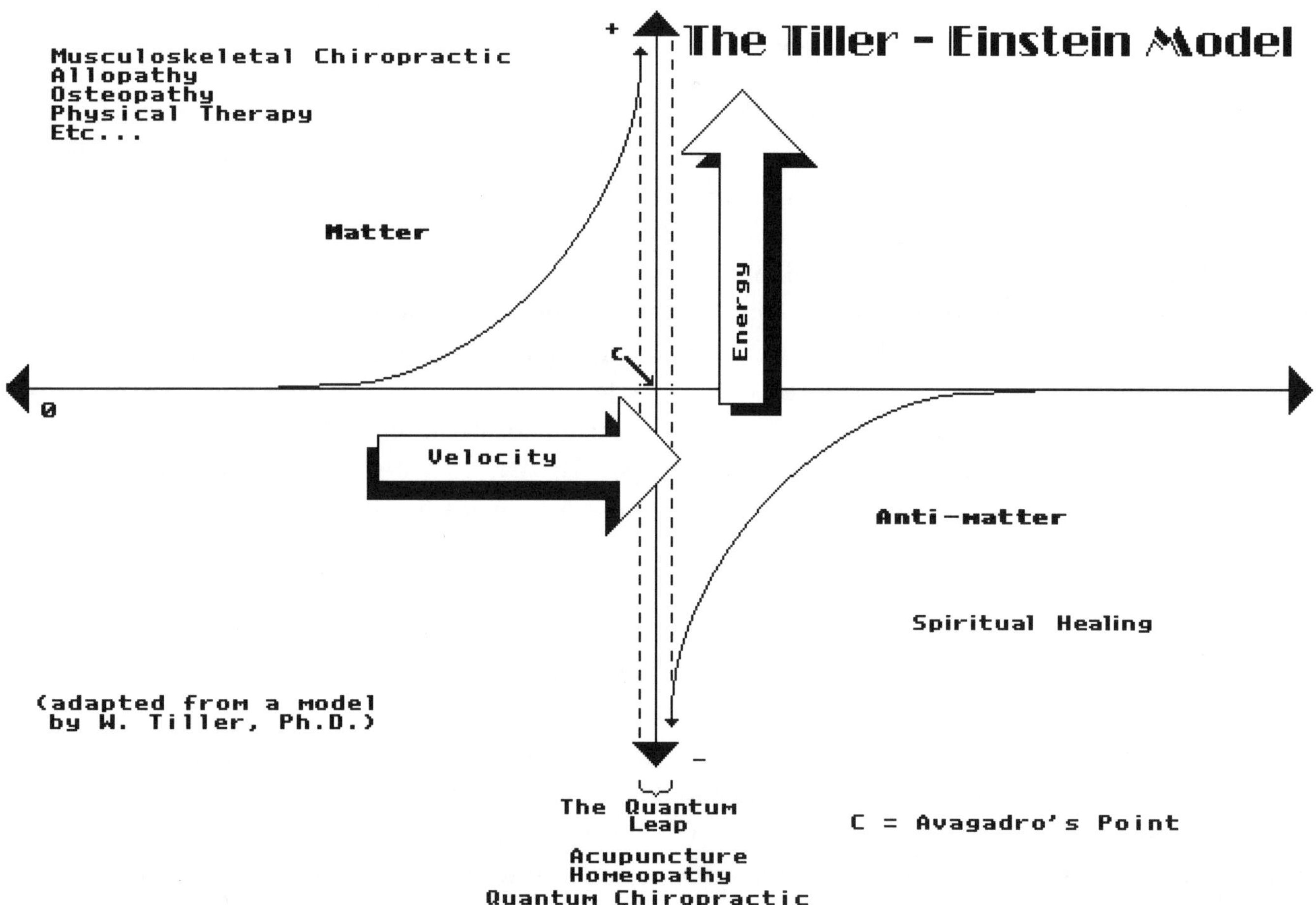


*Figure 18.2 — The Tiller-Einstein Positive/Negative Space/Time Model*

With the Tiller modifications, one arrives at solutions containing the square root of -1. This forces us to accept the parallel universe of -S/T and entities that move faster than light speed. It also mathematically explains the scientific actuality of negative entropy or increasing order experienced by living organisms. This is what D. D. Palmer was referring to when he stated **the dualistic system of the spirit (the non-corporal or anti-matter component) and the body (matter) are united by energy forming the basis of the science of biology.**

## ANOTHER GRAND QUESTION

This magnetoelectric reality creates yet another major quandary. If +S/T, the solid state, upon which western medicine and musculoskeletal chiropractic are currently fixated, is positively entropic, producing **decreasing** levels of order, organization and intelligence, and -S/T, the quantum state, which Native American, African, Oriental, Ayurvedic, and other healing systems utilize but which is ignored by present day western medicine and neuromusculoskeletal chiropractic, is negatively entropic, producing **increasing order, organization and intelligence**, where does that leave western medicine and neuromusculoskeletal chiropractic?

## ENDOCRINE-IMMUNOLOGICAL VECTOR

Endo-immunology requires a paradigm shift within the chiropractic mind set. In D. D. Palmer's day, endocrinology and immunology were terms not yet coined. Therefore, to understand his thoughts we must first come to a knowledge of the terms that he used when attempting to discuss the endo-immuno system. He records, ". . . it is impossible to analyze or compound chemically any part of a living body. That which is referred to - (as) 'chemistry of nutrition' - is metabolism. Metabolism is vital and chemistry non-vital . . . ." Palmer then defines metabolism as ". . . the process by which energy replaces the discarded worn-out tissues, excrementitious products; and constrictive metabolism, anabolism, the change of nutritional substances into body tissue." He adds "The glands secrete bile, saliva, splenic, enteric, pancreatic and gastric juices; products for use in the body economy. Each of these has its special function in metabolism."

Extensive research has documented that neurological, endocrine, immunological and gastrointestinal cells share biochemical and membrane associated properties that **allow them to talk to each other (by non-neural means).** The cell's DNA carries receptors (much like satellite dishes) for different information molecules - such as neuropeptides, neurotransmitters, endocrine secretions (hormones), and so forth - on their surfaces. **When a molecule becomes attached to a cell membrane receptor, the cell receives information that may alter its physiology.** For example, a natural pain-relieving molecule (beta-endorphin), produced in the brain, may attach to immune cells circulating through the brain and inform them of a particular event, perhaps a painful injury or stress, causing a neuropeptide release.

These circulating immune cells may then act very differently, once their opiate-like receptors are occupied, and frequently with greater immunological vigor or, conceivably because certain receptors are occupied, the immune cells "home in" on a certain location in the body. In this way, **mental imagery**, by altering brain biochemistry, can influence or even alter the immune system. It also  has been documented that lymphocytes have become more receptive to antigen stimulation through hypnosis.

As stated earlier, psychoneuroimmunology (PNI) also exhibits a communication system between endocrine and gastrointestinal functions. Cholecystokinin (CCK), a duodenal hormone, stimulates gall bladder constriction and secretion of pancreatic enzymes. It has been discovered that the cells in the hypothalamus have receptors for CCK that, when occupied, produce the mind-body state of appetite stimulation.

The psychological aspect of stress can also be mediated by way of PNI mechanisms. T type lymphocytes have receptors for catacholamines, ACTH, and cortisone. In states of acute alarm or prolonged stress, these receptors become saturated, altering T cell functions, and are thus a critical factor in immune defenses, such as the ability to divide and secrete, causing immune functions to decline.

It is now known that childbirth stress reduces the mother's salivary immunoglobulin A (IgA), a decline augmented by length of labor and the level of anxiety. Another study is examining immunoglobulin concentration in breast milk of pre-term birth mothers. Preliminary results indicate that depression and anxiety in these women seems to lower breast milk IgA, possibly impairing the health of the mother, child or both. **Investigations on how touch influences the immune system (which should be of interest to every doctor of chiropractic and massage) have also been conducted. While touch is known to be soothing and relaxing, the relationship between touch and immunity has not heretofore been studied. One recent study documents that back rubs given by nurses cause a rise in salivary IgA and lower anxiety levels.**

Thus we see that the study of immunology, neurology and endocrinology are inseparable. This is even more evident from the developmental relationship that exists between these two systems. The endocrine system, furnishes the normal chemical control and is older; in fact, in lower life forms, it is often the only control system of activities found in the smooth musculature and secreting glands aside from the normal rhythmic action which is inherent in every cell. As organisms became more complex, however, a more rapid response in the correction of automatic activities became necessary and so the autonomic nervous system was developed.

J. Mackinzie, M.D., in a 1921 article in the *British Medical Journal,* "The Theory Of Disturbed Reflexes In The Production Of Symptoms Of Disease" states that **the endocrine system is the modifier of the nervous system.** F. M. Pottenger, M.D., in his book *The Symptoms Of Visceral Disease* goes even further, stating, **"It is possible that every tissue of the body produces an internal secretion or chemical substance which has some physiological effect."**

Mackinzie adds, **"This effect is usually a modification of nervous function or effect."** This indicates that the endocrine and immune systems also have a dramatic role to play in the control of the living being for Pottenger again comments, **"The chemical control is much slower and a much less efficient control than that produced by the nervous system, yet its action is extremely definite."**

This last statement illustrates the close inter-relationship between allopathy (with its synthetic chemical orientation to health), naturopathy (with its naturally occurring chemical orientation to health) and chiropractic (with its neurological orientation to health). It also illustrates why "scope of practice" is such an archaic and unscientific concept in health care. One discipline is constantly overlapping into another because the living being is an integrated, inseparable whole.

## CANAL VECTOR

To accurately understand this vector, it is necessary to appreciate a lesser known definition of "chaos"; i.e., apparent disorder due to a lack of understanding. R. Bentley of the British Royal Library states, "We ought not to believe that the mountains are out of shape because they are not exact pyramids, nor that the stars are unskillfully placed because they are not all situated at uniform distances. These are irregularities only with respect to our fancies."

Serra adds in the *Introduction To The Physics Of Complex Systems: The Mesoscopic Approach To Fluctuations, Non-linearity, And Self-organization,* "A particular cavity structure . . . functions as an 'ordering principle', but only if one comprehends fractional geometry. Fractional geometry liberates the analysis of natural objects from the tyranny of straight lines, flat planes and regular solids. Order appears to be a compromise between two antagonists. . . . disturbing the delicate balance between these antagonists leads to an 'erratic state' on one hand, or on the other, a 'fossil like state'. . . Therefore, **'at the point of balance, energy flow becomes organized.'** The energy of DNA, proteins, and nerves consists of coherent and organized solitary waves which can only exist at a point of balance." (Emphasis added.) Chaos scientists, ". . . achieve balance and order by adjusting the parameters that govern energy flow." Did not D. D. Palmer specifically state, "Too much or too little is dis-ease."?

R. Serra, et al., continues the concept in these words, "The key parameter is a 'cavity' of a particular size and shape." Therefore, it is the spinal canal not the neural components that guides and concentrates energy flow. In compliance with these laws, Black states, **"Chiropractors produce the coherent flow by fine-tuning the cavity that serves as its 'organizing principle."** This is in complete agreement with D. D. palmer, **". . . vital energy is not transmitted over, thru or by the nervous system".**

It is now clear that **the chiropractic adjustment affects a through-flow system that receives inflow on one end and produces outflow on the other, both of which are also adjustable.** Inflow includes but is not limited to food, water, air, light, sound, information, energy, etc. Outflow includes, but is not limited to mental balance, exercise, talking, working, playing, cleansing, etc.

D. D. Palmer said nerves respond to stimulation according to their habitual function (facilitation). Thus, stimulation of the optic nerve, if sufficiently strong (threshold), results in the sensation of light; of a motor nerve, in contraction of muscles to which it is distributed; of a secretory nerve, in the activity of the related gland. **It depends neither upon any special construction nor activity of the nerve itself nor upon the nature of the stimulus but entirely upon the peculiarities of its central (brain) and peripheral end organs.** See Figure 18.3.

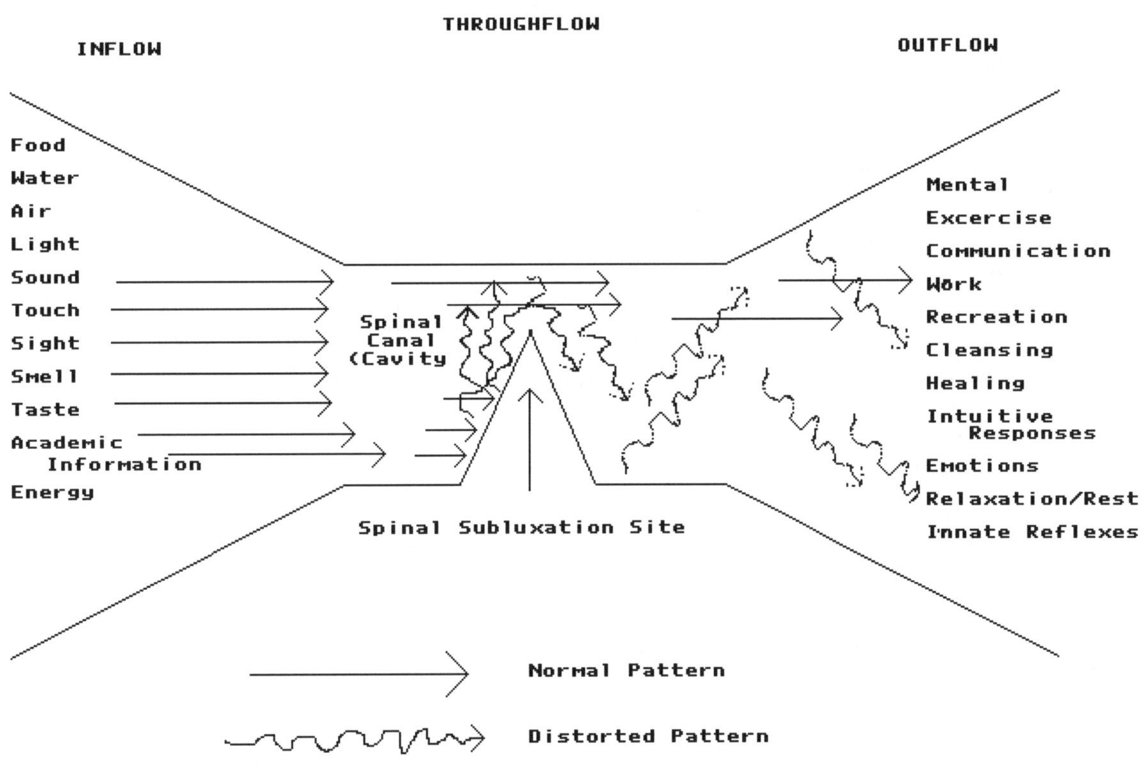


*Figure 18.3 — Spinal Canal Vector*

## MERIDIAN VECTOR

"Too much or too little is dis-ease." This is the ancient principle of Yin-Yang, the universal "Law of Balance" restated. **Evaluation of the energy balance and treatment of the meridians are the only things about the meridian system that are new to chiropractic. Chiropractors, in reality, have been unknowingly affect-**

ing the energy level in the meridians since chiropractic's inception. Along the spine, there are acupuncture points called meridian connectors. By this mechanism, when we adjust the spine, we affect the meridian (energy) system.

F. Stoner, D.C., uses even stronger words, ". . . it is impossible to adjust the spine without affecting the acupuncture meridian connectors. This, in turn, affects the corresponding meridian and its interrelationship with other meridians." If doctors of chiropractic can accomplish so much inadvertently, what is the potential for accomplishing even more if they knew precisely what is being done with an energy adjustment which is what an acupuncture therapy is?

In fact, oriental healers have been aware of this relationship for thousands of years. The chiropractic approach compliments and further extends the treatment of the meridians. Spinal adjustments and muscle relaxation, as well as the application of herbal plasters and compresses (naturopathy), are often utilized as aids in musculoskeletal practice.

In oriental medicine, an imbalance of innate, vital force, ch'i, or life force can develop from many types of stimulus. Again, we must remember that D. D. Palmer wrote that vital energy is not transmitted thru the nervous system or any other system known to him; it is expressed in functional acts. Research to date confirms that this is one of the functions of the non-anatomical, quantum, acupuncture meridians, to adjust the energy flow within the living being.

## HOMEOPATHIC VECTOR

Homeopathic remedies in potencies past Avagadro's Point (the dividing line between matter and energy), like chiropractic adjustments, add nothing material to the living being, as do nutrients and pharmaceuticals, nor do they take anything away, as in surgery.

As represented in Figure 18.4, neuroanatomy documents that there are nine times as many sensory nerves as there are motor nerves. Neuropathophysiologically speaking, this means that what happens to the brain in the sensory side is nine times more important to the body than what happens on the motor side. Yet the vast majority of chiropractic procedures, regardless of whether they are adjusting techniques or modalities, concentrate on the musculoskeletal motor problem.

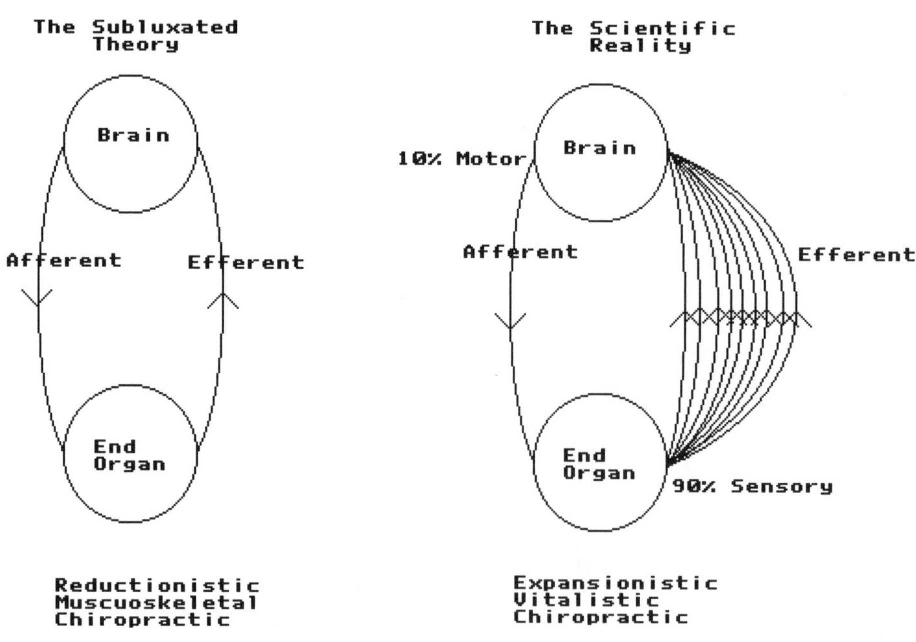


*Figure 18.4 — The Accurate Relationship Of The Safety Pin Cycle*

Homeopathic texts offer chiropractic a vast compilation of detailed neurosensory responses. For the first time, we have a practical means of dealing with sensory nerve interference instead of just the ten percent of the nervous system which is motor. In this new light, pathological reflexes, symptoms and nerve interference take on a whole new meaning. It is now understood that the CSC expands into the ninety percent of the nervous system which is sensory. Chronic subluxation (dis-ease) is in reality a build-up of aberrant neurological dysfunctions that include altered reflexes, incongruous memory patterns and abnormal responses to sensory stimuli. By the process of neurobiotaxis, these neurological abnormalities become pathological reflexes or memory patterns, resulting in abnormal maintenance and defense functions.

We now have a tool to take us into the patient's brain, mind, emotions and spiritual (non-corporal) being. Thus, homeopathy enables the doctor of chiropractic to truly heal from "above down, from inside out"; from the higher quantum to the lower material or physical level. This tool allows the chiropractor to move from the reductionistic, non-vitalistic, solid state concept of treating chronic symptomatic subluxations to the chiropractic practice of dealing with the cause of dis-ease. And this, more often than not, in the CSC, is not at the spinal level but rather at the brain, mental and spiritual levels which can only very indirectly be affected by spinal adjusting.

This is precisely why the mental, emotional and spiritual symptoms are of such profound significance in selecting the proper homeopathic energy template. **We must have a remedy that is capable of permanently altering the QPNIMT holographic engram response within the patient's brain.** C. Prill, D.C., wrote, **"Few chiropractors ever give any consideration to what happens to the brain cells. All of chiropractic discussion is about what happens from the vertebral subluxation down and what happens above the subluxation is totally ignored. In the chronic cases, our attention should be drawn to the brain cell and what can be done to aid its recovery of normal function."**

## GRAVITY WAVE VECTOR

When Albert Einstein originally formulated his "Theory of Relativity", he also predicted numerous phenomena that would prove its validity. Science is currently confirming the last of these criteria, the gravity or standing wave. Gravity waves are energy disturbances emitted by fast-moving objects and/or energies that move through the fabric of time and space like ripples from a pebble dropped into a still pond. This principle is even more readily understood on a larger scale such as a nuclear explosion which sends out shock waves. Vogt, of Cal Tech's Physics Department, says that **we are looking at a whole new force as to transmitting signals.** It has been demonstrated that such action takes place over distances from millimeters to hundreds of meters and that this space has a memory property.

V. Pettibon, D.C., teaches, **"Video fluoroscopy of adjusting forces applied to the spine show that the body is selective in welcoming or rejecting external mechanical forces. Oscilloscope readings further reveal that adjusting creates a wave in the fluids that make up the muscles over the vertebra. This wave can work for or against the adjustment. At least three properly timed toggles are necessary before an adjustment reaches its greatest potential for vertebral correction."**

**Recent evidence shows that our physical body is the mirror image reflection or dense energy pattern manifestation of dynamic actions which take place in our bioenergy field. Since our bodies act as communication devices, we are constantly receiving and transmitting information-coded energy signals; changes in our bioenergy field signal the onset of dis-ease before it occurs physically.**

Living cells, on the sub-atomic level, are composed of particles and/or energy moving in the atomic shells at extremely high rates of speed and therefore producing gravity waves. Quantum physics research is now beginning to document that these "waves" communicate information from atom to atom, cell to cell, and likely from tissue to tissue via non-neural means. Some researchers are even speculating that this phenomenon may transmit data from organism to organism over great distances and could be a scientific explanation for the phenomena of mental telepathy and other parapsychological manifestations.

## 4TH DIMENSIONAL VECTOR

Most chiropractors tend to think of the subluxation complex in only three dimensions; i.e., posterior, right and superior. This is inadequate as the patient actually exists as a six-dimensional being. As many physicists have correctly speculated, time is the fourth dimension; what is today the causative subluxation may not have existed yesterday. **Vastly more intriguing, however, from a QPNIMT viewpoint, is that yesterday's causative subluxation may not even exist today.** Petersen writes that **it is now understood that it is only necessary for the (causative) subluxation (dis-ease) to be present momentarily, from a historical standpoint, to initiate a type of injury to neural elements whose latency of repair of such injury is extended in time beyond the more spontaneous recovery of the musculo-skeletal strain of the articulation.** In fact, F. M. Pottenger, M.D., in his book *Symptoms of Visceral Disease* refers to Sir Charles Sherrington's writings when discussing this principle and A. E. Homewood, D.C., N.D., in his book *The Neurodynamics of the Vertebral Subluxation* devotes an entire chapter titled "Afferents, Time and Trophic Functions" to pointing out that, **"Time is a most important factor in considering the function of the nervous system."** And Stephenson writes in his *Chiropractic Textbook*, **"There is no process which does not require time. . . . Time is an element necessary to the bond between intelligence and matter."**

## LAW OF TIMING AND TRAUMATISM

Every chiropractor has seen the case where an individual stoops over to pick up something as small as a toothbrush and cannot straighten up due to acute lumbosacral pain. This is an inappropriate manifestation of timing. The lumbosacral segmental control responded incorrectly for this particular time and function. It exerted forces required to lift something much heavier such as a bag of cement. With no such weight being present, inappropriate muscle force created a mechanical derangement resulting in Acute Vertebral Subluxation Complex (AVSC).

Timing applies in other areas as well. A person secretes enough stomach acid at 2:00 A. M. to digest a five-course banquet (diagnosed as an ulcer) but produces only one-fourth the necessary amount at meal time (diagnosed as indigestion). The point being, the 2:00 A.M. amount is not an excessive amount for a large meal, nor is the lesser amount abnormal for fasting. The problem once again is one of incorrect timing. **The cause is not the symptomatic mechanical subluxation (dis-ease) but rather it is a matter of incorrect timing.** The chiropractor could adjust this spine until doomsday and not correct the cause of this problem. As D. Tole, D.C., states, **"We cannot treat enough symptoms to get rid of the cause of the problem."**

## 5TH DIMENSIONAL VECTOR

One of the laws of physics states that energy is required to do work. Therefore, energy (the 5th dimension), or quantum factor, is required to achieve a response in chiropractic. D. D. Palmer writes, **"A subluxation does not restrain or liberate vital energy. Vital energy is expressed in functional activity. A subluxation may impinge against nerves, the transmitting channel may increase or decrease the momentum of impulses, not energy. Vital energy is not transmitted thru the nervous system or any other; it is expressed in**

**functional acts.**" It is a well-known fact that force does not become functional until it meets resistance; just as light does not become visible until it strikes an object. Studies indicate this energy, mechanical and/or biodynamic, is the triggering mechanism that activates the innate healing power. Once this "jump start" is accomplished, there must also be energy to move and guide the healing process through the bio-dynamic maze of life. See Figure 18.5.

## 6TH DIMENSIONAL VECTOR

The divergent maze of life (the 6th dimension) is a one-way street. You can never go back and be what you were when you were ten years of age. Once any branch of the maze of life is traversed, the options offered by the other branches up to that point are no longer available. The patterned response, to a great degree, is locked in by each subsequent branch option selected. Therefore, we can never, in the scientific sense, return patients to their pre-injury or pre-illness state. The pathological choices (branches) have permanently altered the QPNIMT engrammimg of the holographic brain and nervous system.

Stephenson writes, "We have no assurance, with ever changing environmental conditions and new subluxations and passing pressures, that the same combination of circumstances will be obtained that existed when we 'sized up' conditions in the first instance." Speransky adds, **"We obtain not a dis-ease in the organism but a new organism, distinguished from the original by a number of constant or accidental features."** (Emphasis added.) D. D. Palmer concurs, **". . . therefore, we never find precisely the same combination with exactly the same symptoms."** (Emphasis added.)

To illustrate, in Figure 18.5, the data stored at point E includes all information stored at point B in addition to data from the B-C-D-E experience which in all likelihood has in some way caused alterations in the point B data. Therefore, points B and E are not identical even though they both lie on the ideal health line.

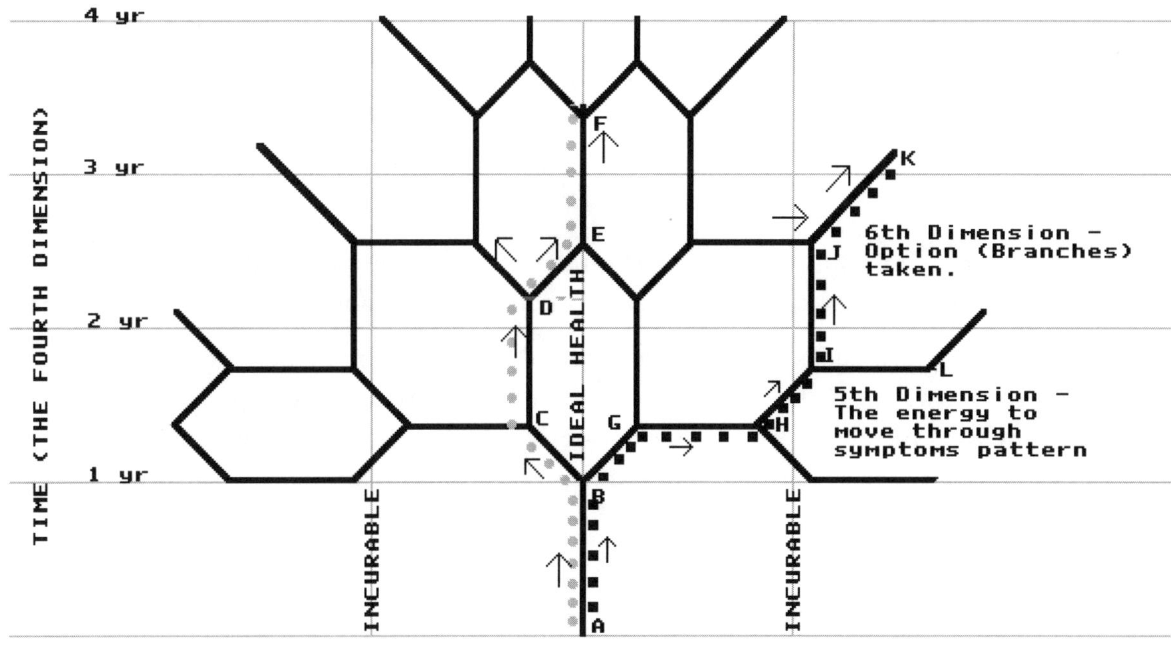


*Figure 18.5 — The Maze of Life*

## LAW OF DIRECT CURRENT VECTOR

R. O. Becker. M.D., extensively discusses this phenomenon. He states the first or primitive living organisms used an analog or direct current(DC)-type of data-transmission that regulates such functions as growth and healing and that also serves as the substrata for our internal control and communications systems while the nervous system is an alternating current (AC) system as exhibited in any physiology textbook under the heading of nerve excitation and conduction.

Becker pointed out that if living organisms used an analog type of data-transmission system and if such a system is still used for injury repair, which his research has proven to be so, then the entire analog system must still be present as part of our entire data-transmission and control system. The brain thus operates as a hybrid computer and forces us look at it in a revolutionary new way as comprising a magneto-electric-brain-mind-body function. What has emerged is a dual nervous system: a primitive analog component that appeared early in evolution, and a more sophisticated digital, nerve-impulse component of more recent origin. It appears that living things have taken advantage of two portions of the electromagnetic spectrum that could be depended upon to always be present: the geomagnetic field and visible light.

Additional research proved that this DC communication system works by using **the perineural cells - in this case, the Schwann cells of the myelin sheath carry the electrical signals that cause fractures to heal. The nerve axon and dendrite have nothing to do with it.** Furthermore, it now appears that the DC system is involved in getting the neuron ready to fire the command to move the muscle and this phenomenon is referred to as the "Readiness Potential"; in other words, **the DC system commands the nerve-impulse system.**

## ADDITIONAL VECTORS?

With the number  of vectors currently known, who is so brash as to deny that there may be additional vectors of the CSC still waiting to be discovered?

## COMMON GROUND

Thus, the old and overly simplistic concept of a subluxation is woefully inadequate in view of the modern quantum understanding of how the living being actually functions and communicates with its various parts.

The eclectic and dynamic principles of the CSC are indeed confirmed by modern science. **A doctor who understands the neurological enervation vector will be consistently more successful than one who snaps and pops vertebrae indiscriminately. Likewise, the doctor who strongly couples other vectors under a favorable set of circumstances will experience massive effects many orders of magnitude larger than those due to the mechanical vector alone.**

Chiropractic, being a part of the dynamic universe, must conform to Stephenson's Third Law and **continually adapt.** Some chiropractors seem unable to make the necessary paradigm shift and have fallen into static reductionist, non-vitalistic, solid state rather than dynamic quantum thinking. This is indeed unfortunate. But as D. D. Palmer wrote, "As soon as the human mind is capable of absorbing a still more refined and advanced method (than neuromusculoskeletal chiropractic) and human aspirations demand it, it will be forthcoming and I hope to be the medium thru which it will be delivered to the denizens of the world."

Yet, even with all of this scientific evidence, many within and without the profession still associate chiropractic with only the mechanical (neuromusculoskeletal) aspect of health care. A careful study of chiropractic, however, reveals that it is **primarily a quantum science,** the purpose of which is to normalize energy flow.

Although D. D. Palmer, the founder, stated that too much or too little (energy) is dis-ease, the majority of practitioners continue to place their primary emphasis on structural dis-relationships forgetting that B. J. Palmer, another luminary of the profession wrote, **"All subluxations are misalignments; but all misalignments are not subluxations."**

Stephenson wrote, **"Chiropractic is based upon the link between mind and matter and it naturally follows that the student is curious to know what that link is. Chiropractic maintains that all phenomena is the result of force in matter and chiropractic maintains that this force proceeds from intelligence. It is called the 'missing link' because it was unrecognized, as the bond between the immaterial and material, until it was discovered by chiropractic and the other quantum healing sciences discussed in this text."**

Some sciences are a study of matter, as chemistry; some are studies of force and energy, as physics; and some are studies of the mental or abstract realm entirely. But it never occurred to any of the western solid states, reductionistic sciences to get together on these until chiropractic put them together, and it is this embodiment of the three in one that is implied in the major premise and the fundamental principle of Chiropractic.

# Chapter 19
# HOMEOPATHIC MEDICINE

*"We put drugs of which we know little, into bodies
of which we know less, to cure dis-eases of which
we know nothing at all."*

— Voltaire

## HISTORY

Many of the laws that govern the present day science of homeopathy are of very ancient origins. By 2,000 B.C., the Ayurvedics of India were discussing the law of similars and minimal dose. The ancient Greeks and Romans also dealt with these issues. In fact Hippocrates (460-377 B.C.) wrote, **"An illness is caused by similar means and similar means cure man of illness"**. In other words, the same agent brings about strangury (slow painful discharge of urine due to spasm of the urethra and bladder) when it is not present, and does away with it when it is. Coughing, like strangury, is caused and is made disappear by the same means. Vomiting is stopped by being made to vomit. But this advanced knowledge appears for all practical purposes to have been lost during the Dark Ages.

After receiving his medical degree in 1779, Samuel Hahnemann, M.D., soon earned the reputation of being one of the most brilliant chemists in Germany. But as he continued to experience the crude practice of medicine, he grew more and more dissatisfied with what consisted mainly of blood letting, purging and forcing the patient to take large doses of mixtures of toxic liquefied heavy metals.

After a few years, Hahnemann gave up his practice and began earning a living translating textbooks from one language to another. In 1790, while translating a book into German, he found that he could not agree with its explanation of the action of Cinchona Bark (Quinine) in the cure of ague (malaria). While in Hungary, Hahnemann had gained firsthand experience with ague fever as it had been epidemic there. As an experiment, he began taking large doses of Cinchona twice a day. He noted that while taking the substance he began experiencing many of the symptoms of malaria, and that these symptoms would go away when he stopped taking Cinchona Bark. **The symptoms, though very similar to malaria, were not malaria but rather an adverse drug reaction.**

After many years of continuing experiments and study, Hahnemann wrote in a leading medical journal that, "Every medicinal substance (is capable of producing) peculiar, marked and violent dis-ease." Therefore, "We should imitate nature, which sometimes cures a chronic dis-ease by suppurating another, and employing in the dis-ease that we wish to cure that medicine which is able to produce another very similar artificial dis-ease, and the former will be cured, similia simibus."

In 1810, Hahnemann published "The Organon Of Rational Medicine". Because of intense protests from allopathic colleagues, it became the "Organon Of Medicine". In it, Hahnemann gave a full dissertation on the principles of his new method of healing, and detailed instructions for the examination of the patient, for proving (testing) of remedies and for the selection of remedies according to the homeopathic principles.

In his introduction, Hahnemann writes, "Hitherto, diseases of man were not healed in a rational way, or according to fixed principles, but rather according to very varied curative purposes, amongst others, according to the palliative rule. In contrast to this is the true, the real way of healing, which I am pointing out. In order to cure gently, quickly and permanently, choose in every case of illness a remedy which can itself arouse a similar malady to that which it is to cure."

From that point on, Hahnemann devoted the remainder of his life to  further documenting the universal Laws Of Healing in a more extensive, orderly and usable format than any other healer had previously done. These universal Laws Of Healing are, in great degree, the genesis of this textbook.

# LAW OF THE MECHANISM OF THE CURE

No amount of solid state research can totally document why a remedy (or any other form of therapy) cures. This is because a therapy does not cure. **The energy (innate, life force, vital force, ch'i, etc.) that causes the being to function is what cures.** This is proven by administering the correct remedy, adjustment, acupuncture, herbs, drugs, surgery, and/or mental therapy to a cadaver with a diagnosed dis-ease. NOTHING HAPPENS! **However, a properly chosen remedy (or any type of therapy) does establish a particular pattern or energy (quantum) template which, when coupled with the life giving vital force, is capable of healing.** In some respects, this phenomenon resembles an algebraic equation in which a minus (the dis-ease) and a plus (the healing energy template of the remedy) cancel each other and return the being to the neutral (ideal state of health).

# LAW OF MIASMA

 The miasmatic principle is the crown jewel of homeopathy, as is dosha in ayurveda, diathesis in chiropractic and phase in oriental medicine. **Without a working knowledge of the miasma (dosha, diathesis, phase) it is impossible to consistently heal.**

Many mistakenly believe that Hahnemann's thinking was only empirical. We must however remember that he was one of the most famous and well respected chemists of his time. What later would became known as the doubling principle was well known to him, as were its many and severe scientific deficiencies. (See Chapter 47, Research.) In the study of miasmas, one thing must be clearly understood. This was the only time when Hahnemann allowed himself to become entirely empirical. That is the reason that so many of his heretofore loyal disciples were unable to accept the miasmatic concept of dis-ease.

In seeking terminology to describe the major patterns of dis-ease, Hahnemann attached to them names of endemic dis-eases of his time. These terms have become standard homeopathic nomenclature. Interestingly, however, recent findings of mummies and texts indicate these same dis-ease traits in societies that according to history had not yet been exposed to gonorrhea and/or syphilis; i.e., Native American cultures who were not exposed to syphilis until contamination from Columbus' crew and subsequent explorers from the old world, the ancient Ayurvedic culture of India, and the indigenous peoples of China. However, the use of these dis-ease nomenclatures by no means negates the validity of the miasmatic concept of dis-ease. In order to make it easier for the neophyte to comprehend the miasmatic concept, I have typed them according to mode of disturbed function. These more modern designations appear in parentheses in the ensuing discussion.

# PERSPECTIVE

In 1676, when Van Leeuwenhoek peered through a magnifying lens and saw "living creatures so small that a hundred lying one against another could not reach to the length of a grain of sand", he had found one of the keys to the mystery of decay, dis-ease and the nature of the living world. But another 150 years passed before Hahnemann became the "Father of Bacteriology" by recognizing the true significance of microbes. **Our vital force, a spirit-like dynamism, cannot be attacked and infected by injurious influences such as microbes unless internal forces are first disturbed** and in like manner all such morbid derangements (dis-ease) cannot be removed other than by the dynamic, alteration of vital force. So it is only by dynamic action of the vital force that remedies or any other form of care are able to re-establish health and harmony after the totality of symptoms have revealed the dis-ease to the carefully observing and investigating physician.

Thus, Hahnemann comprehended that **a miasma is an acquired or inherited constitutional weakness that makes the tissues, emotions, reasoning, energies, etc., more susceptible to certain stresses. It can be either latent or active, acute or chronic and is the underlying cause of dis-ease.** Hence all dis-ease is due to **an irritant** that produces a specific recognizable picture and its origin is due to one or more of the following external disturbances of the physical and quantum components of the patient's being.

# CLASSIFICATION OF MIASMATIC DIS-EASE

I. Acute - **(Functional disturbances), no evidence that it can produce permanent tissue pathology)**
The provoking agent causes a violent flare-up of the underlying miasma and returns to normal after a relatively short period of time. It is most commonly associated with microbes but agents such as intense stress (on any level of the total being), lack of rest, poor diet, lack of exercise, meridian imbalance, subluxations, exposure to toxic chemicals, or a combination of these, can also trigger this response.

    A. By Type

        1) Recurring - i.e., Malaria

        2) Non-recurring - attack only once in a lifetime; i.e., Smallpox.

    B. By distribution

        1) Individual - only a single or very few individuals suffer the symptoms.

        2) Sporadic - small numbers of individuals suffer the same or very similar symptoms without being able to establish a consistent connecting link.

        3) Epidemic - many individuals suffer very similar or identical symptoms with a definite connecting link; i.e., weather, malnutrition, pestilence, war, lack of sanitation, microbes, etc.

II. Chronic

    A. Dis-eases with fully developed symptoms.

        1) Non-miasmatic

            a) Occupational (Homotoxicological) - a vast array of noxious influences, usually presented over a prolonged time frame, eventually causing a derangement in the expression of the vital force. Includes addictions, dietary perversions, allergies, malnutrition, fatigue, worry, dehydration, lack of adequate rest, poor personal and environmental hygiene, radiation, pollution and toxins. Hahnemann prescribed **an improved mode of living or working as one of the essentials for a cure.** In other words, **remove the patient from the causative environment.**

b) Iatrogenic-causes a derangement of the vital force due to **improper and/or excessive care by any health care discipline.**

2) Miasmatic - Hahnemann provided a broad classification of dis-eases naming them after the characteristic skin and/or mucosal changes occurring in the **initial stage.**

A. Single Dis-eases

(1) Psora - (the miasma of deficiency, **parasympathetic) scabrous eczematoid itching.** Psora (from the Latin) is derived from the Hebrew word "Tsorat" meaning a "grove, fault, pollution, stigma, leprous or plague." Kent states, "**All other diseases develop because of this original weakness.**" Its taint goes to the very core of human experience, the primitive wrong, (Biblically, the change that took place due to disobedience in the garden), the universal weakness of the race which has been driven deeper and deeper into the constitution by generations of suppressive care. In other words, Psora is a state of susceptibility which is an outward manifestation of disobedient will and thinking.

The Psoric patient appears timid, reserved, lax, indifferent or even lazy because slight exertions leave him drained, but underneath, he is a bubbling cauldron of emotions. Psoric patients complain of digestive troubles, being cold, of fears. They exhibit defective bone development, find it difficult to concentrate, are often remorseful followed by outbursts of emotions, have poor self-images, are hypersensitive, hyperactive, highly allergic, anxious to the point of fears, and have many ideas that are not followed through to completion.

(2) Sycosis - (the miasma of **excess, sympathetic). From the Greek "Sykon" (fig) for the fig-like **condylomata appearing and proliferating on the mucosal and skin,** the underlying cause being suppression of gonorrhea in the individual or throughout the familial history. Mentally, the miasma revolves around selfishness and covetousness, the desire for pleasure without thinking of the consequences, exploitativeness, daring without reason, excessive feelings of hurry, irritability, restlessness, suspicion, reproductive problems, yellow-green discharges, warts, blood, kidney, liver and lung problems, all "hyper", "osis" and "itis" dis-eases.

(3) Syphilis (Luetic) - (the miasma of destruction, **erratic sympathetic and parasympathetic fluctuations)** with **ulcerations** of the skin, the underlying cause of which is suppression of syphilis. It produces bone and brain problems, violent destructiveness, lack of feelings and disregard for human life. Its victims are spiteful, hateful, revengeful; they rage and are cruel and jealous; they hemorrhage, atrophy, have spasms, and are gangrenous.

(4) One-sided

(a) Only mental Symptoms; i.e., mania.

(b) Only physical symptoms; i.e., headaches.

B) Compound Dis-eases

(1) Tubercular (the miasma of **exhaustion). A combination of the Psoric and Syphilitic miasmas with **night sweats and weight loss.** It produces the cavitation of psora and the exudate of syphilis. The tubercular patient is anti-social, dull of mind, slow, feeble, fatigued, and nervous. He has poor circulation, hot flashes, bruises easily, has rapid pulse, no fear of death, is future-oriented, clumsy, in constant desire of change, has pain of an iron band around the head, craves things that cannot be assimilated, has an empty, all-gone feeling, is allergic to cow's milk, and can be diabetic. His symptoms are aggravated by changes in the weather.

(2) Oncotic (Cancer) - (the miasma of **adaptive failure**). A mixture of Psoric, Sycotic and Syphilitic with **changes in body odor, unusual discharges, intumescences (swelling), changes in warts and/or moles, sallowness of skin hue and sores that refuse to heal.** The patient exhibits neoplasms, bleeding, changes of bladder and bowel habits, hoarseness, coughs, indigestion, tumors, ulcerations, insomnia, fever, diabetes, and AIDS. He frequently presents conditions such as tuberculosis, emaciation, recurrent and/or unremitting infections and fevers, anemia, fear of death, melancholia, loss of appetite, malformations and ulcerations.

C) Duration

(1) Continuous - the condition is constantly present.

(2) Intermittent - the condition comes and goes at periodic intervals.

(3) Alternating - the condition presents itself as one set of symptoms in one locale of the body and/or mind and at a different time and place as a different set of symptoms but with the same underlying cause.

## GRAPHIC REPRESENTATION

Figure 19.1 illustrates the waning vital force as each progression of miasmatic dis-ease is activated. Figure 19.1 also illustrates the acute (functional disturbance) which can happen on any miasma level and the perverted vital force response of homotoxicology which tends to manifest itself most in the psoric (deficiency) and sycotic (excess) miasmas.

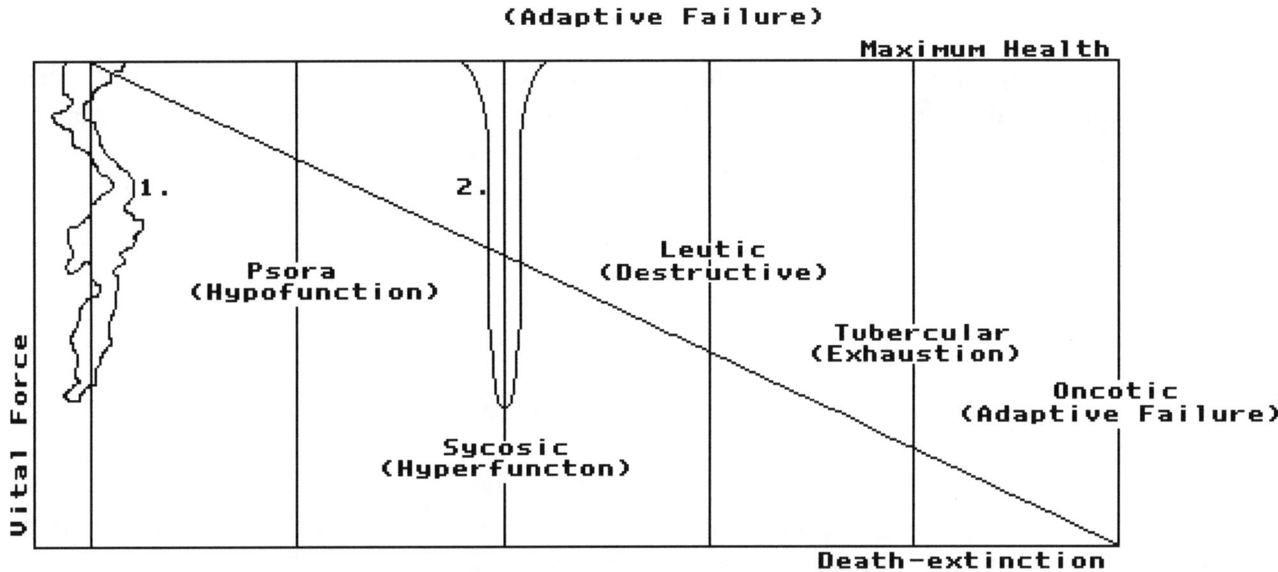


*Figure 19.1 — Miasmatic Relationship To Vital Force*

# FURTHER THOUGHTS ON MIASMAS, DIATHESIS, DOSHA, PHASES

What triggers a miasma, diathesis, dosha, phase dis-ease? Actual dis-ease symptoms produced by these underlying factors can lie dormant within some individuals for many years before being activated. (This is not to say that we cannot determine the individual's miasmatic, diathesis, doshic or phase propensity but rather that there is not active pathology associated with that pre-programmed propensity.) Or this tendency may even remain dormant for an individual's entire lifetime only to emerge in the next generation with great virulence.

Homeopathic philosophy assigns this triggering mechanism to the iatrogenic treatment of the race since time immemorial. Naturopathic philosophy assigns the triggering mechanism to toxic conditions within the body. Chiropractic philosophy regards the triggering mechanism as a lack of proper control by the nervous system. Traditional osteopathy equated the triggering mechanism with disrupted blood supply to the involved tissue(s). Allopathy assigns the triggering mechanism to a chemical imbalance. Oriental medicine regards the triggering mechanism as an imbalance of the regulating Ch'i (Qi) energy. Sufi medicine feels that the triggering mechanism is a lack of harmony with the teachings of Allah (God).

Since these appear to be quite divergent concepts, they cannot all be correct. Or can they? The answer lies in what all of these apparently divergent concepts have in common. **In every case there is a stressor for which the being's defense mechanisms cannot successfully compensate.**

Other mechanisms can fall into this general stressor category. Nutritional imbalances such as excesses or deficiencies of vitamins, minerals, proteins, fatty acids, carbohydrates, can certainly stress a living organism. Severe emotional stressors such as deaths, accidents, job loss, legal and financial problems, anger, guilt, loneliness, fear, moves to new locations, dissatisfaction with employment, marital problems, romantic losses, violence, family problems can likewise stress some individuals beyond their tolerances. Lack of personal hygiene, unhealthy environments, lack of rest, extreme changes of temperature and climate, excessive physical trauma and more can also act as the trigger mechanism in many cases. Limited research has also implicated absence of stress as a potential culprit. **A certain background level of stress seems to be necessary in order to maintain the being's normal QPNIMT defense mechanisms at an optimal level.**

# LAW OF HYDROTHERAPY

Hahnemann states there is a palliative usefulness in this modality when purpose, temperature, duration and frequency are properly taken into account. Temperature ranges suggested are from 7 to 13 and from 31 to 34 degrees centigrade depending upon the results desired. He recommends the use of concurrent massage in many cases. **A major caution is given by Hahnemann regarding mineral baths which can antidote other therapies.**

# LAW OF HYPNOSIS

According to Hahnemann, hypnosis affects the patient by balancing the num, kundalini, vital, innate, life, ch'i force where it has been causing vegatonia. In view of the knowledge amassed since Hahnemann's time, there is far more than just the effect of the Vagus nerve upon the total being.

# LAW OF MASSAGE

Hahnemann states that massage is especially beneficial to the chronically ill and weak patient. He writes that massage **causes the vital principle to be stimulated,** restoring tone to muscles, blood and lymphatic vessels. He cautions against the excessive stimulation of massage, especially in hypersensitive patients.

# LAW OF NUTRITION

Over-cooking, fermentation, salting, and use of alcohol and vinegar destroys medicinal and nutritive qualities of foods.

# LAW OF ORGANOTHERAPY

All crude animal, mineral and vegetable substances have medicinal  virtues and can alter the state of the patient's health, each in its own unique way.

# LAWS OF PHARMACODYNAMICS

1. The sap (juice) of a plant can be stored indefinitely without deterioration of its medicinal qualities when it is mixed with an equal part of grain alcohol if the container is properly sealed and stored away from intense light and heat.

2. For plants high in mucilage, two parts of 90 to 95 proof grain alcohol to one part of sap is the desired recipe. This latter proportion is also needed for plants of a very dry nature.

3. Exotic plants, barks, seeds, roots, and animal components should not be accepted in powdered form by the homeopathic pharmacist because they tend to deteriorate in medicinal qualities during long-term improper storage.

4. If no options are available, the pharmacist must guarantee her/himself of the freshness of the plants, immediately dry them until the particles no longer stick together and store them in an airtight opaque container.

# LAW OF DYNAMIZATION/POTENTIZATION (TITRATION AND SUCCUSSION)

Potentization releases the latent quantum (energy) of substances even those which in the crude state do not have the slightest medicinal qualities. There is within an iron bar or steel rod a slumbering trace of magnetic force. When either has been left standing upright immediately after being forged, the lower end repels the north pole of a magnetic needle and attracts the south pole. But this is only a latent force; not even the finest iron filings can be magnetically attracted to or held by either end of such a rod. Not until we have dynamized a steel rod, by rubbing it strongly in one direction with a blunt file, does it become a true, active, powerful magnet capable of attracting iron and steel and of imparting magnetism to another steel rod not only by contact but even at some distance.

Similarly, by the titration of a medicinal substance and the succussion of its solution (dynamization, potentization), the medicinal forces lying hidden in it are developed and uncovered more and more and its material is spiritualized (non-corporeal).

In quantum physics terminology, this is not difficult to understand. Solid state physics cannot even agree about the nature of a substance as basic as water. Solid state science knows that water is H20 but understands very little about the weak hydrogen bonds that hold the molecule together. Quantum physicists, on the other hand, know that these bonds transform water into a crystal-like formation or polymer. **This means that information can be "written into" water, or any other bond-oriented substance, by slightly changing the orientation of the molecules.** In fact, this is precisely what takes place when we record on an audio or video tape. The metal oxide molecules on the tape's surface are re-oriented as we record data. In like manner, information can be recorded as homeopathic remedies are titrated and succussed by subtle changes of global molecular arrangement.

Therefore, this transformation increases the power that these substances have to affect humans and animals in their state of health. In this refined condition, when they touch or closely approach sensitive living tissue, just as a magnet can magnetize a steel needle without changing any of the steel's other physical or chemical properties. And just as the magnet cannot magnetize non-magnetic metals, such as brass, so also dynamized remedies do not affect non-living things.

Homeopathic remedies frequently are incorrectly referred to as "dilutions" when in fact they are exactly the opposite: titration and succussion that unlock the healing energy of the substance to be used by the body to "jump start" its own innate healing power. This is in complete harmony with the laws of quantum physics which state, "You can neither create nor destroy anything, only change it." If there is less matter present, there must be more energy and/or antimatter present. Thus, potentized remedies are actually **energy templates** rather than molecular substances such as are found in pharmaceutical drugs and/or phytotherapeutic agents (herbs) or nutritional substances. The dynamic forces of mineral magnetism, electricity and galvanism act homeopathically on the being's vital principle.

Additional extensive quantum physics research regarding this topic is presented in Chapter 35 of this text.


# LAW OF HORMESIS

Paracelsus (1493 - 1541), the greatest scientific mind of his age, wrote, **"All things are poison, nothing is without poison: the Dosis (dose) alone makes a thing not a poison."**

Smith-Sunneborn's research at the University of Wyoming confirms this principle. She has been able to document that very small doses of radiation, certain antibiotics and heavy metals significantly extend the life expectancy of insects and animals. She states, "It (hormesis) is a biphase response, where at low doses you get a beneficial response and at high doses you get a detrimental response to the same agent. . . (Arndt-Schultz Law). Hormesis (appears to) increase DNA repair." Smith-Sunneborn also says, "It may stimulate higher levels of protective responses in the cell, such as production of antioxidants. . . . It may also be that hormesis stimulates the immune system, giving the organism greater protection."

Nor is Smith-Sunneborn alone; Neafsey's work at Tufts University, School of Medicine, and Boxenbaum's at Merrill Dow Research Institute have concluded that, "Assessment of mortality data from modern-day bioassay studies indicates that low-dose animal exposure to a variety of toxic agents can, through an unknown mechanism, induce beneficial changes which promote health and longevity."

Benveniste of INSERM, the French Medical Research Institute, has documented similar findings. Additionally, his work has been duplicated at major universities in Canada, Israel and Italy. Fornter, at the University of Toronto, states, "It is unbelievable and breaks all of the rules. . . . We all assumed that where there are no molecules present, nothing will happen. This has really shaken up our world. Even people who have seen this phenomenon find it hard to conceive what could be happening here."

Yet, Hahnemann had gone far beyond mere conception or even a working hypothesis of this phenomenon. By 1810, he had developed a consistently reproducible clinical therapy, homeopathy, which he organized and set down in very concise laws (aphorisms) of application in his classic textbook, the *Organon Of Rational Medicine.*

## PROCESS OF DYNAMIZATION

1. Powder/Pellets -  Place 1/3 of 100 grains of powdered milk sugar in a glazed rough-bottomed mortar, add 1 grain of the mother substance. Mix with a porcelain spatula, then titrate with a rough-bottomed porcelain pestle for 7 minutes. Scrape from the mortar and pestle for 3 _ minutes and stir to a homogeneous consistency. Again, without adding additional material, place back in mortar and titrate for an additional 7 minutes. Again, scrape the mortar and pestle for 3 _ minutes. At this point, add the second third of the milk sugar, stir with spatula and titrate as with the previous 1/3. Follow the identical procedure with the last 1/3. The powder thus prepared is stored in an air-tight container and is labeled the 1/100, C1 or 1st centesimal potency.

To prepare the 2C 1/10,000 potency, place 1 grain of the powder from the 1C preparation in the mortar with 1/3 of 100 grains of powdered sugar and follow the identical steps for preparation of the 1C potency. For the 3C 1/1,000,000 potency place 1 grain of the 2C potency in the mortar and rehearse the entire titration procedure. It will take approximately one hour to prepare each potency.

2. Liquid - 1 grain of the mother substance is dissolved in 500 drops of a mixture of 1 part grain alcohol and 4 parts distilled water. A **single** drop of this preparation is placed in a vial, add 100 drops of grain alcohol, **which will fill the vial to the 2/3 level,** cap and succuss 100 times against a hard but elastic (usually leather covered) striker. Sugar globules, of a weight of 100 globules to a grain, are thoroughly moistened with the vial contents and immediately spread out to dry on filter paper. This is the 1 LM 1/50,000 potency. When this is completely dried, store the globules in an air-tight container.

To prepare a 2 LM 1/5,000,000 potency, 1 globule in taken from the 1 LM container and dissolved in 1 drop of distilled water. To this is added 100 drops of grain alcohol, filling the vial to the 2/3 level, and it is succussed 100 times. Again, it is spread on filter paper to dry and stored in an air-tight container.

## KIRLIAN PHOTOGRAPHY AND HOMEOPATHY

Kirlian, a Russian scientist, developed a specialized photographic  procedure in which the film is exposed with a 25Kv current flowing through it. See figure 19.2. Such a procedure allows the magnetoelectric energy field or "aura" which surrounds an entity to expose the photographic plate. It also is capable of documenting the deterioration of the energy field as a living entity dies and the alterations in the field with dis-ease and the re-establishment of the normal field as healing takes place.

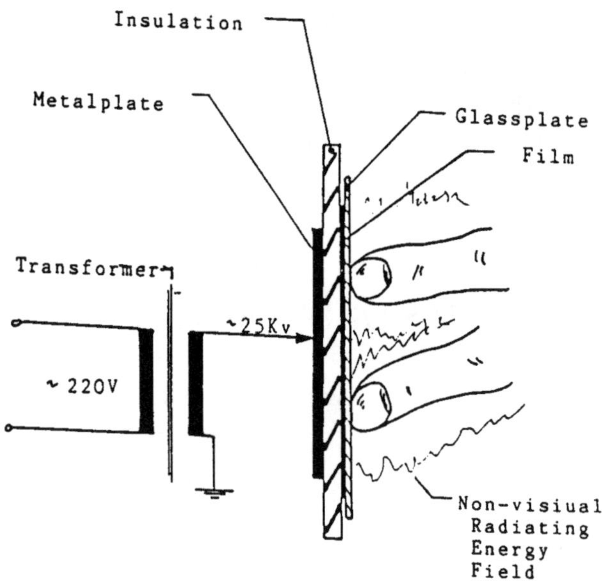


*Figure 19.2 — Illustration of the Kirlian photographic process*

## KNAPP'S WORK

Knapp, a German Ph.D., slightly modified this Kirlian process in order to photograph the magnetoelectric energy templates of homeopathic remedies. See Figures 19.2 and 19.3. **Knapp was able to document that each remedy has its own unique energy "fingerprint" or pattern and that each potency of each given remedy also exhibits its own energy template which is just as individualized to that remedy and potency as fingerprints are to a particular person.** See figures 19.4 - 19.7.

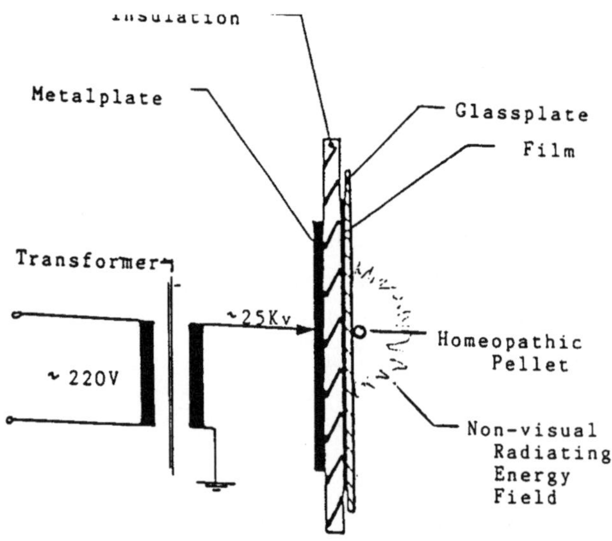


*Figure 19.3 — Modified Kirlian photographic process of Knapp*

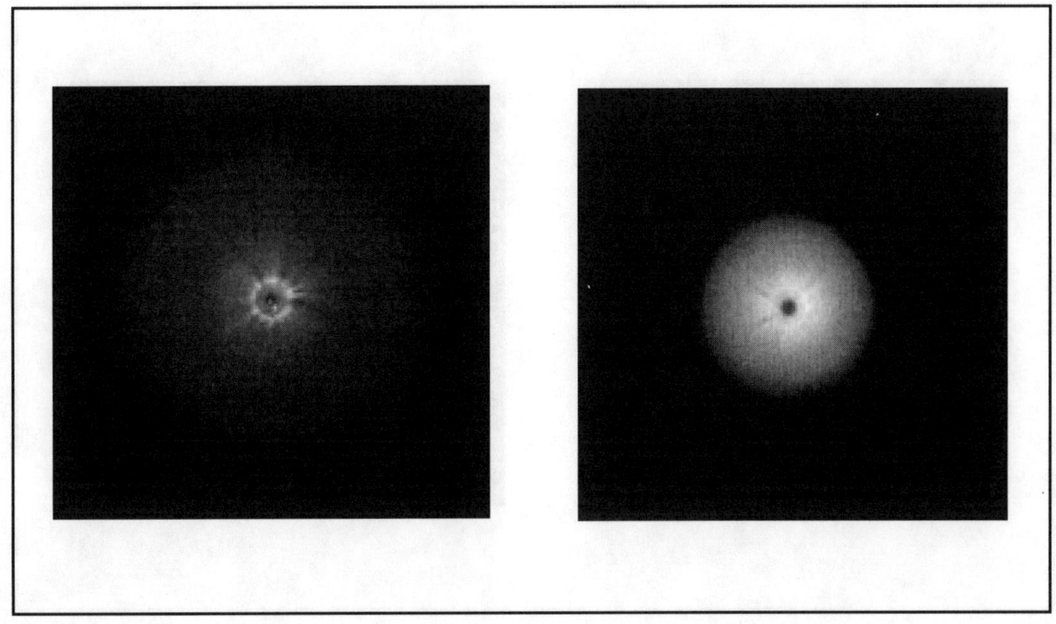

*Figure 19.4 — Comparison Of Arnica 30X (left) and Belladonna 30X (Right)*

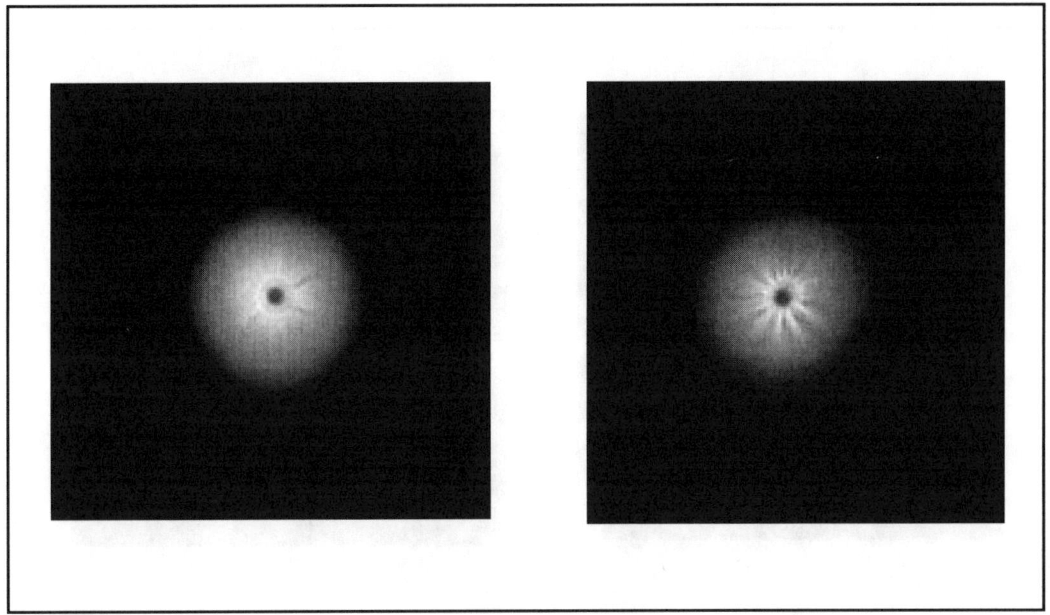

*Figure 19.5 — Comparison Of 30X Belladonna (left) and 200X Belladonna (Right)*

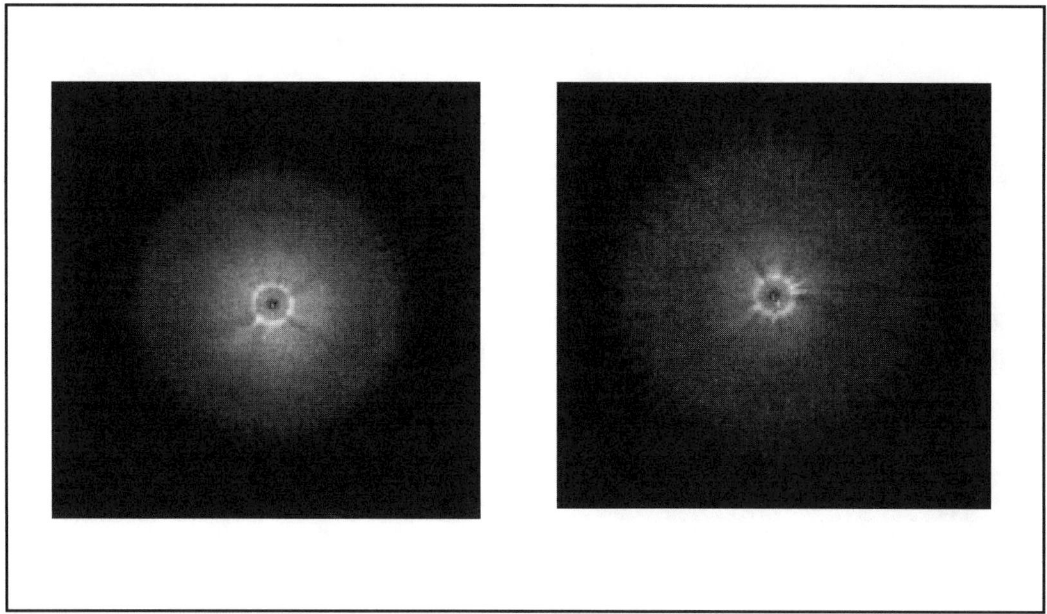

*Figure 19.6 — Unique Templates Of Arnica 6X (Left) and Arnica 30X (Right)*

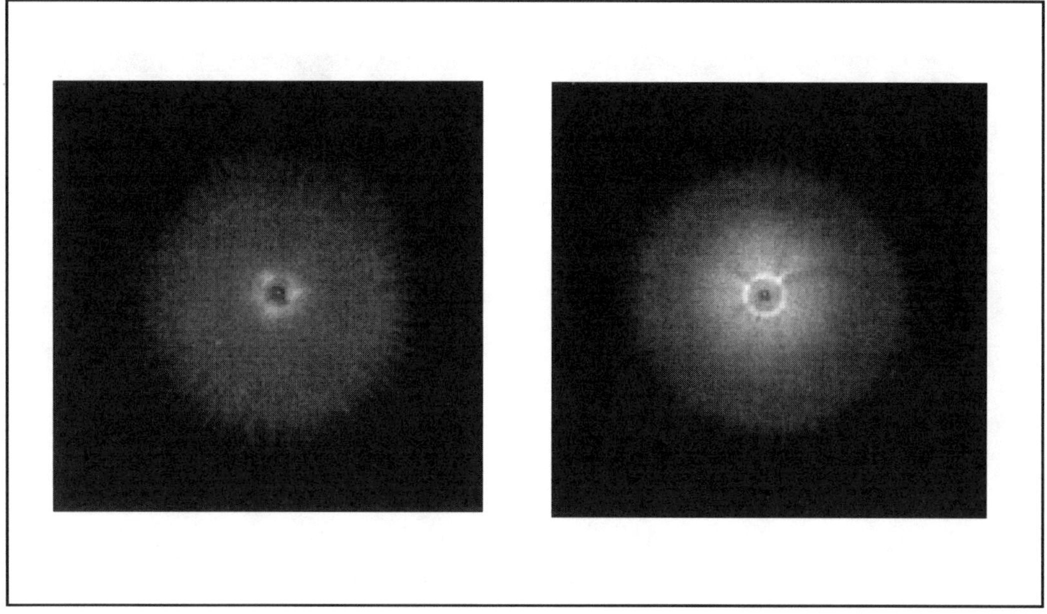

*Figure 19.7 — Comparison Of Thuja 12X (Left) and Arnica 6X (Right)*

## LAW OF SHELF LIFE

Controlled double blind studies have confirmed that 110-year-old remedies prepared in this manner produce responses that are comparable to recently manufactured remedies. For all practical purposes it can be concluded that the shelf life of a properly manufactured homeopathic remedy when properly protected from excess light, heat and moisture is **indefinite.**

## LAW OF MODE OF ACTION

One globule placed on the tongue results in only a very few nerve endings being affected by the remedy. But extensive research has proven that an identical globule dissolved in water and shaken before being administered produces a polymeric or holographic pattern involving all of the water molecules in a magnetic, semiconductor, nanocrystal, quantum dot cluster and, therefore, has a far more dramatic result because many nerve endings are affected by it. Current quantum physics research is documenting that, through contact with the dissolved substance, the remedy's "information" is transmitted even when molecules of that substance are no longer statistically present in the solution. In fact, many quantum physicists now agree that "water, which is of decisive importance as a transmitter of information in material dilutions, has the "memory of an elephant".

## LAWS OF DOSAGE

**Practitioners of homeopathy must have at their command a mastery of the full range of potencies.**

In acute dis-ease, the 6X to the 200C potencies and occasionally the 1M potency prove to be the most successful. In chronic dis-ease of the hypersensitive patient, the 30C to the 10M potencies, as a general rule, prove the most reliable. In chronic dis-eases, of the normally sensitive patient, the 10M and greater potencies usually prove to be the most effective. In prescribing for constitutional and miasmatic cases, potencies frequently begin in the LM or MM ranges.

**In all types of dis-ease, the initial potency should be continued as long as improvement is noted.** As progress with a particular potency comes to a standstill, the next higher potency should be prescribed, working through increasing potencies until a cure is obtained. **At that time, prescribing should cease.** If the remedy is not the similia, it generally will act in only one or two potencies and then there will be a change of symptoms indicating the need for a new remedy.

**A major error is to suppose that increasing the potency of the dose makes it more "therapeutic".** For ideal responses, the attenuation (potency) must be similar to the plane of the disruption in the patient's being. **Excessive increases in the potency and/or unwarranted frequency of prescribing can completely disrupt the case or temporarily and dramatically aggravate the symptoms. With the correct potency and frequency, we obtain healing  without aggravation.**

**For maximum results, all remedies should be in wet administrations of a single pellet. In chronic, constitutional and miasmatic prescribing, the remedy's duration of action must also be considered. The duration of action forms a guideline for future frequency of prescribing.**

## LAW OF SERIES IN DEGREES

Kent writes, **". . . One potency is not sufficient for chronic diseases. It will generally do for acute sickness. Many chronic sicknesses are cured by keeping the patient under the influence of the one indicated remedy for two or more years. But this cannot be done, with continuous curative action, unless the doctrine of series in degrees is fully understood and used."** He then adds, **". . . The degrees must be far enough apart to represent an octave, or failure follows. . . . I have settled (after much research) upon the octaves in the series of degrees as 30th(C), 200th(C), 1M, 10M, 50M, CM, DM, and MM."** Kent then cautions, **"The very high potencies seldom require repetition, if clearly indicated, to produce a long curative action in chronic cases, but in severe acute sickness in robust constitutions** several doses in quick succession are most useful." Kent continues, "Each change of potency brings new and deeper curative action."

## ILLUSTRATION OF THE HOMEOPATHIC PRINCIPLE

Medical literature presents a confounding set of articles which are easily explained by the principles of homeopathy. In a letter to the *New England Journal Of Medicine*, published on July 16, 1981, various studies from the 1950s were cited to show the benefit of vitamin E in preventing post-traumatic or post-surgical blood clots in the lungs and/or legs. The evidence was quite convincing. Yet, in the *Journal of the American Medical Association,* published six days earlier on July 10, 1981, a warning about the use of vitamin E was sounded. In an article entitled, Perspective on Vitamin E as Therapy, the author presented a list of the known side effects of prescribing high doses of vitamin E. The first side-effect listed was blood clots in the lungs and legs! The article continued by listing most of the symptoms that vitamin E is supposed to help according to the *New England Journal of Medicine* article.

This is yet another example of standard allopathic medical literature reaffirming the basic principle of homeopathy, that **ALL substances act by the Law of Similars. Medicines cure the exact symptoms in the ill that they produce in the healthy.** This also confirms that even vitamins, when taken in very large doses, act not as a vitamin but instead as a drug that produces adverse side effects.

## DIET, MAGNETISM, ELECTRICITY AND MINERAL BATHS

Homeopathy recognizes the value of other agents in addition to homeopathic remedies. Hahnemann indicates that the use of baths, electricity, magnetic fields and diet are especially **useful for dis-eases of sensibility or irritability, abnormal sensations and involuntary movements.** He states, "The dynamic forces of . . . magnetism, electricity and galvanism act no less homeopathically and powerfully on our vital principle than . . . actual homeopathic (remedies) . . . The dose can be regulated by increasing or reducing the duration of application."

## DRAINAGE FORMULAS

Some companies sell combination formulas that they refer to as "homeopathic drainage remedies". Unfortunately, the manufacturers of such products are completely lacking in an understanding of the principles (aphorisms) of homeopathy. **Any properly selected remedy IS the simillima for the case and is therefore always the drainage remedy best suited for that case. This is true because the simillima deals with the totality of the symptoms including any weakness and/or dis-function of the organs of drainage such as the liver, lungs, kidneys, skin, or lymphatics.**

## INSTRUMENT TESTING AND COMPUTERS

In recent years, some enterprising firms have been in the process of trying to develop electronic machines with which to test homeopathic remedies. While theoretically an intriguing concept, the actual results fall far short of the stated goal because **to date no one has succeeded in programming a machine to understand**

and reason through the application of the universal laws of healing in each and every situation and no one ever will be able to do so. Therefore, the results of such machine testing are erratic at best.

Because the vast majority of instrument-oriented practitioners have failed to take the necessary time and effort to master the universal laws, they are incapable of recognizing when the instrument is giving invalid and/or conflicting findings. Thus, they frequently become an iatrogenic danger to the very patients they are supposed to be aiding. In the vernacular, "They are flying blind."

Additional data regarding other questionable assumptions of instrument testing are similar to those discussed under the heading of "Kinesiology" in Chapter 17. In summation, A poor homeopath with an expensive instrument is still a poor homeopath. A good homeopath with an expensive machine may save time.

# Chapter 20
# MASSAGE

*"Miracles do not happen in contradiction to nature,*
*but only in contradiction to what*
*is known to us in nature."*

— St. Augustine

## REDUCTIONIST CONCEPT

Reductionistic masseurs traditionally list the purposes of massage as:

1. Increasing the blood supply to a treated part

2. Increasing lymphatic drainage and venous return

3. Joint drainage decreasing periarticular swelling

4. Muscle relaxation

5. Prevention of or resolution of fibrosis and adhesions

6. Prevention of muscular atrophy.

## EXPANSIONIST CONCEPT

To clearly understand the full quantum range of massage's effects it will be necessary to study the chapters 17 and 18. Many, if not all, of the extra-neural concepts discussed there also apply to a full understanding of the science of massage.

## INCREASED ACCEPTANCE

In 1995 G. Kamps, et. al., reported that The State University of New York at Syracuse documented that 54 percent of primary care and family practitioners said they would encourage their patients to pursue massage therapy as a treatment and 34 percent indicated they were willing to refer their patients to a massage therapist.

We must, however, remember that this study only documented allopathic usage of massage therapy. Because of massage's inherent compatibility with the philosophies of chiropractic, naturopathy and oriental medicine it is likely that a far higher percentage of these practitioners utilize the professional services of masseuses. In fact, many such practitioners not only refer but also maintaining in house masseuses.

# NEURAL AND QUANTUM RAMIFICATIONS

Massage provides a dramatically increased bombardment to the nervous system with afferent impulses and also to the other communication systems within the living being. Since 90 percent of the nervous system is afferent (input or sensory) and only 10 percent is efferent (output or motor), this form of therapy has profound and far-reaching effects. In reality, a proper massage should balance the energy of the entire body. In most situations, therefore, it should be a rejuvenating experience.

# Chapter 21
# MENTAL HEALTH AND HYPNOSIS

*"A human being is a part of the whole called by us 'Universe,' a part limited in time and space. He experiences himself, his thoughts and feelings, as something separated from the rest, a kind of optical delusion of this consciousness. This delusion is a kind of prison for us, restricting us to our personal desires and to affection for a few persons nearest to us. Our task must be to free ourselves from this prison by widening our circle of compassion, to embrace all living creatures and the whole of nature in its beauty."*

— Albert Einstein

## THE PHYSICAL BACKGROUND OF EMOTIONS

It has been said that an emotionally dominated person thinks through his body; an intellectually dominated person, through his brain. **From a functional (solid state) point of view, the brain is but another organ of the body and, as such, can become sluggish and can malfunction the same as any other organ.** If a person eats wrong foods, wrong food combinations, introduces drugs and other accumulative toxins and has poor elimination, the body can become clogged with toxins. Dr. Wilson's work at the Spear's Chiropractic Hospital also documented that a systemic alkalinity in combination with these toxins lowers the functional capacity of the brain and thereby affects the thought process.

The United States is acknowledged to have the most over-medicated, over-operated on and over-inoculated population in the world. We routinely impose drugs, surgeries and techniques intended for serious or life-threatening dis-eases and which may have no scientific validity, on minor, even trivial, illnesses such as the common cold, illnesses that are self-limiting and that, except for symptomatic relief, do better without interference from the physician. We think of health as something that can be bought, rather than a state to be sought through an accommodation to the norms of nature. All of these unnecessary treatments form internal pollution which affects the living brain and nervous system.

## THE INTERFACE

Compton, a Nobel prize winning Ph.D. in Physics, writes, **"If freedom of choice is admitted, it follows by the same line of reasoning that one's thoughts are not the result of molecular reactions obeying fixed physical laws. For if they were, his thoughts would be fixed by the same physical conditions, and his** choice would be made for him. Thus, if there is freedom of choice, there must be some thinking possible independently of any corresponding cerebral process."

This simply means that thinking does not come from the brain "secreting" thoughts as the liver secretes bile. If thoughts were the product of such a process, their formation would be as circumscribed as the formation of bile and therefore could not exceed their boundaries. If it were true that thoughts couldn't exceed their boundaries any more than bile can, we would have had no progress, no civilization, no modern comforts and would still be eking out an existence with stones and clubs for weapons, caves for shelters, skins for clothes and bed, the flesh of animals and wild vegetables for food.

But since thought does exceed its boundaries, it proves, as Compton said, that thinking is at least partially if not completely divorced from brain activity. It strongly indicates that man thinks through the brain and it further indicates that thought involves far more than the brain.

## THE MENTAL BACKGROUND OF EMOTIONS

It is true that universal intelligence started the development of our personal characteristics; it is also true the we were left to our parents and grandparents, our environment and our own wishes and desires to complete our development. Seabury, the noted psychologist said, "What a person is an hour after birth constitutes the sum of his inherited intelligence and is the 'real' man."

To date, it has been demonstrated that a child's inherited intelligence is capable of only a 10 to 19 percent improvement. Gesell states, "Environmental factors inflict, support, and modify, but they do not generate the progressions of development. They do not establish the primary potentialities of either physical or psychological growth."

The num, kundalini, innate, vital, life, ch'i insures, Compton writes, "everything is directed toward a definite end. This concept throws new light on the evolutionary process and gives meaning to life. In this view, the world and mankind are not developing at random out of atomic chaos. On the contrary, I believe I have found evidence strongly suggestive of a 'directive intelligence' or a purpose back of everything, with the creation of intelligent beings as its reasonable goal."

J. A. Widtsoe, past president of the University of Utah, adds, "Associated with universal energy that vivifies universal matter, and possibly is identified with it, is universal intelligence, a force which is felt wherever matter and energy are found, which is everywhere. The forces of the universe do not act blindly, but are an expression of a universal intelligence. That a degree of intelligence is possessed by every particle of matter cannot be said; nor is it important. The great consideration is that, since intelligence is everywhere present, all the operations of nature, form the simplest to the most complex, are products of intelligence. . . . We may conceive that energy is only intelligence, and that matter and intelligence, rather than matter and energy, are the two fundamentals of the universe."

Smuts, past president of the British Association For The Advancement Of Science, agrees, "The old science tried to reduce life to terms of matter and the result was a materialistic view of the world. The new science, coming from discoveries in relativity, has destroyed the old concept of matter. . . the world evolves on three levels: matter, life and mind; which can be roughly translated into organization, organism and organizer." This is the same thought Voltaire had when he said, "If a direct intelligence didn't exist, we would have to invent it in order to explain the workings of nature."

Sir James Jeans, another eminent scientist, has gone so far as to say, "The universe begins to look more like a great thought than a machine and . . . mind is not the intruder in the realm of matter, but is its creator and governor."

K. Menninger, the noted psychologist, in *The Vital Balance* continues the concept, ". . . back of all life there is an energetic drive to accomplish certain ends, which brings about a state of tension within the individual until its gratification is achieved." This "drive" has been variously explained as "the will-to-do," "the will-to-be-superior," "the desire to excel," "an upward-striving tendency" or "the will to survive." To Freud, this drive is the sex instinct; to Trotter, the herd instinct; to Varonoff, the influence of the glands; to Ley, conflict; to Woodworth, instinct; to Jung, intro- and extra-version; to Adler, the inferiority complex; to Sadis, fear; to McDougall, hunger; to Eatson, distress; to Link, service; to Trow, a primitive urge; to White, the libido; and to Seabury, the impulse for love, for comfort and for amusement. Regardless of what it is called, one fact consistently comes across. **The governing force of the universe is an immaterial entity.**

L. Rhine and J. Rhine, former professors at Duke University, after reviewing the concepts of the above authorities, and others not mentioned, continue our discussion, **"Yet, oddly enough, no one even claims to have proved that the mind is physical. There is no physical theory of conscious mental process on record. It is astonishing that a branch of science gives acceptance to a view of the mind not only without positive proof but without even so much as an untested hypothesis to account for it. Such an act can only be characterized as one of pure belief, as an act of 'faith'. Yet it has become almost as typical in scientific circles and classrooms as the belief in the soul has been in schools of theology."**

This argument presented by the Rhines has never been successfully answered, or even directly challenged. Together with the other facts presented, it stands as an indictment against the so-called reductionist, solid state, scientific concept of life which says man is no more than a machine, controlled by laws of chemistry and physics.

## THE EXPANSIONISTIC APPROACH

**Thus, chemical drugs can never be more than a control mechanism for mental conditions. They lack the ability to cure because they fail to deal with the quantum component of mental health. Only forms of healing that deal with the non-material (quantum and anti-matter) aspect of the mind can produce a cure.** Soli put this concept into a philosophical setting by stating, **"Illness is communication from your higher self. And until you understand that communication, there cannot be healing. It is impossible because the communication is the dis-ease.**

## HYPNOSIS

The history of hypnosis or the **ability to control one's own mind and body** is long and involved. The art was practiced by the ancient Egyptians, Greeks, Indians, Druids, Incas and numerous other cultures. Yet, as B. Inglis writes in *The Case For Unorthodox Medicine*, "For some reason, no method of disciplining mind and body comparable to Yoga ever established itself in the West." Therefore, it is extremely difficult for the reductionistic mind to accept the non-corporal therapeutic value of hypnosis.

Hypnosis found only limited acceptance in 18th and 19th century western medicine as a means of anesthesia and with the advent of modern chemical pain killers it was, for all practical purposes, abandoned.

## LAW OF FOCUS

The prevailing notion among novice practitioners is that hypnosis has much in common with sleep. But the patient's behavior under hypnosis is quite different from his behavior while in a deep sleep. **During hypnosis,**

**the mind is focused rather than diffused as in deep sleep.** Therefore, hypnosis must be categorized as **a third state of mind in which the individual retains most faculties without being fully conscious and readily accepts and assertively acts upon suggestions.**

The question is frequently asked, "How effective is hypnotherapy?" The classic laboratory experiment is to tell the subject under hypnosis that he or she is being touched with a red-hot probe at a specific location on the skin. The subject withdraws from the probe, cries out in pain and the skin in that specific location blisters even though the probe is cold. Furthermore, there are documented changes in respiration and heart rate that are characteristic of such physical insults. Conversely, when the individual is told the probe touching the skin is cold when in fact it is red-hot, there is no withdrawal response, no pain, no blistering, no heart rate or respiratory changes. Other studies reveal similar changes in blood sugar levels, gastric secretions levels, and other bodily activities when the subject is told her or she is being touched with a red-hot probe or subjected to pain.

But the results are even broader in scope. Hypnotic suggestion is effective for extended periods of time. Delayed physiological changes can develop days, weeks and even months after the original hypnotic suggestion(s) is (are) given. This implies that the mind concentrated by hypnosis is capable of virtual reality (VR).

In hypnotic VR, all experiences are in the holographic *now*. Details are vivid and concise, even though the incident may have occurred years ago and has been consciously suppressed. This includes the patient's physical, mental, emotional and spiritual responses as well as his conscious and/or unconscious reasoning for adopting a particular survival strategy. Once these causative factor(s) are identified, they then can be successfully dealt with.

## LAW OF CAUSE

It all seems so basic; hypnotize the patient and by suggestion remove the social, physical, emotional and/or spiritual symptoms. But we MUST realize **we can never treat enough symptoms to remove the cause.** Therefore, hypnotherapy's great contribution is to enable the patient and healer to identify the true underlying cause(s). Once the cause is identified, hypnotherapy generally reduces the time and amount of care necessary but does not necessarily alter the nature of the care.

## CONCERNS

There is no evidence that reputable therapeutic hypnosis controls the will or changes the basic character of the patient. Nor is there any scientific documentation to lend credence to the idea that a professional hypnotherapist can exploit the patient for non-therapeutic purposes. Yes, on a theatrical level, hypnotized subjects may embarrass themselves but on a clinical level, **there is no evidence to show that they can be led to commit deeds that are repugnant to their nature under hypnosis.**

The great **potential** danger would seem to lie in the dastardly combination of an unscrupulous practitioner and a patient without morals, convictions and conscience (the syphilitic miasma in homeopathy). Unfortunately, there appears to be little or no research confirming or refuting this position.

## LAW OF EXPECTATION

An individual's ability to perform is significantly improved by praise and reinforcement.


## INTER-RELATIONSHIP OF TIME AND ETERNITY

R. Hulbert, Ph.D., in *The Sun Is Always Shining* discusses C. S. Lewis' concept of time, a reductionist concept, and eternity, an expansionist concept, intersecting in the present. In fact, Hulbert quotes Lewis' book *The Screwtape Letters* as follows: "The present is the point at which time touches with eternity. . . ." As the present slips into the past, opportunities are lost. **We cannot go back and make changes in the past but making changes in the future can and does profoundly alter our future.** See Figure 21.1.

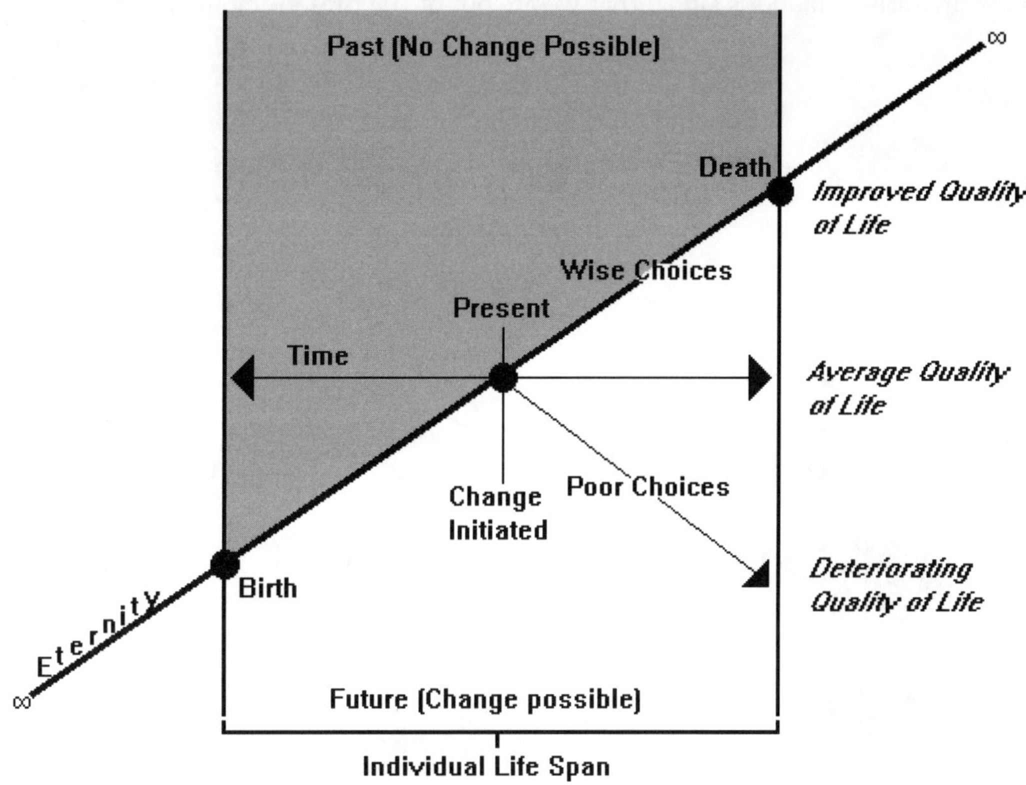


*Figure 21.1 — Inter-relationship Of Time And Eternity With Regard To Mental Health*


## LAWS OF MENTAL, EMOTIONAL AND SPIRITUAL HEALTH

Hulbert's text can be summarized into the following core issues for achieving mental, emotional and spiritual health. See Figure 21.2.

1. **Universal Intelligence's (God's) influence can never diminish and is the source of all life, truth and understanding. What we think and do can and does, however, add to or detract from our physical, mental, emotional and/or spiritual well-being by placing ourselves in a position of greater or diminished harmony with the Universal Intelligence.**

2. **There are different levels of "awareness" or learning. When our mood deterio-rates, our understanding and harmony diminishes,** usually without our initial recognition of the fact.

3. **All memories have an emotional holographic component that  determines how negatively or positively such memories will impact our total being and health but they especially affect our self-worth and self-image.**

4. **We learn, function and progress most efficiently and effectively by experiencing opposites, and with a regular flow of sensory input, rather than by reprocessing old data.**

5. **We function at our optimum and are the most easily enlightened when in the present mode.** We cannot successfully live in the past or the future and be well-adjusted individuals. **Being preoccupied by past or future obsessions, fears, phobias, thoughts, emotions, and daydreams is generally counterproductive.** As a rule, pleasant, calming feelings signal that we are in the present moment and unpleasant, irritating emotions signal that we are out of the present moment.

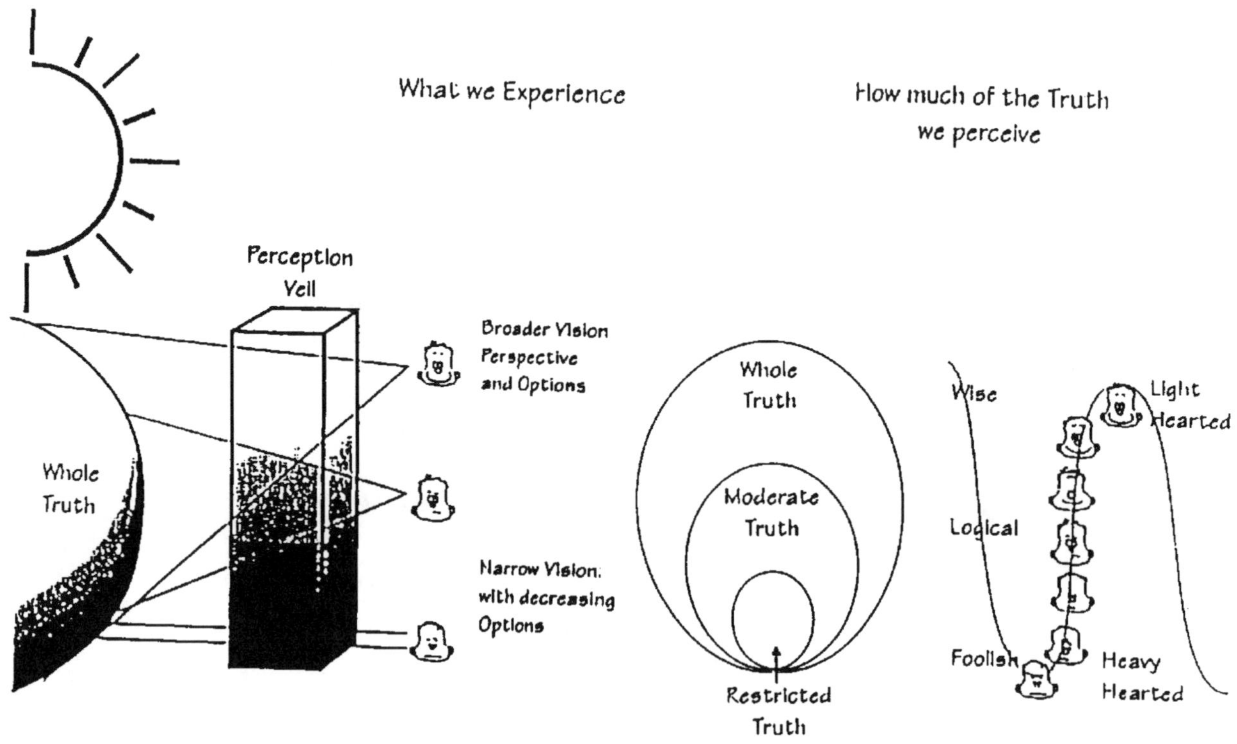


*Figure 21.2 — How Much Of The Truth We Perceive*

# Chapter 22
# NATIVE AMERICAN AND OCEANIC MEDICINE

*"In the native American tradition, diseases and their
cures are inseparable from the larger scheme
of things. Medicine is a ritual matter. . ."*
— Gordon Brotherson
Images of The New World

## LAW OF ONE

To the Native Americans and Pacific Islanders, **there is no separation of the spiritual, physical and nature. One is the logical extension of the others. Nothing material takes place that does not affect our natural and spiritual worlds, and there is nothing spiritual that does not have physical and natural implications. Life and health are the result of living in harmony  with this natural physical-spiritual balance and dis-ease is the result of violation of these natural physical-spiritual laws of balance.** This is an ancient, and yet advanced, philosophy dating back to approximately 2250 B.C.

## LAW OF SONG AND SPEECH

This intertwining of concepts is nowhere seen more clearly than in the Navajo Indian language's term for Medicine Man; "Hataalii" means "The Singer", referring to the chants that are employed in the healing ceremonies. The Navajos believe that without these spiritual chants (prayers), the full healing power of the phytotherapeutic and other agents cannot be achieved. Dis-ease is understood to be a manifestation of an imbalance within the quantum or spiritual (Yin) component as well as the physical (the Yang), to borrow terminology from oriental medicine.

Native peoples comprehend song and speech to be an energy generation force producing a vibration that once set in motion continues to vibrate indefinitely. Thus, a word or chant uttered a thousand years ago is still reverberating through the universe. The prayer of a millennium ago is just as valid today as the day it was pronounced. This concept is supported  by strong scientific documentation. Light from a distant star may have traveled for hundreds of millions of light years to reach our Earth but it still exists even though its generating star may have ceased to exist millions of years ago.

The quantum paradigm of modern quantum physics is not new to these  indigenous peoples. The quantum link between observer and observed and the basic holism of all phenomena are long-cherished knowledge. Modern quantum physics also teaches the indigenous ancient principle that the holographic concept of the whole being is contained within each of its parts.

In modern physics, the essential building materials of the universe cannot be reduced to atoms, but exist as relationships and fluctuations at the boundaries of matter, energy (Avagadro's Point) and anti-matter. Native scientific knowledge has taught for thousands of years that all that exists is an expression of and an inter-relationship between anti-matter (spirits), energy and Matter.

Leading edge thinkers in modern quantum, theoretical and astrophysics now teach that the universe is not a collection of objects in steady state but rather a system in constant flux. The concept of constant flux within creation is so basic to Native American and Oceanic philosophy, arts, science and culture that it is no longer even questioned.

## LAW OF TIME

Realizing that ancient chants and words, as well as light from distant stars, all still exist, then in a very concrete sense **all time is present time.** Since all time can be present time, one does not have to rush and it becomes more important to perform ceremonies, healings, chants, prayers, and rituals properly, to live our lives and even to die properly. Thus, indigenous peoples are far more concerned with the right time for healing rather than healing on a specific day and a specific hour (the appointment). If the time (circumstances) is not correct, native healers simply will not see the patient.

## LAW OF CATEGORIES

The reductionist thought process tends to categorize. For example, birds fly. But indigenous peoples reason such **categorizing leads to   scientific inconsistencies and mistakes.** For example, insects also fly but they are not birds. Nor are airplanes birds but they also fly. Mammals such as bats fly but they are not birds.

**The mind of a true healer must not be locked into a particular mind fix but must be fluid in order not to overlook therapeutic possibility.** Therefore, the study and use of phyto and other native therapies are not normally categorized by the dis-eases they treat. Rather, the individual with the dis-ease is the primary consideration. Thus, we find an almost homeopathic concept of the patient's individual need rather than the dis-ease's need. In indigenous healing, two individuals with similar dis-eases may be cared for according to very different protocols.

## LAW OF LOGIC

Solid state logic teaches that an object cannot simultaneously be a member of two categories at once but native logic has not accepted this limitation. An electron can be both a wave and a particle depending on the circumstances. **The world at the sub-atomic level definitely does not act according to solid state laws. Therefore, in indigenous healing it is scientifically illogical to believe that a therapy must act exactly the same under every set of circumstance and in every patient. If a patient has a particular physical dis-ease, a specific remedy may be indicated but if the patient has the same physical dis-ease and a mental dis-ease concurrently, a different remedy may be necessary because the original remedy may not possess the same healing power on** both the physical, quantum energy and anti-matter level.

# LAW OF TRUE SCIENCE

**Solid state definitions of science are inadequate in the quantum healing arts.** Speaking of the uncompromising solid state "scientific" attitude, Eysenck said, "The fact that my mother did not love me is not important, because such a thing cannot be measured. It is very difficult to see how a mother affects her child. If it cannot be tested, it does not exist."

To the truly educated, such a statement is sheer scientific nonsense. Of course, love for an infant affects the child. Repeated studies have documented that infants deprived of all affection die. Therefore, it is scientifically unacceptable to believe the solid state myth that if it cannot be measured, it is not science. Science is an attempt to understand reality, discover our relationship to the cosmos, and provide a rationale for our actions and the structure of our society that satisfies ALL levels of our beings.

Unfortunately, current reductionist, solid state science is not making any significant attempt to come to reality with these issues. But, fortunately, expansionist, quantum scientists are finding the traditional native scientific concepts necessary in order to understand the realities of our dual existence. Quantum and theoretical physicists now consider the elemental particles merely as dense representations of something deeper. In fact, Peat, one of the greatest theoretical physicists of our day, said, ". . . 'the building blocks of matter' is a confusing misrepresentation of the nature of quantum reality. Rather, they are the surface manifestations of underlying quantum processes. In other words, reality lies not in the elementary particles, nor in the surface forms we see around us, but with relationships that exist within the flux of energy and processes of quantum nature." This is exactly how indigenous healers see the scientific position of their healing mission.

One cannot completely and accurately measure the effects of poetry, drama, music, religion, near-death experiences, combat, grief, hate, envy, anger, elation, loneliness, mental abuse, and even inanimate objects such as "pet rocks" upon an individual but it is unscientific to believe that such effects do not exist in the presence of such overwhelming evidence.

# LAW OF PREDICTION

Prediction of outcomes in science and healing is, in many cases, confirmation of a closed loop thought process. **True science and healing must be capable of producing aberrant results in order to progress.**

# LAW OF ECOLOGY

Modern ecology stresses the basic interconnection of all living things but to the native of America and Oceania this is indeed an ancient principle. And it is not limited to just the external environment but applies also to the internal environment of the individuals. Intensive "spiritual" cleansings were and are still undertaken by native peoples. In fact, the peoples of these races appeared to have experienced far less dis-ease prior to the arrival of the Europeans.

One of the greatest dissertations ever delivered on ecology was spoken by Chief Seattle in 1854:

". . . Every part of this earth is sacred to my people. Every shining pine needle, every sandy shore, every mist in the dark woods, every clearing, and humming insect. . . . We are a part of the earth and it is part of us. The perfumed flowers are our sisters; the deer, the horse, the great eagle, these are our brothers. The rocky crests, . . . the meadows, the body heat of the pony, and man - all belong to the same family. . . . This shining water that moves in the streams and the rivers is not just water but the blood of our ancestors. . . . The water's murmur is the voice of my father's father. . . . It carries our canoes, and feeds our children. . . . And what is there to life if a man cannot hear the lonely cry of the whippoorwill or the arguments of the frogs around a pond at night? . . . .The Indian prefers the soft sound of the wind darting over the face of the pond, and the smell of the wind itself, cleansed by rain. . . . The air is precious to the red man, for all things share the same breath; the beast, the tree, the man, they all share the same breath. . . . air shares its spirit with all the life it supports. The wind that gave our grandfather his first breath also received his last sigh. . . . What is man without the beasts? If all beasts are gone, man would die from a great loneliness of spirit. For whatever happens to the beasts, soon happens to man. All things are connected. . . . Whatever befalls the earth, befalls the sons of the earth. Man did not weave the web of life, he is merely a strand in it. Whatever he does to the web, he does to himself. . . . Teach your children what we have taught our children, that the earth is our mother. . . ."

# LAW OF DELIBERATION

There is an old saying "A politician thinks of the next election while a statesman thinks of the next generation." While this is wisdom it is inadequate to the Native American and Oceanic mind. Their higher level of understanding is exemplified in *The Great Law of the Iroquois Confederacy* which states **"In our every deliberation, we must consider the impact of our decisions on the next seven generations."**

In the past seven generations may have been adequate but as we shall learn when we begin studying Chapters 32 through 39 **we are now forced, as a matter of survival, to think in terms of the next one hundred thousand or even the next million generations. To do less is to be totally irresponsible and therefore unscientific.**

# PHYTOTHERAPY

Certainly no group of people has ever mastered the medicinal use of more phytotherapeutic agents than the indigenous peoples of the Americas and Oceania from the arctic to the tropics, from desert to rain forest, from alpine to submarine. Some authorities suggest that as much as 70 to 75 percent of our current allopathic materia medica, and 85 to 95 percent of the homeopathic materia medica, is derived from the knowledge of these indigenous peoples. The same authorities suggest as much as 50 percent of the allopathic materia medica currently comes from tropical South and Central American jungle plants.

1) One great weakness, however, is that the vast majority of this pharmacological knowledge has never, other than orally, been recorded for posterity.

2) A second weakness is that there is no single repository for this vast knowledge so that one species of plant can be compared with another.

3) Third, since this voluminous knowledge has traditionally been passed on orally, much will be irretrievably lost with the deaths of those individuals who have mastered this knowledge.

4) And lastly, even that which has been preserved is catalogued primarily as pharmacological data which completely ignores the spiritual and, in many cases infinitely more significant, the inter-relationships needed for its use by these indigenous peoples.

The great challenge now before us is that many phytotherapy agents are being lost as their natural habitats, the virgin deserts, rain forest, wetlands, prairies, barrier reefs, shorelines, old growth timber, and fisheries are being eliminated.

## SARCODES

Sarcodes consist of various parts of animals, insects, reptiles, fish, crustaceans, and birds prepared for therapeutic purposes. All naturally occurring glandular therapies, hormone therapies, vitamins from fish liver, and so on, fall under this heading. It is doubtful that any cultural or ethnic group ever amassed such an extensive knowledge of these healing agents including so many life forms from so many climatic, geographic and specialized ecosystems as did the Native American and Oceanic peoples. Unfortunately, as with the phytotherapeutic agents, volumes  of healing knowledge are being lost as indigenous peoples lose their native life styles.

## SURGERY

While it may be difficult to envision major surgery being performed in a tepee, hogan, igloo, long house or grass hut, but archaeological findings among the more advanced cultures of Central and South America provide evidence that ancient Andeans were skilled in surgery. Skulls show where operations have been successfully performed in the Americas thousands of years ago. The difficult surgical procedure known as trephining, (i.e., cutting away a part of the skull of the living person) was brought to a high state of perfection by the ancient people of the Andes. Again, such skills have not survived the cultural destruction that faced these Indian societies and this surgical knowledge has been lost.

## THE LAW OF FLUX

The shifting of perspective is difficult for reductionist thinkers to comprehend but is second nature to expansionist thinkers. Where solid state scientists have been trained to seek fixed laws and ultimate explanations, **the science of indigenous peoples has for thousands of years dealt primarily with the laws of a fluxing, changing, transforming, and transmutating universe.**

For example, natives are known to change their names because they desire to absorb particular animal characteristics such as "Strong Bear" into their constitution; or to enhance personal attributes such as the personal courage of "Stands Alone". Moreover, the indigenous peoples freely did and do change their names and, in their minds, their thought processes and relationships. Therefore, their identity changes as they move through different phases of life.

Indigenous culture and mythology also preserves this quantum fluidity. The oral literature and theology includes stories of humans changing into animals, birds, fish, trees, rocks and, conversely, of objects taking on human form. This fluidity of the thought process is vital in understanding quantum, theoretical and astrophysics. Some of our greatest quantum, theoretical and astrophysicists should be coming out of native cultures because members of these groups have been trained for generations to think in the fluid concepts necessary to excel in these sciences.

## EXAMPLES

At the beginning of the 20th Century, scientists were perplexed by irregularities in the newly emerging study of atomic structures. Einstein and Planck realized that the old solid state laws could not account for the apparent irregularities of action of sub-atomic components. Under some conditions, they acted as particles (matter) and under others, they acted as energy and under yet other circumstances, they acted as anti-matter. Physicists found that they had to re-formulate the solid state laws and develop new laws to explain what they were observing.

By the third decade of the 20th Century, Heisenberg had developed a new "Quantum Theory." But even he was reluctant to completely trust in this new flux, change and transformation concept in thinking. At this point, Bohr commented, "You are still clinging to classic (solid state) ideas. . . . It's obvious in the very language you speak. When you say that the electron has a position and a speed which is disturbed by the act of measurement, you mean that in some way the electron possesses a position and speed, that it has a reality of its own that is independent of the observer."

The idea that electrons and other quantum components "possess" intrinsic properties, Bohr argued, is in reality a holdover from the old solid state way of thinking. He then explained that, in the quantum mode, such characteristics are ambiguous. **At the level of sub-atomic components, "position", "speed", "direction" and "mass" are relative and, therefore, unreliable methods of measuring and calculating sub-atomic characteristics.**

# LAW OF THE NATURE OF KNOWLEDGE

To native peoples, knowledge does not represent a destination or an entity that can be accumulated like money in a bank account. To the indigenous peoples, **knowledge is a dynamic, constantly changing action verb not a static, unchanging noun.** Anciently, such concepts were also part of the early European cultures. In medieval English, the word "knowledge" was used much like our modern word "knowledgeable", meaning that the one who possessed such wisdom had a "working understanding" of the subject. In turn, the origins of knowledge lie in the even more ancient Germanic verb "to know" which conveyed the idea of having the correct perception of a concept or accurate recognition and the ability to distinguish and correctly apply such wisdom."

Modern European languages have developed as noun-oriented languages. They divide the world into physical objects (nouns) and thinking into separate concepts (nouns). Most indigenous languages and thought processes do not work in this manner. They are verb-based. For example, the word "medicine" in western terminology denotes a pill, a mechanical procedure to adjust bones, a specific herb or herbal formula, a specific surgical procedure. But in the indigenous concept, it denotes energy, power, spirit, relationships, balance, a way of life and yet, at the same time, very specific phytotherapeutic agents (nouns) may be used.

Thus, indigenous medicine is not the "either/or" philosophy but rather the "totality" of the universe that controls the individual. In his book *Synchronicity: The Bridge Between Matter And Mind*, F. D. Peat says that in western science a molecule is a geometrical arrangement of atoms. But in indigenous science, it is an alliance of spirits (intelligences) which maintains the integrity of molecules; once taken into the body, this alliance dissolves and takes up new configurations as its elements are utilized by the living being.

The native idea of using herbs to heal dis-ease at first may appear similar to western pharmacology suggesting that the "power" of plants and animal substances lies in their biological molecules. But this certainly cannot be the entire concept of medicine as understood by native peoples. For example, the time of year or time of day that a phytotherapeutic agent is collected can have dramatic effect on its usefulness. The manner of preservation likewise has its effect. The vitality of the living being and its ability to absorb, rearrange its constituents and utilize them affects the therapeutic outcome. How the agent is combined with other phytotherapeutic agents may change its properties. To illustrate, Peat states, "I buy brand-name non-drowsy hay fever tablets at my local drugstore. . . . Next to them is a 'no-name' generic package whose active ingredient is chemically identical. According to our current view of science, a molecule that has been synthesized in one laboratory is identical in its effects to the 'same' molecule made in another laboratory, even when the two manufacturers have synthesized their products through totally different chemical reactions." And most westerners find both will work equally well to relieve their hay fever.

To a native, on the other hand, the medicine may contain the same biologically active molecule but yet not be identical. In addition to the specifically active biological molecule, the remedy may contain a wide variety of other active biological molecules that interact with the specifically identified "active molecule" thus enhancing, decreasing, modifying, or antidoting its action in a non-linear mode

Additionally, indigenous peoples assert that chemicals, plants and animals have a "spirit" that can be affected by their environment. For example, a pharmaceutical worker who hates the unjust work demands of his cartel will impart a different "spirit" to the manufactures than an individual who feels fulfilled in his chosen occupation. Such a "spirit" will dramatically affect the results of the drug being manufactured.

Another example is the use of a forest plant that has grown in a logged area. It will not have the same "spirit" growing in full sunlight as the same species of plant growing in the deep shadows of the primeval forest. Plants grown in depleted soil do not have the same "spirit" as those grown in nutrient-rich soil.

Even the healer affects the phytotherapeutic remedy. Some healers *give* energy to the herbs they prescribe while other healers *take* energy from the medicine. The latter may not necessarily be undesirable. A weak patient may not be able to handle a "strong" medicine which could overtax a weak system.

The true nature of indigenous healing lies in substance (molecules), ceremony (the way it is gathered, prepared, stored, and utilized) and energy (the non-material influences of the substance, the healer, interested parties, etc.). Such energy, innate, kundalini, ch'i, vital or life force concepts have special scientific significance in the homeopathic context of Avagadro's Point, the dividing line between matter and energy

## LAW OF CHAOS

Chaos is the science of non-linear systems. In the western, solid state, reductionist, Newtonian mind fix, order is considered the norm and chaos the breakdown of the norm. Thus, chaos is equated with lawlessness. This is not so among the native peoples of America and Oceania nor, interestingly, among "modern" quantum, theoretical, astro and chaos physicists. For them, **order always emerges from chaos and chaos always emerges from order.** It is the ancient oriental Taiji principle appearing yet again that **there must be opposition in all things.** See Figure 22.1. The chemist, Ilya Prigogine, in his study of dispersing systems ranging from cells, to periodic chemical reactions, to growth of cities and traffic patterns, found in each and every case order emerging from chaos and flux and that excess order, control and rigidity produces revolution, chaos and change.

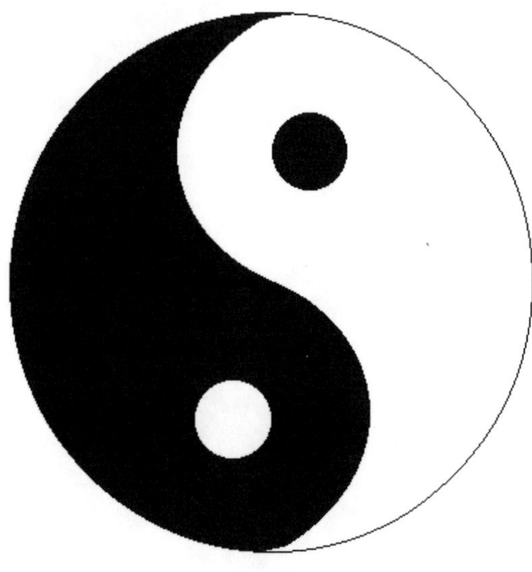

*Figure 22.1*

## THE GREAT GIFT

Only a few laws relating to indigenous healing have been discussed in this text. While they definitely do exist and are compatible with the other branches of complementary healing, these laws have never been clearly codified and written down. This makes the task of comparing them extremely challenging. Far more importantly, the natives of America and Oceania, to an extent greater than any other peoples, have bequeathed to us **a dynamic way of thinking that is vital to our comprehension and application of quantum healing, a thought process that allows for change without having to abandon previously acquired laws and knowledge.**

## HOW IT CAME TO BE

How have the American and Oceanic indigenous peoples come to this dynamic quantum understanding of and respect for the universe? They came to respect the worlds they lived in by making disastrous mistakes.

On certain islands in the Pacific, species of birds were hunted to extinction. On Easter Island, the forests were completely felled so that there were no materials left with which to build boats to leave the island. Overpopulation produced starvation and collapse of the indigenous culture. In South and Central America, many huge cities and empires lie in ruins, reclaimed by the jungle. Things went terribly wrong; groups were no longer able to sustain their civilizations because they built their cities on the prime farmland. The marginal land that was left could not sustain the population. In short, these native peoples learned the hard way from their mistakes. They failed to live in harmony with the laws of the universe and the laws destroyed them.

Is modern man capable of learning from history or must we be taught the same lessons? If we follow the same suicidal pattern depicted by the histories of the native peoples, then we have not acquired dynamic knowledge but only static learning.

# Chapter 23
# NATUROPATHIC MEDICINE

*"Until man duplicates a blade of grass, Nature
can laugh at his so-called scientific knowledge.
Remedies from chemicals will never stand in favorable comparison with the products of Nature — the
living cell of the plant, the final result of the rays of
the sun, the mother of all life. When correctly used,
herbs promote the elimination of waste matter and
poisons from the system by simple, natural means.
They support Nature in its fight against dis-ease;
while chemicals, not being assembled, add to the
accumulation of morbid matter and only simulate
improvement by suppressing the symptoms."*
— Thomas A. Edison

## THE HISTORY

Naturopathy is the oldest of all healing arts and the root of all other forms of medicine. Prehistoric sites have yielded numerous medicinal herbs; cave paintings in France demonstrate early spinal manipulation; over 5,000- year-old Chinese writings describing the energy flow through the living body became the basis of acupuncture; by 2,000 B.C., Ayurveda (natural medicine of India) was firmly established; a 50-volume materia medica, completed during the Ming Dynasty (1644-1368 B.C.), contains over 12,000 medicinal formulas; in 300 B.C., the great natural medical school was founded in Alexandria, Egypt. In 377 B.C., the Queen of Ireland, Macha Mong Ruadh established the first Druid hospital called Broin Bherg (House Of Sorrow) at Emain Macha in which there was extensive use of naturopathic methods. During the dark ages, natural (Sufi) medicine was alive and well in the Islamic world. In the 1790s, Hahnemann established homeopathy using many of the laws found in Ayurvedic medicine; in 1895, Palmer re-established chiropractic.

But naturopathic medicine is much more than a system of healing; it is the philosophy that teaches we have the power or energy within to heal ourselves if we live in harmony with basic laws. Hippocrates stated two of these laws of naturopathic medicine: **"Let your food be your medicine."** and **"Do nothing to harm the patient."** Twenty-three centuries later, naturopaths still practice and live by these same laws.

Allopathy (M.D.s) broke away from naturopathic medicine when its practitioners began using strong and often harmful synthetic drugs as well as more and more invasive surgery instead of concentrating on good nutrition, healthful living habits and prevention of dis-ease. While allopathy stresses drugs and surgery, naturopathic medical doctors specialize in treatments that strengthen the body and aid it in healing itself without adverse side effects.

Naturopathic medicine's emphasis on proven natural remedies is sometimes misunderstood by the uninformed. They mistakenly assume that today's naturopathic doctor is not taking full advantage of the latest scientific developments because he continues to utilize old, but well-proven, therapies. Naturopathic physicians, as part of our Hippocratic Oath, reaffirm, "I consider for the benefit of my patients, and abstain from whatever is deleterious . . ." At the same time, every safe means is used to fully understand the patient's current health status and the possibilities of success of prescribed care.

Willian Tiller, Ph.D., Chairman of the Material Sciences and Engineering Department at Stanford University, writes, "It is clear that we are going out of the age of chemical and mechanical medicine and into the age of energetic and homeopathic medicine." Truly, naturopathic medicine is the medicine of the past, present and the future.

Today, naturopathy's greatest shortcoming is that the vast majority of its practitioners have allowed themselves to be seduced by the reductionistic, non-vitalistic, solid state mentality of **treating symptoms with natural substances. This prostitution of the naturopathic principles has left very few true naturopathic physicians who care for the cause of dis-ease.**

# LAW OF DIS-EASE

**Dis-ease is an attempt by the being to rid itself of the morbid products of incorrect living. Acute dis-ease is a cleansing process while chronic dis-ease is caused by suppression of the cleansing, thereby resulting in destruction of tissues and functions by the accumulated waste products.** In short, dis-ease is the result of man's own follies which nature is doing its best to rectify for him.

# LAW OF CURE

**The ability to heal is found within the patient's being and not in the doctor, procedure, adjustment, modality, remedy, herb, medicine, or surgery.**

# LAW OF PRACTICE

The twin purposes of naturopathic practice are to bring about self-healing of the being and to teach the patient how to maintain the state of health.

# LAW OF MICROBES

Microorganisms may be the *apparent* cause of dis-ease and people may "catch" dis-eases from each other but *only because they have within their system the nursery for the genesis of these dis-eases in the form of accumulated toxins and/or malfunctioning systems. No one who is truly hygienic in body and mind and possesses a well-functioning system can be adversely affected by microbes.*

## LAW OF CAUSE OF DIS-EASE

1. **Incorrect diet**

2. **Improper personal, mental, external and internal hygiene**

3. **Lack of health education**

4. **Improper living habits** (i.e., exhaustion, worry, fear, overwork, lack of exercise, excesses, environmental causes, drug usage, etc.)

5. **Hereditary weaknesses** (Miasmas, diathesis, dosha, phase). No dis-ease can be cured if the cause is ignored.

## LAW OF INFLUENCES

1. **The physical body must be looked upon as something that is part of a much greater whole and is linked to other bodies that act upon it and react to it.**

2. **The physical body is subject to the influences of energies that are brought to bear on it and flow around it and into it from other bodies and from outside influences.**

## LAW OF UNIVERSAL INTELLIGENCE

Sub-atomic factors are magneto-electrically charged. Magneto-electricity is a form of energy. It is intelligent energy; otherwise it could not act with precision in the atoms of the universe. This intelligent energy can have but one source, the Universal Intelligence. If this supreme intelligence should withdraw its creative and governing influence, the electrical charges (forms of energy - quantum energy), the atoms, and the entire material universe would disappear in the flash of a moment. From this, it appears that crude matter, instead of being the source of all life (as reductionist, non-vitalistic concepts proclaim) and its mental (non-corporal) phenomenon, is but an extension of the Life (Vital Force, Spirit), itself a manifestation of a great creative intelligence (-S/T, negative entropy) which some call God, others Nature, the Oversoul, Brahma, Prana, or The Great Spirit.

## LAW OF HARMONY AND RESONANCE

As early as 1863, John Newlands discovered that when he arranged the elements of matter in the order of their atomic weight, they displayed the same relationship to one another as do the tones in the musical scale. Thus modern chemistry appears to demonstrate the variety of the "music of the spheres" and how the entire sidereal universe is built on the laws of harmony and resonance.

## LAW OF CAUSE AND EFFECT

Allopathic medicine attributes dis-ease largely to accidental causes: to chance infection, or to drafts, chills, wet feet, and other external influences. The religiously inclined frequently attribute dis-ease to the retribution of God or the Gods or errors of the mortal mind or the product of a dis-eased imagination. Naturopathy, on the other hand, presents a more rational cause, namely: **that dis-ease is brought on by violation of laws; and that it is corrected by compliance with those laws.** There is no reprisal, no ill luck or misfortune, only suffering brought on by transgression of law. This transgression may be due to ignorance, willfulness or viciousness. The effect is always the same. This places the responsibility of dis-ease, except for truly unavoidable accidents, squarely upon ourselves. Dis-ease is nothing but cause and effect.

## LAW OF INTERVENTION

Intervention is **a copious influx of quantum life, vital, innate, ch'i force and an adequate nerve supply from the organic (solid state) headquarters in the brain and spinal cord.** The freer the inflow of num, kundalini, life, vital, innate, ch'i force into the organism, the greater the vitality and the more strength available for positively resisting the dis-ease and the greater the recuperative power. Also, anything that interferes with the nerve connection of the cell to the sympathetic, parasympathetic and central nervous systems lowers the vitality of the cells, tissues and organs and of the organism as a whole, and interferes with transmission of afferent and efferent nerve impulses.

## LAW OF NUTRITION

Proper nutrition results in the normal composition of blood, lymph and other bodily fluids. Dis-ease can be the result of excess or deficiencies. This includes not only normal vitamin and mineral levels but also normal hormone levels, and normal cell counts.

## LAW OF ELIMINATION

**The accumulation of waste and morbid materials poisons tissues and interferes with normal nutrition and function, venous and lymphatic circulation.** This can take place due to under-activity, over-work, irregular schedules, weakening habits, excesses and over-indulgence, drugs and other poisonous substances, ill-advised surgery, mechanical factors and wrong thinking and feeling.

## LAW OF MIASMAS (DIATHESIS, DOSHA, PHASE)

In creating abnormal hereditary tendencies, the parents, or earlier ancestor, must have unknowingly ignored or wantonly violated natural laws, with such violation resulting in lowered vitality and the transmission of specific weakness from generation to generation.

## LAW OF EPIDEMICS

It is common for the majority of individuals in a certain locality or area to be addicted to the same bad habits of living, the same ethnic and cultural norms, and of treating and mistreating their ailments similarly, producing in themselves the same kind of morbid soil (dosha, miasmatic, diathesis weakness) which allows them to become the favored host for similar forms of microbes producing similar symptoms (dis-ease).

## LAW OF MICROZYMES

**Microorganisms develop from microzymes, the primal unit of living organisms, but this occurs only under morbid, mutant, pathogenic (dis-ease) conditions.** (This concept has been repeatedly substantiated by the research of Bechamp and V. Livingston.) These microbes feed on and decompose the morbid wastes that allow them genesis. When the morbid food supply has been exhausted the microbes then devour their own protoplasm and in conjunction with the body's QPNIMT responses are destroyed. As long as the morbid food supply exists, the microbes are practically indestructible but in sterile (non-morbid or sanitary) conditions, they are incapable of pathogenesis.

At first glance, it may seem that this concept does not differ materially from the germ theory of allopathy. On closer examination, however, it is found that there is a vast difference. According to allopathy, microbes are special entities which of their own accord create dis-ease. If that were true, then "killing germs" would make sense. On the other hand, if microzymal mutation is correct, we must prevent the development of morbid host conditions and the microbe will cease to be generated. Killing the scavenger microbes will not remove the morbid host soil but only provide temporary relief while a new generation of facilitated (further mutated) microbes grows on the antibiotically altered morbid soil. This is the reason so many patients take one antibiotic after another without permanently curing the "infection".

## LAW OF BIOLOGICAL TOXINS

Today's natural healer is confronted by a challenge that previous generations have never had to consider let alone actually have to contend with in practice. Genetic engineering has produced tens of thousands of mutant or designer organisms annually. These organisms are in the forms of microbes, plants, animals, fowl, insects, and even human alterations. They have been purposefully engineered to overcome specific weaknesses or to create specific weaknesses. Unlike any other challenge in human history, they also have the ability to reproduce themselves. **Chemical pollution will eventually bio-degrade but biological pollution can continue to increase in numbers as it reproduces itself and can take over and destroy other life forms.**

This situation obviously has the potential for dramatically altering, and in many cases irreparably damaging, the balance of nature. Entire species can potentially be wiped out by more virulent species. Our food supply can be dramatically and possibly permanently altered.

## LAW OF ALTERED FOOD SUPPLY

An excellent example of altered food supply is hybrid garden plants. Almost all of these hybrid strains have been developed since World War II. With plants such as corn, new strains are developed almost yearly. That

means that we can have 50 or more generations of change by the end of the 20th Century and yet many of the individuals consuming these altered foodstuffs are exactly the same individuals who were living in 1945 and who have not experienced even one generation of change. In other words, the food supply can be mutating at a rate 50 times faster than any change in those consuming it. This being so, horticulturists are concerned that we may digest and assimilate our foodstuffs less and less efficiently with each subsequent biologically-induced mutation. **This literally produces the potential for starving to death in the midst of plenty because we are unable to process and utilize the nutrients in mutated plant and animal foods.**

# LAW OF FEVER

Hippocrates stated, **"Give me fever and every dis-ease can be cured."** The most advanced works in pathology admit the constructive and beneficial character of inflammation. Each degree of fever increases metabolism by approximately 7 to 10 percent. Such increased metabolism allows the body to eliminate toxins at a 7 to 10 percent greater rate. Thus, a fever of 103.6 increases metabolism by 50 percent. Naturopathy regards inflammation and acute dis-ease (i.e., vomiting, diarrhea, rashes, perspiration, etc.) as a forceful house cleaning which is necessary as long as human beings continue to disregard and violate the natural laws of health.

# LAW OF DUAL EFFECT

Every agent, drugs, surgery, phytotherapeutics, vitamins, minerals, adjustments, physical therapy, or acupuncture affecting the human organism produces two effects: a first, temporary response, and a second, lasting effect. **The second, lasting effect is always contrary to the first transient effect** which is usually due to the effort of the organism to overcome and eliminate the effects of therapy. The second long-term response is due to the retention of the adverse effect by the organism and produces a destructive action. In theory and practice, most authorities on the subject consider the first short-term effect and ignore the secondary lasting effects. Almost all forms of so-called "health care" administer therapies whose primary effect is opposite to the dis-ease condition. Therefore, in accordance with the law of action and reaction, the long-term effects of such therapy must be similar to the dis-ease condition. Common, everyday experience should teach us that this is true; for example, laxatives and cathartics produce chronic constipation if used excessively. The secondary effect of prolonged use of stimulants and tonics is increased fatigue, weakness and lethargy.

Every therapy when used indiscriminately produces new dis-ease. Therefore, the only scientifically rational approach is to administer therapies whose first temporary effect is similar to the dis-ease condition. In accordance, then, with the law of dual effect, the secondary long-term effect must be contradictory to the dis-ease condition. Only this method is capable of effecting a true cure.

# HOW SAFE IS PHYTOTHERAPY?

W. Walup of Health Canada, Bureau of Drug Surveillance reported in the *Therapeutic Products Directorate* that there have been **only 90 reported adverse side effects and one death attributed to the use of herbal products since 1990. Furthermore, there had been no reported adverse reactions or fatalities from the use of nutritional supplements during the eight years studied. For comparison, during the same time frame there were approximately 28 million adverse reactions and 850,000 deaths from prescription drugs.**

# LAW OF SUPPRESSION OF ACUTE DIS-EASE

Acute dis-ease, when cared for in harmony with nature's intent, always proves beneficial. If, however, through neglect or wrong care, the inflammatory processes are not allowed to run their course, if they are checked or suppressed, or if the dis-ease conditions in the system are so far in the ascendancy that the healing forces cannot react properly, then the constructive forces may be overwhelmed and the dis-ease may take a fatal course or develop into chronic ailments. **Only in the latter critical situations should suppression be considered and then the practitioner should constantly keep in mind that as a result of suppression, toxins must be dealt with for they form the basis of chronic dis-eases. This is accomplished by facilitation and recruitment of new tissue by way of the nervous system.**

The reason for this is that organs of depuration are so constructed that they eliminate only waste materials of comparatively simple chemical construction. Pathogens, however, make highly complex substances that cannot be eliminated through the organs of depuration unless they are first broken down into simpler compounds which are chemically adapted to the organs of detoxification and elimination. **This decomposition can only be accomplished in the presence of inflammation. This is why aggravations (healing crisis/retracing) are necessary in the initial stages of healing.**

# LAW OF IMMUNIZATION

Between July 1990 and November 1993, the National Vaccination Information Center (NVIC), located in Vienna, VA, reported 54,072 severe reactions to immunization, resulting in 471 deaths. These iatrogenic reactions normally occurred within seven days and consisted of paralysis, convulsions, nausea, extremely high fevers, hysteria, chronic nervous system disorders, acute encephalitis, diarrhea, learning disabilities, hyperactivity, permanent brain damage and death.

**Vaccinations are administered to the general population without any consideration of individuality and susceptibility.** When a vaccine is administered, it changes the magneto-electric (-S/T) vibrational rate in the same way as severe illness does. A *mild reaction* to vaccination indicates that the patient is indeed susceptible to the disease and, consequently, the defense mechanism is creating a *local* inflammation, itching or pain, or perhaps even a little pus. This reaction indicates that the defense mechanism is *not strong enough* to fully nullify the adverse results of the vaccination.

If the vaccine produces *systemic* reactions, such as fever, malaise, headaches, anorexia, muscle aches, or flu-like symptoms, then the *defense mechanism is quite strong* and is counteracting the morbid influence of the vaccination.

*A very strong reaction* indicates that the susceptibility of the organism is extremely high but that the *defense mechanism is too weak to counteract the morbific influence of the inoculation.* This is the most dangerous situation because it can be fatal. If the patient survives, the inoculation produces *chronic* dis-ease which can be traced in its development to the date of immunization. It may take years to regenerate the patient's health.

# LAW OF THE CARNIVORE

Every serving of animal, fowl and fish is saturated with the excrement of its cells in the form of uric and many other kinds of acids, alkaloids of putrefaction, xanthins, ptomaines, and other toxic substances. **The organism of the meat eater must dispose not only of its own impurities produced in the process of diges-**

tion and of cell metabolism but also of the morbid substances contained in the animal flesh consumed as a food source.

# LAW OF FASTING

In many cases of lowered vitality and weakened powers of resistance, the problem is due to the accumulation of morbid matter. If the encumbrances consist of superfluous accumulations of waste materials, fasting can be successful in eliminating the impurities. **If, however, the dis-ease has its origins in other causes or if it is due to a weakened constitution or miasmatic (diathesis, dosha, phase), fasting may aggravate the condition.**

During a prolonged fast, the functions of digestion and assimilation come to an almost complete stop. Suppression of these physical functions allows heightening of the spiritual (non-corporal) components. This explains the importance given to fasting among many religious sects. This is also why **during a well-conducted fast, one should experience Hering's Law or aggravations of the symptoms taking place from the quantum (spiritual) to the physical, from the most to the least vital organs, from above down and from inside out and old symptoms may temporarily return in the reverse order of their original development.**

# LAW OF VIBRATORY PLANES

**The higher the degree of complexity, refinement and vibratory activity of a compound or substance, the greater its potential energy.** On the lowest plane is the electromagnetic spectrum binding together the elements into the simple inorganic compounds of the mineral plane. In the intermediate vegetable kingdom, the phytochemical life element with the aid of the sun's energy builds up the elements of air, water and minerals into more refined and complex living molecules. Still higher is the spiritual (non-corporal) life element governing the animal kingdom which further refines the living matter of the vegetable plane, organizing and vivifying it to potencies of vital force and creative energy. Next comes the increasingly intellectual plane which is not restricted by the instinctive capacity of animals. The highest plane of energy is the spiritual (anti-matter); it is capable of learning, development and expansion beyond instinctive limitations until it has assimilated all there is to be learned and experienced in the sidereal universe.

Up to now on this earth we have become acquainted with only four kingdoms of nature and their corresponding life components; it is anticipated, **based upon intellectual speculation, that there may be as many as seven planes of life and action,** each leading to yet higher planes of magneto-electric generation or negative entropy.

# LAW OF ACID-BASE

Physiologically, science now admits that almost all cell waste is chemically acid and that it must be neutralized by alkaline elements as quickly as it is formed in order to prevent the accumulation of damaging morbid waste products (i.e. free radicals, etc.). Thus, the salts eliminated through the kidneys and skin are neutralized acid residue.

Interestingly, **we are learning more and more about the role that acids and alkaline substances play in the vital generation of electricity and magnetism in and around the living organism.** Preventive and recuperative therapy must therefore revolve around detoxification of the patient through proper eating, fasting, bathing, dressing, breathing, exercising, working, resting, thinking, and spirituality.

## LAW OF CONSERVATION

Acute dis-ease represents a *temporary* increase of activity of the num, kundalini, vital, innate, life, ch'i force in order to overcome the obstructions in the system caused by pathological conditions. Chronic dis-ease is a *permanent* obstruction to the activity of num, kundalini, vital, innate, life, ch'i force.

**Excess in any form is detrimental to the functions of the living being. Excesses rob the organism of vitality instead of supplying it.** Excessive fuel smothers a fire but excessive restriction of fuel also causes the fire to fail. **Habitual desire grows with indulgence and, through such indulgence, the being who should be the master becomes the slave.**

## LAW OF ADJUSTING/MANIPULATION

How would you resolve a puddle of water produced by a leak in the roof? Most would say, "fix the leak". But if that is all you do, any water damage that has occurred will remain. Would not the rational individual also wipe up the standing pool of water? Would he not also check the roof for other likely trouble spots that might leak in the next storm? Might it be necessary to re-roof the entire building? When the chiropractor or osteopath merely plugs the leak (the pain) by adjusting/manipulating the spine, he allows the previous damage to continue and the danger of future damage to continue unabated.

Naturopathy, in addition to adjusting the pain (plugging the leak), wipes up the puddle (removes the morbid waste) and re-roofs the house (uses principles of correct living - proper nutrition, exercise, breathing) to strengthen and repair the structure. **In order to do justice to patients and their health, healers must use all that is good in healing to return the patients to health, as quickly, as cost-efficiently, as permanently as possible. To do less is to neglect their responsibility as healers.** Progressive chiropractors and osteopaths are using naturopathy without realizing it!

## LAW OF MAGNETISM

All healers are aware of the polar valences at work in chemistry.

What they do not address is what takes place at death. We still have the identical elements with identical valences composing the tissues but lacking the vital, innate, life force, or ch'i. Thus, quantum magneto-electric activity exhibits an additional principle of vital life force which is lacking in solid state electro-magnetic chemistry. It is this additional principle of life force that is the key to successful magnetotherapy. **It is never found in bio-static bar or other solid state magnets making them poor candidates for magnetotherapy. Nor is it present in electro-magnets. Only biodynamic living organisms produce it and the higher the order of the healer, the more refined and precise it seems to become. It would also appear that the higher and more refined the patient, the more successfully magneto-electric therapy will be.**

# LAW OF CHROMOTHERAPY

The higher the degree of velocity and refinement of the num, kundalini, vital, innate, life, ch'i force, the higher it manifests in the vibratory range (Hz) of the color scale in Figure 23.1.

Blue - 250 - 275 Hz

Green - 250 - 475 Hz

Violet - 300 - 400 Hz

Yellow - 500 - 700 Hz

Violet - 600 - 800 Hz

Orange - 950 - 1,050 Hz

Red - 1,000 - 1,200 Hz

Blue - 1,200 + Hz

Violet - 1,000 - 2,000 Hz

White - 1,100 - 2,000 + Hz

*Figure 23.1 — Hertz Ranges For Color Therapy*

From work in Kirlian photography, it appears that the color of the aura or energy field of the living being can also vary with emotions being experienced; i.e., anger shows as red, envy or jealousy as green, etc.

# LAW OF CHRONIC DIS-EASE

**Chronic dis-ease is of a functional nature and develops when an otherwise healthy organism becomes saturated and clogged with poisons to such an extent that these encumbrances interfere with the cells, organs, and tissues, especially of the circulatory and nervous system.** Such cases resemble a watch that is losing time because its workings are filled with dirt. Frequently, this situation can be resolved by conditions of right living; i.e., proper mental attitude, exercise, proper diet, ventilation and respiration, and sanitation. **By far the greater part of chronic dis-ease is the result of improper hygiene.**

# LAW OF ORGANIC DIS-EASE

**In dis-eases of an organic nature, good results are not easily achieved.** A being affected by organic dis-ease resembles a watch whose mechanism has been injured and partly destroyed by corrosion. In organic dis-ease, the time has passed that right living can fully resolve the problem. **The body is no longer capable of completely repairing itself by normal physiological means. Frequently, however, it is due to a lack of knowledge on the practitioner's part regarding how to activate the self-healing mechanism within the patient's being.** Such cures require miracles in which lower order laws are suspended by higher order laws. Surgeons may remove the damaged parts but they are not and never will be capable of replacing them with new parts of like quality.

## LAW OF PLANES

Humans live and function on distinct planes of being; the physical, the mental, the emotional, and the spiritual. The true healer must look for the cause of dis-ease on all of these planes in order to heal the total patient.

The purely reductionist mechanic in healing is like the musician who says, "My instrument is all that counts." He consistently keeps the instrument in excellent condition but neglects to practice on it, to master technique, harmony, rhythm, counterpoint, theory, harmonics, melody, and interpretation.

The purely faith healer is like a musician who spends all of his time dealing with the spiritual theory and academic aspects of music but at the same time allows his instrument to fall into severe disrepair.

**The true healer is the great master who is balanced and well-rounded** both in the care of his physical instrument and in the spiritual theory and academia of music. **If natural healing teaches nothing else, it emphasizes the strengthening of will power and self-control. This is the very purpose of life. Upon it rests all further achievement. Self-control is the "master key" to all higher development on the mental, emotional and spiritual planes of being; but before we can exercise it on the higher planes, we must have learned to apply it on the lowest physical plane of our existence by managing to control our physical appetites, desires, passions and habits. To learn how to accomplish this is one of the purposes of religion.**

## LAW OF LIFE PATTERN

In reductionistic medicine it is generally assumed that degenerative dis- ease will limit us more and more as we age. In today's hostile environment the quality of life slowly begins to ebb as we enter our 30s and 40s. But this need not be so. Dr. R. Walford of UCLA recently states that our bodies should last a minimum of 120 years according to genetics and development patterns in vibrant good health. Interestingly, 120 years is the life span allotted to Moses in the Bible and the wording is very revealing, we read, ". . .his eye was not dim, nor his natural force abated." In other words he remained ruggedly handsome and well developed, mentally and physically active and spiritually alert to the end. There was no degenerative dis-ease at work in his being. He lived a rich, full life which ended, as R. L. Wysong, B.S., D.V.M. so poetically describes, "like a leaf falling from a tree" in the last few days of autumn. Such a life is the result of living in complete harmony, on all level of our being, with universal law. See Figure 23.2.

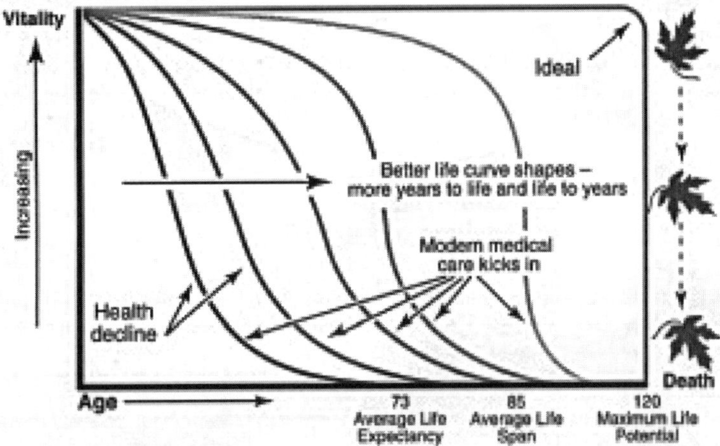


If we chart health and vitality against age, the curves to the left on the chart represent typical loss of health and languishing for decades under medical care. The goal should be to maintain optimal health and vitality right out to our genetic limit (squaring the curve) with life ending like a leaf falls from a tree.

*Figure 23.2 — Degenerative Life Pattern vs. Healthy Life Pattern*

# SURGERY

Surgery is beneficial to the infirmed when a tissue or an organ has been so badly damaged that it no longer has the ability to repair itself. At this point it has moved beyond the "Limitations of Matter" and becomes a liability to the living body. Its retention causes a perpetual drain on the num, kundalini, innate, ch'i, life, vital force resulting in a slowly weakening patient.

# Chapter 24
# NUTRITION

*"We live not upon what we eat but upon what
we can digest and assimilate into the
living tissues of our bodies."*

— A. Atwater

## LAW OF CELLULAR FUNCTION

Ultimately all nutrition takes place across the cell membrane (nutrition in, waste out). Each hour of the day one billion of the body's 300 trillion cells are replaced. This process of constant repair and generation requires all the elements, not just those currently acknowledged by so-called "nutritional science". "Advanced formula" and other sales promotions sound impressive and sell products to the under-educated but how can humans with an incomplete knowledge of human nutritional needs (we are still discovering essential elements) compete with nature's complete knowledge?

To illustrate this lack of knowledge, one technical article tells us condition X-Y-Z responds to vitamins A-B-C. But another article, from an equally "prestigious journal", reveals that too much vitamin A-B-C is responsible for condition X-Y-Z. Still another article tells us we are deficient in vitamin N-O-P, but only brand H of these vitamins can be effectively absorbed and assimilated into the human body. Where does the truth lie?

## LAW OF SUB-GENETICS

As early as 1944, Dernan determined that the cell should not be considered the functional unit of living matter but a complex organization of even more minute living units. He and others suggested that an organizing "skeleton" for specific protein molecules has the unique function of creating and maintaining the specific character and physical form of living organisms. This provides an explanation for all of the characteristics (genetics) passed on from previous to new generations of living organisms.

The 74th United States Senate document #264 reads as follows, **"Certainly our physical well-being is more directly dependent upon the minerals we take into our systems than upon calories or vitamins or upon the precise proportions of starch, protein or carbohydrates we consume. . . . A marked deficiency in any one of the more important minerals actually results in disease. . . . It is not commonly realized, however, that vitamins control the body's appropriation of minerals, and in the absence of minerals they have no function to perform."**

But DNA/RNA sub-factors such as chromosomes which are responsible for determination of characteristics of the species and of individuals had to be further subdivided. Further sub-factors such as genes needed to be identified to determine the specific characteristics of individuals within the same chromosome pool. **This still did not provide for all of the necessary sub-factors. Genes must contain sub-factors that determine individual cell morphology.**

For example, why does one of two siblings have diabetes while the other does not? R. Lee, D.D.S., called the determinants that are responsible for this phenomenon "cytomorphogens". But even this does not provide a complete answer. Carrying this one step further, we arrive at a sub-sub-factor which determines the make-up of biological proteins. These, Lee determined, were the **trace and micro-mineral components of the living body. These form complex but highly stable protein molecules linked together by the chemical affinity of the micro-minerals in question, which by reason of their physical and chemical structure determine the exact pattern in which the component parts of a specific protein are combined.** Thus, these "protomorphogens", as Lee called them, exert a profound influence upon the mitotic activity and vitality of every living cell. **The mineral constituents are the organizational components or "links" for the protein molecule and control all growth and repair in the living being.**

This leads to a startling conclusion. **In the absence of minerals, vitamins have no physiological activity. Minerals, in the absences of vitamins, continue to exert a lesser degree of physiological activity. Thus, the trace and micro-minerals are one of the secrets of life.**

## ANTIGEN PROPERTIES

Since the specific serologic reactions of proteins are due to their molecular geometry, it follows that the antigenic properties of a protein are derived from that protein's protomorphology. The absence of even one of the mineral elements going into the complex structure of the mineral-protein seriously impairs or prevents its determinant action in organizing specific proteins.

## TOXIC EFFECTS

**Excessive amounts of incomplete nutrient complexes do not go into the building of necessary mineral-proteins, and may cause a toxic pharmacological result characteristic of overdosing as found in research and clinical literature. This is true because the body metabolizes isolated, high potency nutrients like a drug, with resultant side-effects, nutritional interferences and all. No longer are we within the safe world of nutrition; we have instead entered the realm of sledgehammer pharmacology.** In other words, a megadose vitamin produces a pharmacological not a nutritional effect. **While nutritional pharmacology may be beneficial for one function, it very frequently causes simultaneous iatrogenic dis-ease at another level.**

## LAW OF REGULATION OF CELLULAR VITALITY

**The dynamic state is a state of matter requiring a constant input of energy for its maintenance.** This is the characteristic difference between living and dead protein molecules. **Such an understanding required no further necessity for simpler units of physical organization beyond the mineral-protein.** This also makes the living mineral-protein the basic framework for all viruses.

Thus the mineral-protein possesses chemical, physical and quantum (energy) components as follows:

1. They are one of the keys linking the solid and quantum state

in all living organisms because they form a chain-like (DNA/RNA helix) molecule.

2. Their structural characteristics and morphogenetic influences depend upon the moiety of the nucleoprotein (amino acid) molecule.

3. The mineral content of the protein moiety is the stabilizing influence on its structure.

4. The molecular size, different degrees of composition of their molecules, and thermo-stability of mineral-proteins have different biological effects depending upon the phase of their biological cycle; they are thermo stable up to 700 degrees C if the mineral framework and its protein synthesizing influence is considered but are destroyed at 100 degrees C if growth influences are considered.

5. **Oxidation destroys some of the growth-influencing potency of mineral-proteins, thus anti-oxidants must be considered.**

## LAW OF ALLELOCATALYST

The vitality of the cell is controlled by dynamic vital balance (force) and if external stimuli are added during favorable periods, large populations may be obtained. This is the homeopathic principle by which many investigators have found the growth-inhibiting substance to be a growth-stimulating substance when diluted.

All animal cells secrete such allelocatalysts into their surrounding medium and are in a constant reciprocal relationship with the intercellular concentration of this substance. This relationship is the basic influence over the division (growth and repair) rate of the cell; it is primarily responsible for the degeneration process of senescence (old age). **Therefore, mineral-proteins are as much a growth factor as they are a determinant of morphology.**

## LAW OF BIOLOGICAL DETERMINATION

The attempt to synthesize biological products in the laboratory has often resulted in a product with an activity very similar (but not identical) to the one being attempted to duplicate but differing very slightly in its chemistry. The slight difference may be (and frequently is) that of structure rather than content. For example, Vitamin B12 has a cyanocobalamin, a hydroxycobalamin and a nitrocobalamin form, i.e., AC or adenylcobamide, BC or bensimidazolcobamide and DBC or 5,6-dimethalbenzimidazolylcobalamide configurations with the possibility of the less functional forms comprising 48 to 72 percent of the total cobalamide forms in the human liver.

It is this positioning of elements on the molecular structure that alters function. In fact, it is the entire chemical basis for the synthetic drug industry. Change the position of even one molecule and the nature and physiological function of the drug can be changed allowing a new patent to be issued and a financial monopoly on the "new" drug to be granted to its developer.

Thus, **a naturally occurring and a synthetically produced vitamin may have close but not identical physiological functions in the living being.**

# LAW OF BIOLOGICAL TRANSMUTATION

In 1822, Prout documented that the amount of calcium in a newly hatched chick was four times that of the egg from which it came. Because the egg is a closed system, this four-fold increase or "creation" of calcium could not be explained until 1935 when Kervran successfully produced dozens of different biological transmutations of one element in abundance to one in deficiency.

Kervran states of his work, "The reluctance of some physicists to admit that not all their laws are applicable to biology, comes mainly from those university professors . . . who have lost sight of original principles on which the laws were founded. They declare that negative entropy, the force which in biology would build up matter, is an impossibility. For them there is only . . . positive entropy, in accordance with the second law of thermodynamics . . . would imply an endogenous production of energy. . . . These physicists do not deny the presence of an energy which maintains life, but for them this energy comes from what the organism takes in from its surrounding outside medium. They do not realize the great flaw in their argument! If energy comes from outside, it is a mistake to represent it as justification for applying (the second law) to biology. This principle has never been applicable in such cases. It was formulated only for closed systems having no exchange with the outside; therefore, the concepts of entropy and negentropy have no significance when there is an exchange with outside medium."

The core of Kervran's work is that the mechanism of transmutation occurs when **equal numbers of protons or neutrons are present simultaneously to yield a biological transmutation.** For example, sodium (Na) (11 protons) combines with oxygen (O) (8) to form potassium (K) with (19) protons. He also recognized that this method can produce "incompatibilities", and he emphasized, one must not "manufacture nonexistent elements from written equations. The reverse also occurs as with bacterial action on limestone where calcium (Ca) (20) minus hydrogen (H) (1) forms K (19). A third option for production of K is aluminum (Al) (13) plus carbon (C) (6) which forms K (19).

This provides vast potentials in body chemistry. A Na (11) plus H (1) yields manganese (Mg) (12). Then Mg (12) plus O (8) produces Ca (20). Naturopaths know that Equisetum Arvense (Horsetail) is high in silicon (Si) (14) and has traditionally  been used for re-calcification of bones and to hasten calcification of the lesions in tuberculosis patients. In fact X-ray examinations demonstrate the re-mineralization with Equisetum Arvense actually takes place faster than with calcium supplementation. Si (14) plus C (6) yields Ca (20). Of course, if circumstances permit, C (6) plus O (8) yields Si (14). Other of Kervran's experiments include putting fresh water fish in salt water (NaCl) and after 72 hours documenting an increase in NaCl and the presence of a substantial amount of KCl. Na (11) plus O (8) produces K (19). Kervran studied the formation of crustacean shells (conch) and documented that the shell is formed by Mg (12) plus O (8) yielding Ca (20). Germinating seeds took manganese (Mn) (25) plus H (1) and produced Iron (Fe) (26).

# LAW OF VALENCE SHIFT

Poly-valent elements such as Fe with +2 (ferric) and +3 (ferrous) forms exhibit one form that is more easily assimilated by organisms. Plants possess the ability to trans-valence such elements to their easiest metabolized forms. Therefore, **plant sources of these minerals are generally superior forms of supplementation.**

# LAW OF BIO-AVAILABILITY

**All nutritional products are not created equal.** If we knock rust off of rusty nails and encapsulate it as a nutritional supplement, it will not perform with the same ease as iron that has first been absorbed by a living plant and then administered to a patient. The biological change that takes place makes the latter far easier for the living being to incorporate into its cellular structure.

Unfortunately, the first could label its product as having a very impressive amount of iron being present but it may be of little or no value if the living system cannot easily assimilate it. In fact, a person could expend even more energy trying to assimilate the inferior product than the product will produce. This would leave the patient's system with a deficit state and, thus, that inferior product would actually be a liability. A product with a much lower label amount may, in fact, be a much superior product based upon how readily the patient's system can utilize it. This concept is termed "Bioavailability".

## LAW OF POTENCY

Lee documented in the 1940s that, "High potency is a much abused term. **Test animals on a 'High Potency Enriched Diet' do not live as long as those on the same low potency vitamin diet without enrichment."** Again, we see in operation the universal law of too much or too little being the cause of dis-ease. Therefore, the proper potency, not mega-potency, is the critical factor in supplementation.

## LAW OF SYNERGISM

Lee was able, as early as the 1940s and 50s, to document that **the various components of naturally occurring vitamin complexes, in conjunction with their naturally occurring trace mineral factors, have an effect upon each other which dramatically increases their physiological activity. This is quantum physics at work again; the effect of the whole being greater than the sum of the parts.**

The problem is that no matter how many components of whole food modern nutritional science isolates, we do not have the capacity to recombine them in a synergistic manner that is equal in effectiveness to that of nature. Nearly all vitamin supplements are synthetically manufactured. Raw products for hundreds of brands are supplied by five major chemical companies, including Kodak and S. Denko. This is done because vitamins extracted from plants or animals cost more to manufacture. For example, Roger Williams spent $20,000 in 1948 to extract 10 mg. of vitamin B5 (Pantothenic Acid) from beef liver. Once the chemical structure was identified, Kodak initially produced the same amount of B5 for $20.

The lesson to be learned from all of this is that **potency, or nutritional effectiveness, is not necessarily measurable by milligrams or international units, but rather by amount and synergistic qualities.**

## LAW OF pH

**A shift in the body's pH can dramatically enhance or diminish its ability to carry on physiological reactions.** Proper pH (5.0 to 6.5 of urine according to Wilson) is just as important as the presence or absence of particular nutrients. Acid dominance produces sympathetic (stimulating or yin) responses while alkaline dominance produces a parasympathetic (sedating or yang) response. **It is extremely difficult to have a high vital force without being slightly acid, while a low vital force generally is indicative of an alkaline system.**

Instead of being a set chemistry as in a test tube, living chemistry is dynamic based upon many factors. The body is more acid in the afternoon, in summer, when fasting, following physical activity, with menses and in health. It is more alkaline in the early morning, in winter, after eating, from inactivity and in sickness, especially in chronic dis-ease. Disappointment, shock, emotional upsets, fear, worry and stress produce an alkaline shift.

## CLASSIFICATION OF FOODS

Alkalizing foods are high in one or more of the following elements: calcium, magnesium, potassium and sodium. In short, any element that forms hydroxyls. Fruits are among the most alkalizing foods in this category.

Acidifying foods are high in the elements: chlorine, iodine, iron, nitrogen, phosphorus and sulphur or any other element that forms carboxyls. Proteins from meat, nuts, grains and legumes form this category.

In his research at Spears Chiropractic Hospital in Denver, Colorado, G. Wilson, D.C., documented that foods such as green leafy and root vegetables can be consumed with either of the above groups without significantly altering the body's pH. Tubers should be eaten with green vegetables by alkaline individuals.

## LAW OF COMPLETE COMPLEXES

The rationale is often used that there is no difference between the chemical structures of synthetic and naturally occurring substances. This does not correlate with the scientific facts. For example, the argument that synthetic and naturally occurring vitamin C are identical is based only on the observation of the ascorbic acid component of the entire vitamin C complex. In figure 24.1 we can clearly see that naturally occurring vitamin C has far more to its architecture than just ascorbic acid. The same is true of the vitamin E complex illustrated in Figure 24.2. Unfortunately, reductionist science tends to disregard what it doesn't adequately understand.

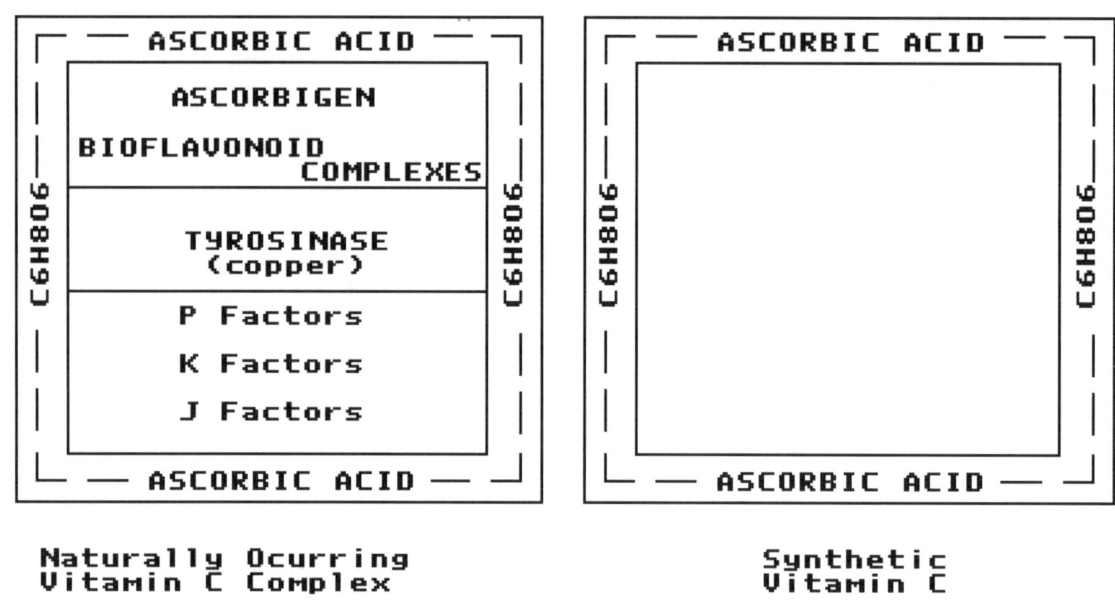



*Figure 24.1 — The Functional Architecture Of The Vitamin C Complex*

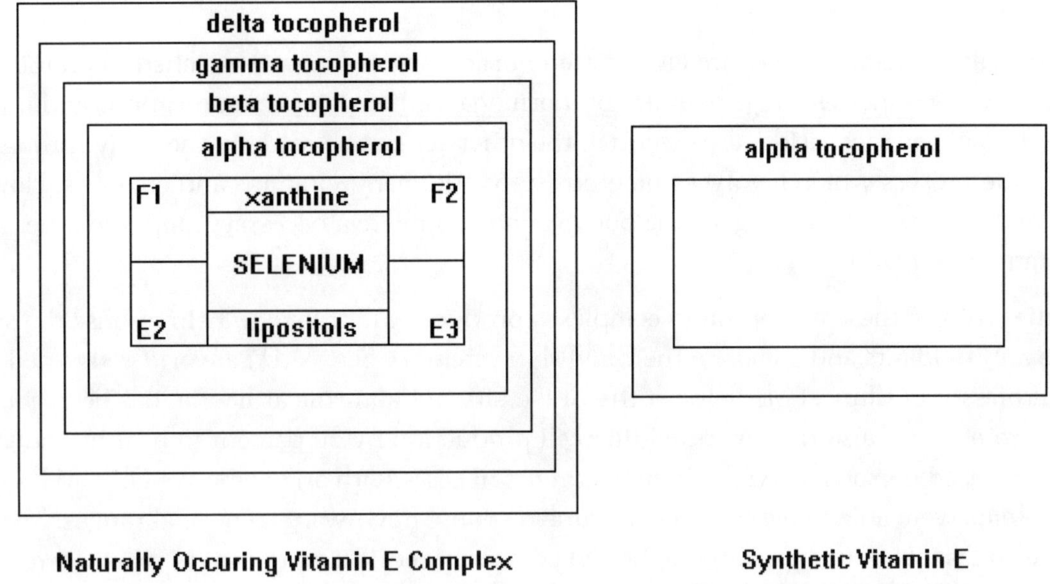


*Figure 24.2 — The Functional Architecture Of The Vitamin E Complex*

## LAW OF RACEMIC MOLECULES

Many hydroxy acids and nearly all of the amino acids obtained from protein and various other compounds are capable of forming asymmetrical molecules that rotate the plane of polarized light. These substances contain exactly the same elements attached to the central carbon atoms but have a different arrangement of these elements, thus forming mirror-image molecules designated (D) dextra and (L) levo in chemistry. See figure 24.8.

## PHYTOCHEMICALS

Presently there are over 106,000 chemically active compounds that have been identified, only a few hundred of which have been studied in detail, in every category of plant foodstuffs. These substances dramatically aid and regulate the use of vitamins, minerals, fatty acids and proteins in the living tissues. They have been documented acting as stimulating, altering, blocking and suppressing agents. Literally thousands of recent studies have demonstrated that individuals who consume adequate amounts of foods containing plant foods have markedly reduced incidents of colon (40 to 60 percent less) and breast (25 percent less) cancers.

Additionally, phyto chemicals, many of which are brightly colored and help give plants their vivid hues, are key components of the antioxidant defense system. They also guard against a vast array of adversities including viral attacks, harsh weather and insults in the handling of the foodstuffs.

# GLUCOPROTEINS

Glucoproteins as the name implies are eight different saccharides (sugars) attached to protein molecules which are necessary substances for non-neural, non-hormonal cell-to-cell communications and intracellular functions. Only two of the saccharides are essential, the other six can be made in the body through a very complex and fragile process which involves numerous steps and many vitamins and enzymes. However, if any of these vitamins and enzymes are lacking, or the body cannot complete a necessary step, the other six glucoproteins cannot be made.

Among other things, these glucoprotein complexes produce glutathione to help cleanse the system of toxins, work as anti-oxidants and stimulate the QPNIMT system. D. See, M.D., a world-renowned immunologist and Associate Professor of Clinical Medicine at the University of California at Irvine, has been able to document that such glucoproteins can also raise natural killer cell production by 50 percent in healthy individuals and by 400 percent in dis-eased persons. Even more interestingly, in cases with an overactive QPNIMT system such as in Lupus, glucoproteins were able to regulate the immune response downward to normal ranges. Speaking of his research, Dr. See states, "No vitamin, mineral, herbal or pharmaceutical drug can do what the gluconutrient complex can do . . LACK OF UNDERSTANDING

Unfortunately, the reductionist mentality has corrupted the thinking of many causing them to miss the greater concept. They prescribe isolated phytochemicals (also termed "nutriceuticals", nutrients + pharmaceuticals or "nutribiotics", nutrients + life) not understanding that **plants commonly contain dozens of interacting substances. When segregated from their companion phytochemicals they can and frequently do act in erratic and/or altered manners producing adverse side-effects.**

# ANTI-OXIDANTS

When the fats and oils in as living organism go rancid they produce free radicals which are extremely damaging to the tissues. Anti-oxidants prevent the fats and oils from going rancid and producing free radicals. The naturally occurring vitamin C complex (see Figure 24.1), which contains copper, the naturally occurring vitamin E complex, which contains selenium (see Figure 24.2), beta carotene and zinc and manganese are among natures best anti-oxidants.

Some firms which sell anti-oxidants claim they have products which are "50 times more efficient anti-oxidants than vitamin E". This is a true statement when they are comparing their product to alpha tocopherol but a false statement if we compare their product to the complete vitamin E complex. (See the Law of Synergism in this chapter.)

Even in their isolated synthetic forms anti-oxidant factors are so effective that a study published in the June, 1997 *American Journal of Cardiology* indicates that the doctors surveyed took anti-oxidant supplements 44 percent of the time as compared to 42 percent taking aspirin for cardiovascular protection. Sadly, only 37 percent of these same practitioners recommended anti-oxidants for their patients cardiovascular protection preferring instead to prescribe the more dangerous aspirin.

# ADULTERATION OF FOODS

H. W. Wiley, M.D., the first head of the Food and Drug Administration, in his book *Foods and Their Adulteration* describes in great detail the origins, manufacturing and composition of food products; a description of common adulterations; and a listing of food standards, national food laws and regulations. He also discusses simple tests for adulterations, food values, effects of storage and standards of purity.

R. Lee, D.D.S., commenting on Dr. Wiley's book said that any poison put into food, no matter how small the amount, is excessive. It's like putting Emory powder into the gear box of a car. The gears will have their teeth ground away by abrasive action but there won't be any warning until the damage is past the point of no return.

D. T. Quigley, continues to develop the unsavory picture in *Notes on Vitamins and Diet,* stating, "The most common non-vitamin foods are sugar, white flour, white rice, and macaroni products. These have become common foods; in fact for the average civilized American individual they constitute from sixty to ninety percent of the total food intake. These have become common foods because of a commercial reason. They can be stored and shipped because of the fact that they are devitalized and demineralized. They do not furnish a proper food even for insects or germs and so may be handled commercially with considerable ease and profit. The economic situation here involved has forced foods into general use in the civilized world which, if continued, will mean the destruction of those who consume them. A very great number of interlocking organizations connected with the manufacture and distribution of pernicious and unfit food materials has come into existence. They will do everything in their power to continue to sell their goods."

# CHROMATOGRAMS

A chromatogram is an analytical technique that identifies components of a solution by means of colors and patterns absorbed by filter paper.

Synthetically produced or nutrient-depleted foodstuffs and soils do not produce chromatographic finger-prints that are characteristic of foods and soils with complete complements of nutrients. Therefore, it is scientifically impossible for them to be representing identical substances. See figures 24.3 - 24.7. The chromatograms presented here represent only a fraction of the voluminous research extending over more than 40 years conducted by E. E. Pfeiffer.

But the problem is even more far reaching. R. Murry, D.C., writes, "**A fraction of a vitamin whether natural or synthetic at best is a drug and can only have a drug effect in the body - not a physiological or curative benefit.** The literature is abundant with studies demonstrating that large or megadoses of ascorbic acid can and do create serious problems in the human biochemistry. Some problems reported include: Collagen disease; rebound scurvy, a vitamin C deficiency disease; imbalance of other vitamins like vitamin A and B; formation of some types of kidney stones; and diabetes mellitus. In matters of diabetes, keep in mind that synthetic ascorbic acid is hexose-derived and that hexose is a six-carbon sugar, a monosaccharide." (Emphasis added.)

Even Nobel prize-winning L. Pauling, Ph.D., recognized this problem. He said, "Pure crystalline ascorbic acid is made from glucose (corn sugar). What is called rose hips vitamin C is the same pure crystalline ascorbic acid with a pinch of rose hips powder added."

In today's high pressure Madison Avenue advertising environment, we are victims of degenerative dis-ease resulting from scientific malnutrition and poisoning. Even those who superficially appear well nourished are starving for complete vitamin and mineral complexes. These poor souls cry for life-giving bread and instead advertising gives them a dis-ease producing, nutritionally deficient stone.

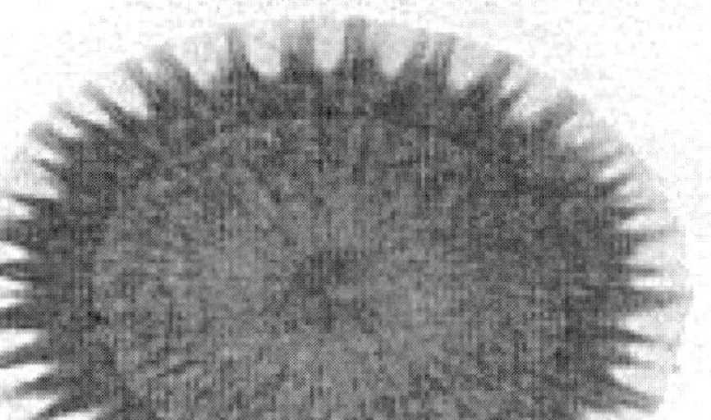
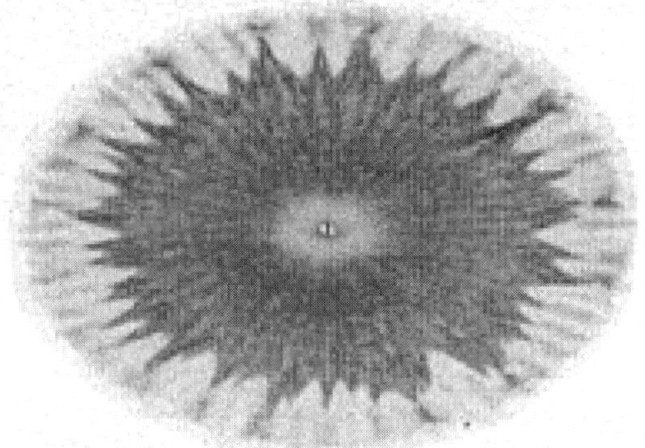
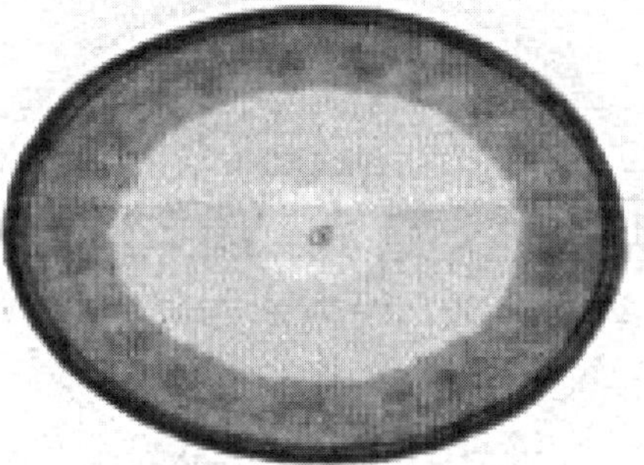
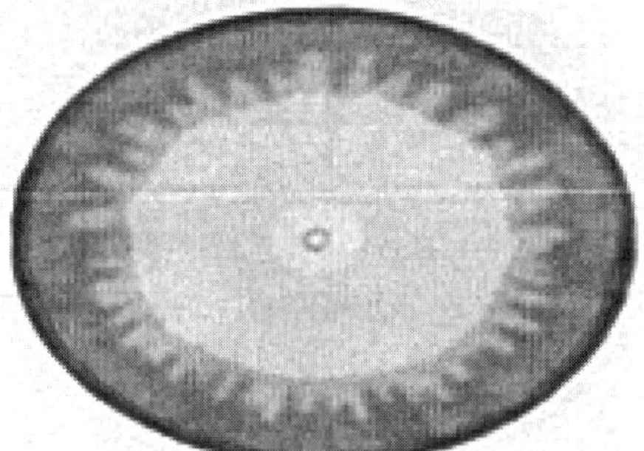
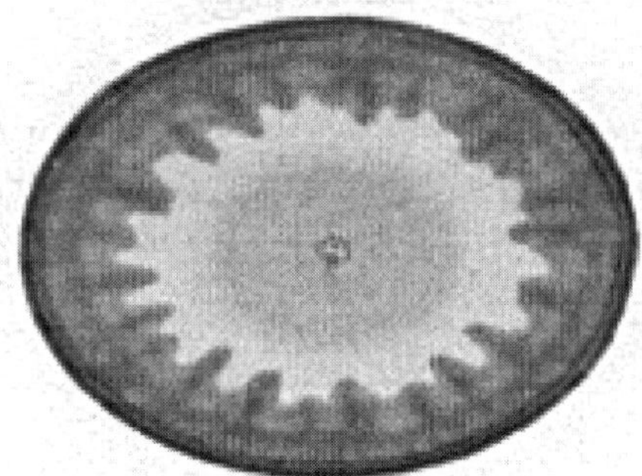
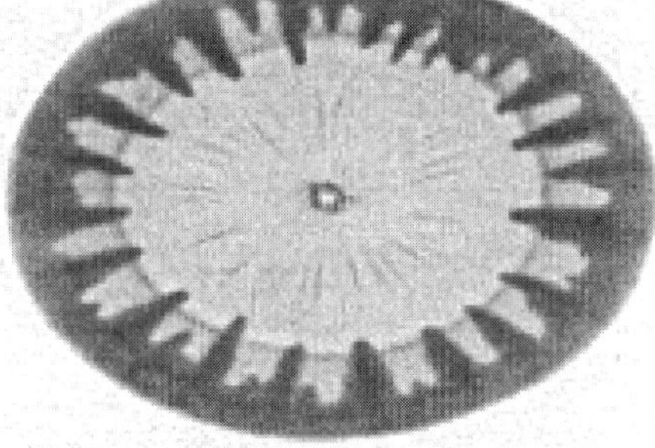



*Figure 24.3 — Comparative Chromatograms*

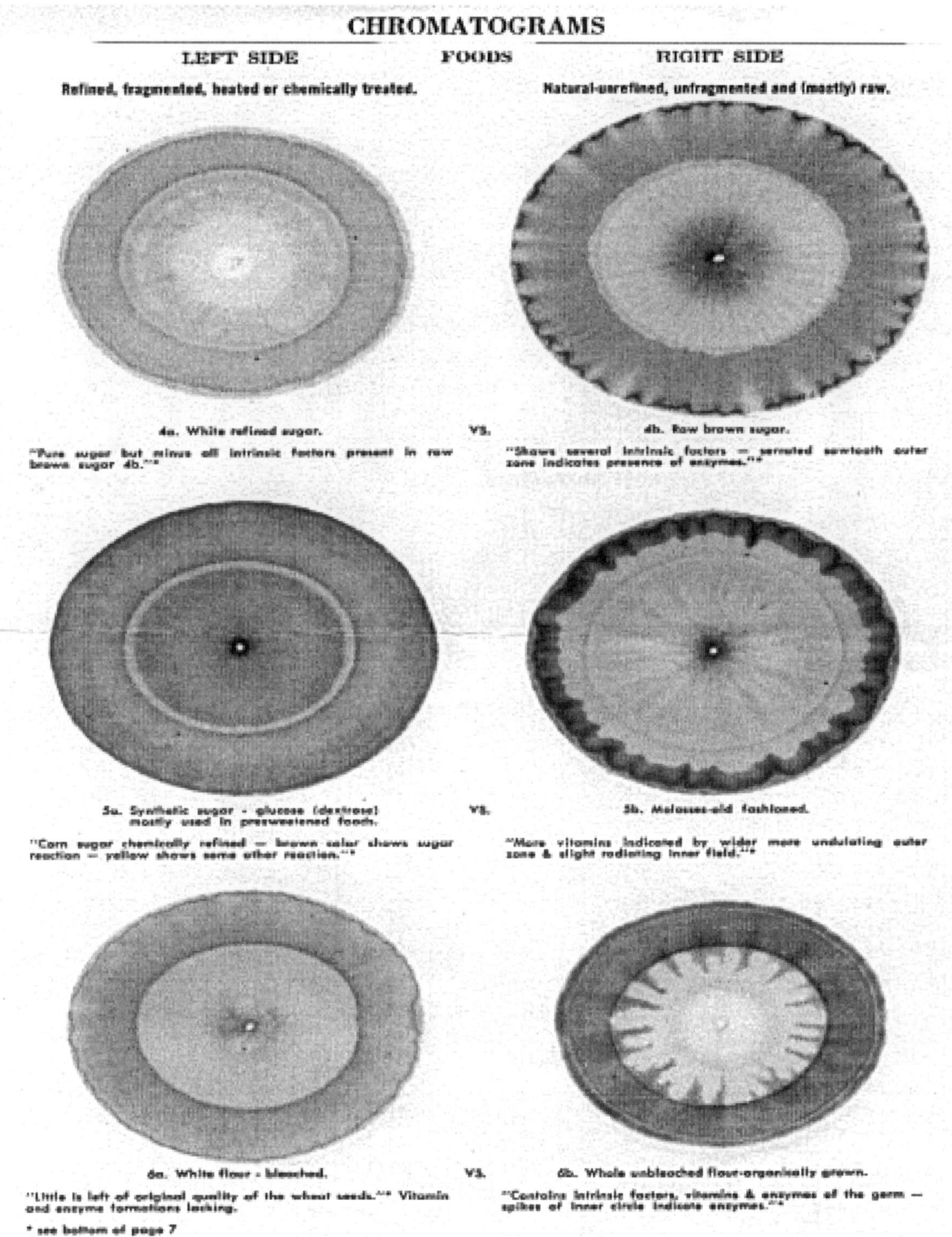


*Figure 24.4 — Comparative Chromatograms*

## CHROMATOGRAMS

**LEFT SIDE** — FOODS-cont'd — **RIGHT SIDE**

Refined, fragmented, heated or chemically treated.  Natural-unrefined, unfragmented and (mostly) raw.

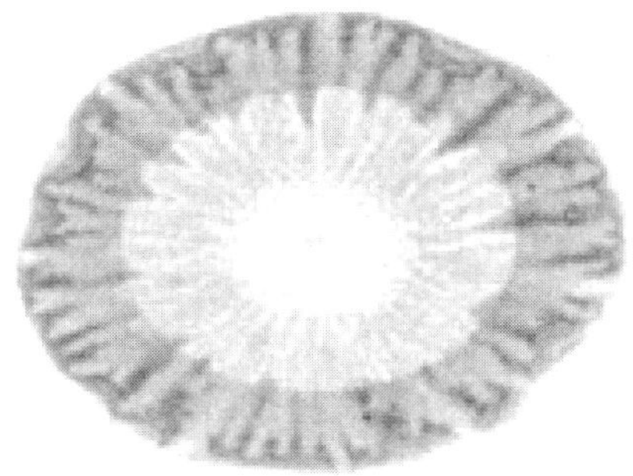

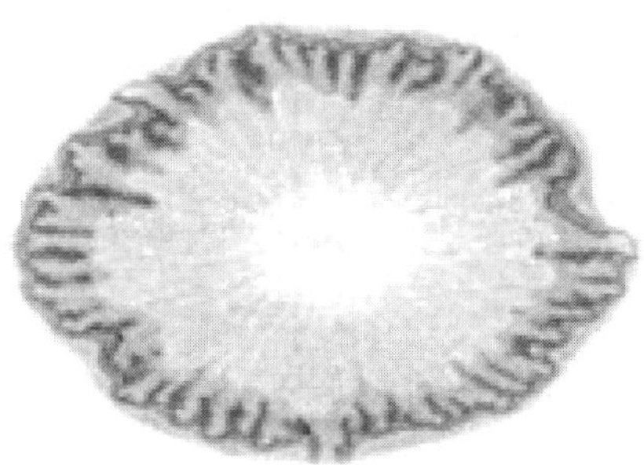

7a. Pasteurized milk-whole.  VS.  7b. Raw milk-whole.

"Paler, less definite formations than 7b indicating some loss of factors."*  "Patterns of outer edge & protrusions from edge to center indicate proteins, vitamins & minerals."*

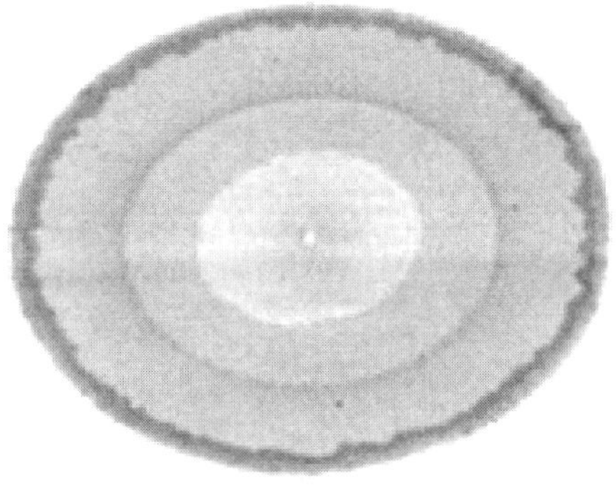

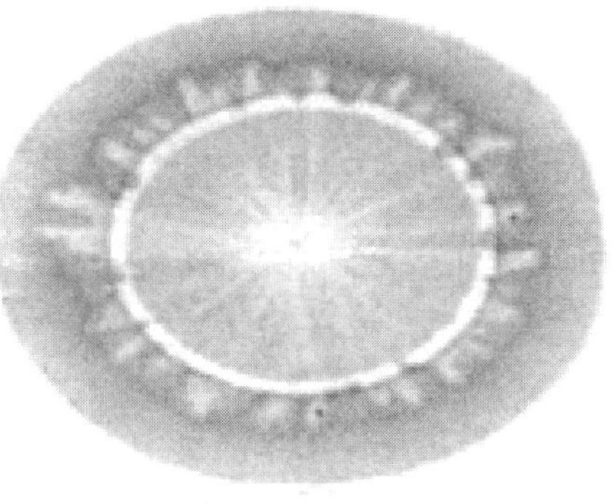

8a. A popular soft drink.  VS.  8b. Fresh orange juice organically grown.

"Outer edge shows the sugar — other factors not identified."*  "Outer zone indicates presence of enzymes & Vit. C, latter shown, also by color of inner circle."*

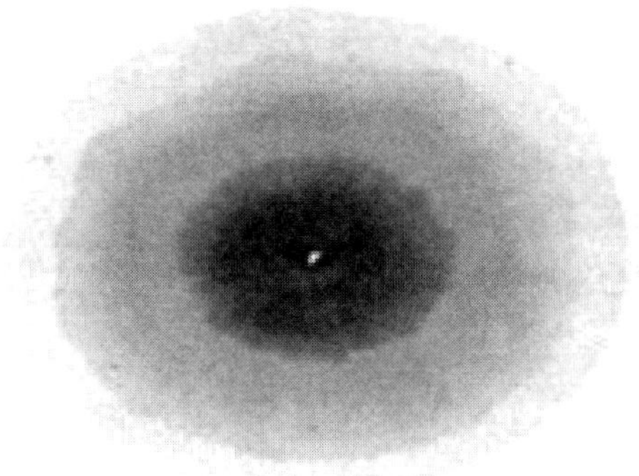

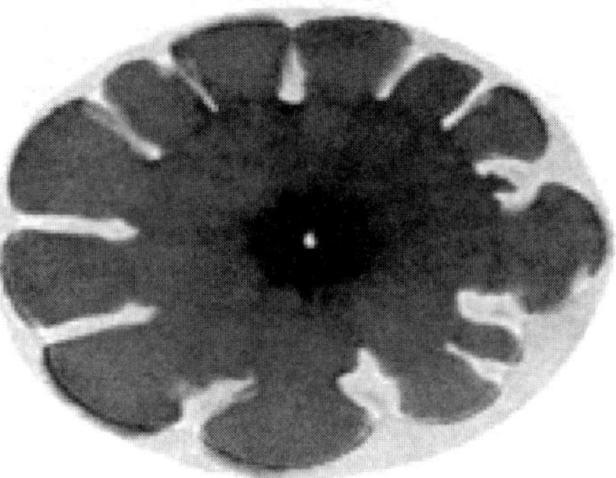

9a. Margarine.  VS.  9b. Butter — fresh home-made from unpasteurized milk.

"Lacks vitamin & enzyme formation — its value best judged by comparison with butter 9b."*  "See the winged pattern and color of many intrinsic factors and vitamin influences."*

* see bottom of page 7

*24.5 — Comparative Chromatograms*

## CHROMATOGRAMS

**LEFT SIDE**       **VITAMINS and FOOD SUPPLEMENTS**       **RIGHT SIDE**

Synthetic Vitamins and inorganic minerals-inert.       Unrefined vitamins and minerals as found in Nature.

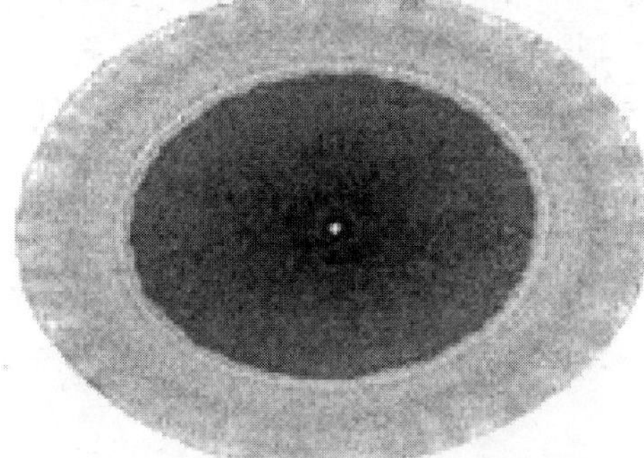

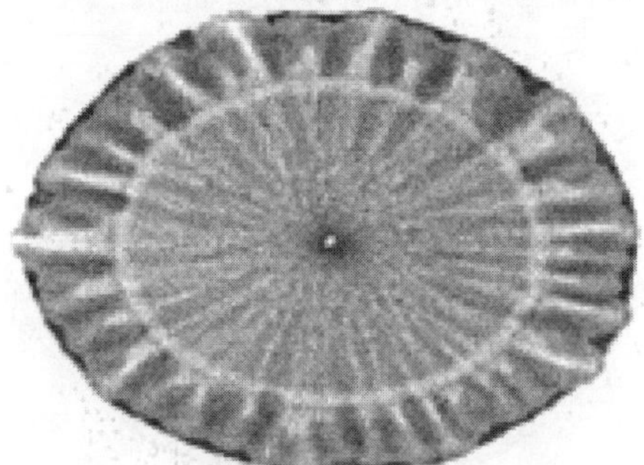

10a. Pure Commercial Vitamin C (ascorbic acid)       VS.       10b. Acerola — a tropical cherry — Natural C — used in Vit-Ra-Tox #17, Springreen #17 & Sonne's #17.

"Typical color and rings of ascorbic acid but no biologically active ingredients."*       "Jagged border & strong radiations indicate intrinsic factors, vitamins & enzyme activity."*

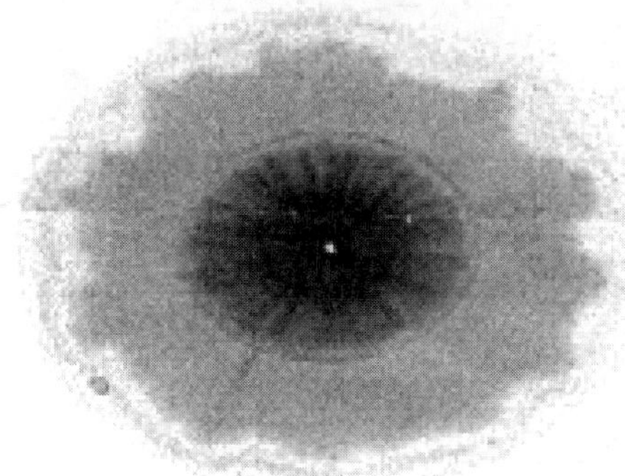

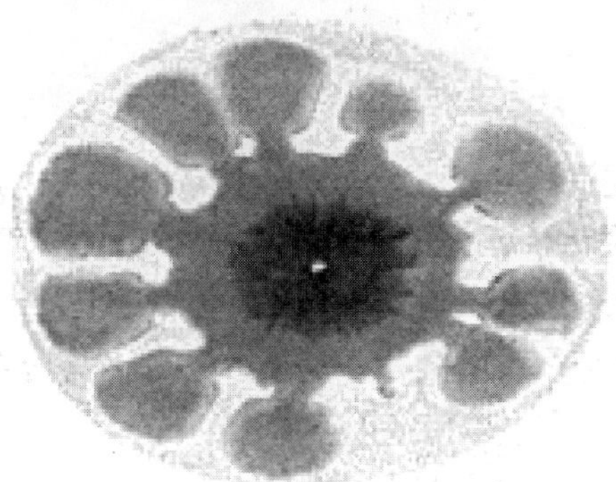

11a. Alpha — tocopherol commercial Vitamin E only a part of complete E complex.       VS.       11b. Wheat Germ Oil unheated encapsulated in Vit-Ra-Tox #23, Valox #83 and Sonne's #3.

"Intrinsic factors cannot show up because of refined state."*       "In addition to Alpha-Tocopherol other fatty acids and enzymes indicated — note similarity to butter."*

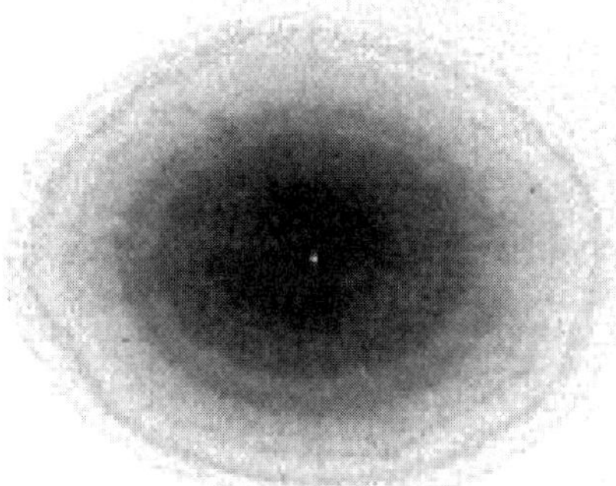

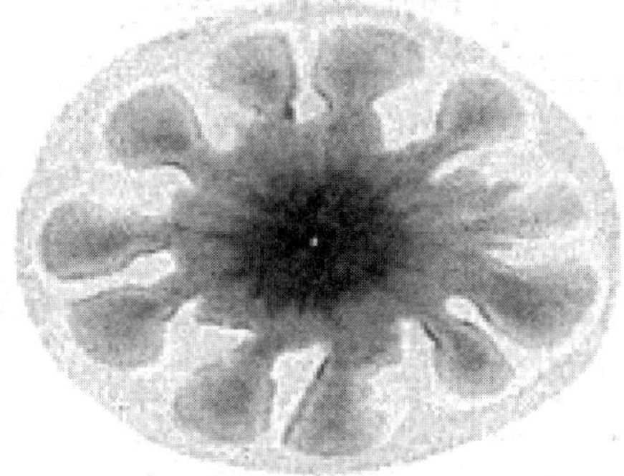

12a. Synthetic Vitamin A made from refined and chemically altered lemon grass root.       VS.       12b. Cod Liver Oil — unrefined specially made for V. E. Irons, Inc. — excellent source of Vit. A & D.

"We miss here the winged or leaf pattern which shows up in natural products."*       "Note wings or leaf pattern found in all natural oils or fats as butter and wheat germ oil above."*

* see bottom of page 7

*24.6 — Comparative Chromatograms*

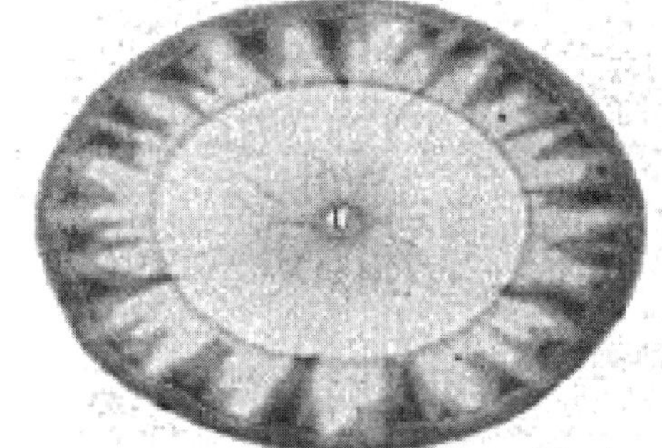
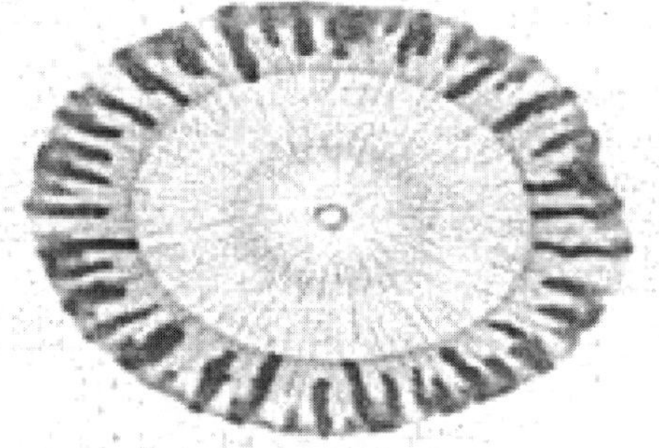



*24.7 — Comparative Chromatograms*

Naturally formed molecules produce L configurations while synthetically produced products produce both L (left) and D (right) molecules. The living body has a strong disposition for L molecules and uses them with far greater ease. Giving the living body D molecules is like wearing a right-hand glove on the left hand. It is functional but not nearly as comfortable and functional as wearing the correct left-hand glove. See Figure 24.8.

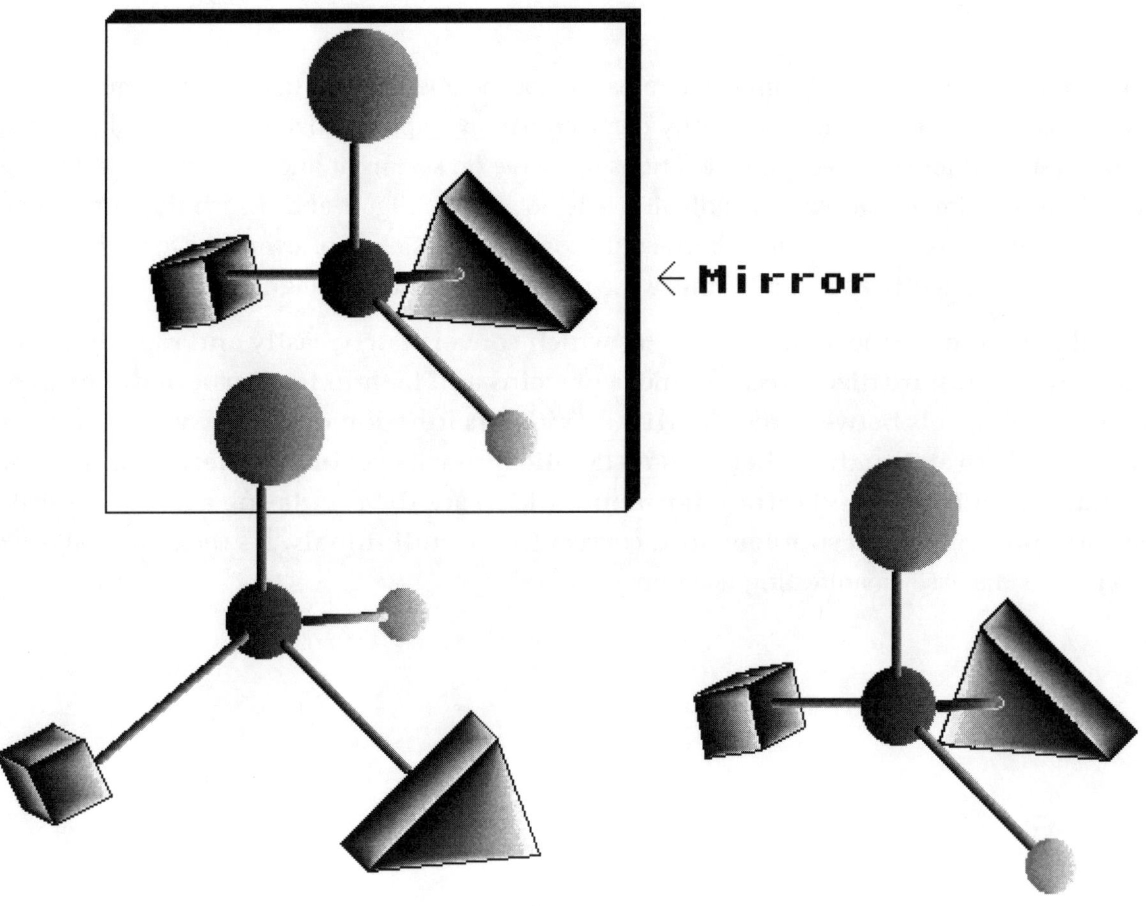


*Figure 24.8 — Racemic Molecules*

In short, synthetic D racemic molecules are much more of a challenge for the living body's chemistry to utilize than are naturally occurring L molecules. This is one of the reasons why synthetic vitamins, the D and L mix, cannot work as efficiently in the living being as naturally occurring L substances. It is possible to convert D to L configurations but the conversion, like all processes, requires additional and unnecessary expenditures of time and energy.

The vital question healers must ask themselves is, "Is it wise to take patients who may already be suffering from a depletion of their vital healing energy and require them to do additional and unnecessary work that will further deplete their energy reserves? Will that restore health in the most rapid, gentle, permanent and least demanding and harmless manner? If not, then why would healers even consider such an inferior approach? **The rule is that natural food and natural supplements are preferable.**

## LAW OF METABOLIC TYPES

**Everyone is not created equal metabolically.** The ideal nutritional complement for one can be a nutritional disaster for another, just as a high-performance gasoline engine will not run well on diesel fuel.

Some individuals oxidize (burn) their foods faster than others. Thus, an ideal diet for a slow oxidizer will leave a fast oxidizer without sustainable energy levels. Another analogy of this is building a fire; the tinder (carbohydrates) used to ignite the fire is consumed fairly rapidly, the kindling (proteins) builds the fire and the logs (fats) burn for long periods of time and give off considerably more heat (energy) than the other two types of fuel.

Humans are genetically pre-programmed to a particular metabolic type, fast, slow or mixed (balanced) oxidation, and that cannot be quickly and easily changed. An example of this would be an Eskimo who has been genetically programmed for hundreds of generations to thrive on seal meat and whale blubber who marries a girl from Tahiti who feeds him mangos and breadfruit. He is not able to digest and absorb the nutrients from her native diet as well as she is and vice versa. Each could conceivably sicken or even starve in the midst of plenty because they do not efficiently absorb and utilize the nutrients from the foreign diet.

**Slow oxidizers require more carbohydrates which convert fairly easily and rapidly into energy and less protein and fats; fast oxidizers require more proteins and fat and less carbohydrates in order to sustain their energy levels between meals. Mixed oxidizers function optimally with more protein and less fats and carbohydrates in their diet. The metabolic types also exhibit different optimum requirements for vitamins, minerals and certain hormones which are the regulating agents of cellular combustion. Therefore, no single food supplement is correct for all individuals.** It's the universal law of "Too much or too little is dis-ease" manifesting itself once again.

# Chapter 25
# ORIENTAL MEDICINE

*"Each thing exists to nourish all others and in turn
to be nourished itself. In this manner, each kingdom of nature serves, to receive and transmit life. . .
These forces are not all material, but include
subtle energies of. . . a spiritual nature. . . ."*
— Vasant Lad and David Frawley

## HISTORY

The saga of oriental healing can be traced back approximately 4,500 years. During that time many great authors documented much of this science in various texts. Some of these texts still survive, others are referred to extensively by later authors so we know a great deal of their content even if they no longer exist. Unfortunately, it is difficult if not impossible to find a single text that concisely details all of the laws identified during this extensive time frame. This fact, more than anything else, makes the study of oriental medicine a challenge. The contents of this chapter is an attempt to rectify that shortcoming.

## LAW OF MAINTAINING ORDER

Maintaining order rather than correcting disorder is the ultimate principle of oriental healing philosophy. To cure dis-ease is like setting out to dig a well only after one is already thirsty. The true physician teaches "Tao" - or how to live a healthy, happy life. **Humans are nature manifesting itself in the form of people; therefore, natural laws must be obeyed.**

## LAW OF CH'I

The (quantum) force that creates, animates and regulates all material matter and life is called Ch'i (Qi). **Matter is ch'i, num, kundalini, innate, vital, life force (energy) that is compacted into a tangible form; therefore, matter is an extension of energy and is controlled by energy.**

# LAW OF ADAPTABILITY

**Healthy organisms adapt to altering environments.** Dis-ease is an inability to adapt to the constantly changing environment.

# LAW OF YIN-YANG

**There must be opposition in all things.** Cause and effect are inseparable. Without cause, there cannot be effect. Without effect, cause cannot be expressed.

# LAW OF INDIVIDUALITY

**Illnesses may be identical but the persons suffering from them are different. The emotions and the excesses affecting people are not the same. Some people may be strong and others weak as far as their Qi (ch'i) or the condition of their body is concerned. One's nature may be tough or soft, one's sinews and bones may be firm or brittle. There are patients who suffer in their hearts from grief and others who enjoy happiness. If a practitioner treats all those patients who appear to suffer from an identical illness with one and the same therapy, that practitioner may hit the nature of the illness but the approach used may still be exactly contraindicated by the influence of Qi (ch'i) that determines the condition of the individual patient's being.**

# LAW OF ORGAN STRENGTH

**When an organ has excessive energy, the cause of the dis-ease usually involves organs that are affecting related weak organs (which are being drained of num, kundalini, ch'i, innate, life, vital force). When the organ is deficient in energy, the symptoms usually involve the organ itself and/or the one succeeding it in the destructive Sheng cycle of the five phases.** See Figure 25.15.

# LAW OF MERIDIANS (ENERGY PATHWAYS)

**An acupuncture meridian controls what it is named after, such as liver, heart, lung, and the parts of the body that it passes through; i.e., the liver meridian controls the eye, large intestine and the nose.** See figures 25.1 - 25.14.

# THE LAW OF FIVE PHASES

**Each entity exists to nourish others and, in return, to be nourished by them.** Thus, there are definite consistent inter-relationships in the living being. These relationships can be utilized to determine where dis-ease began, what it will next affect if not resolved and how best to resolve the case. See Figure 25.15.

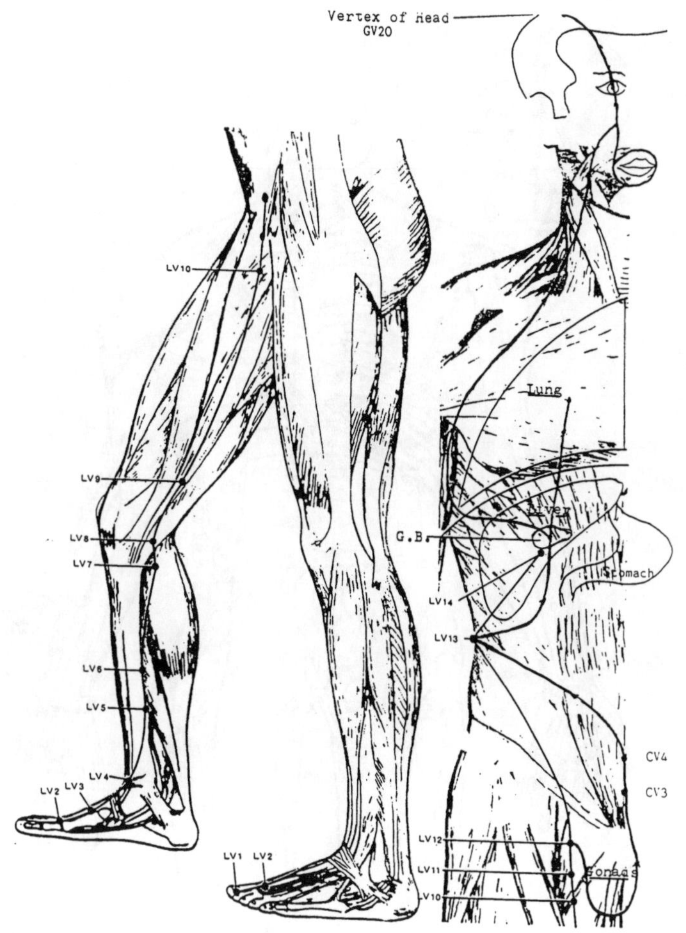

*Figure 25.1 — Liver Meridian With Internal Pathways*

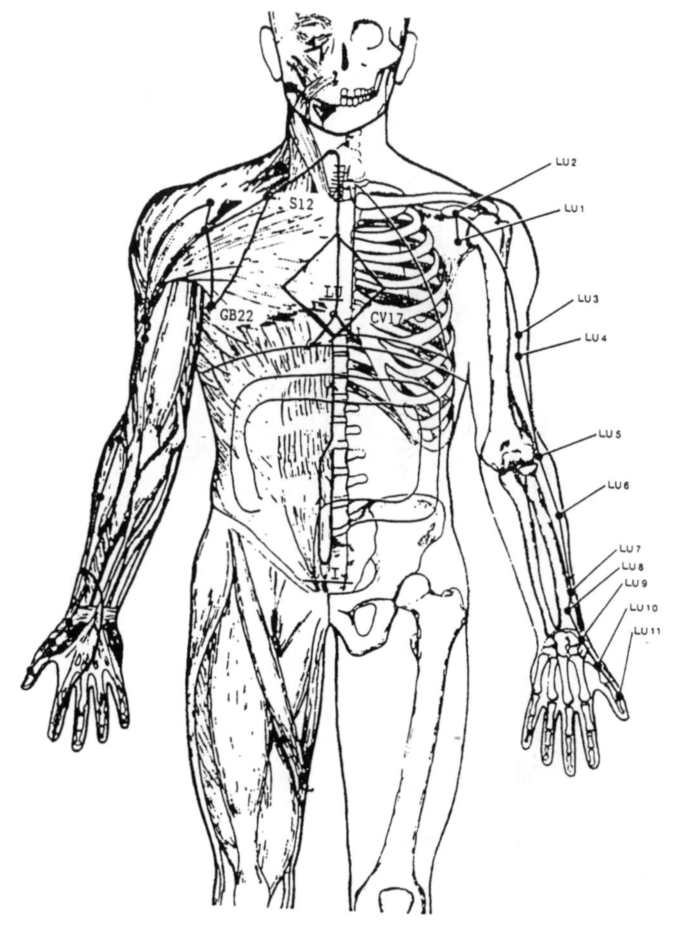

*Figure 25.2 — Lung Meridian With Internal Pathways*

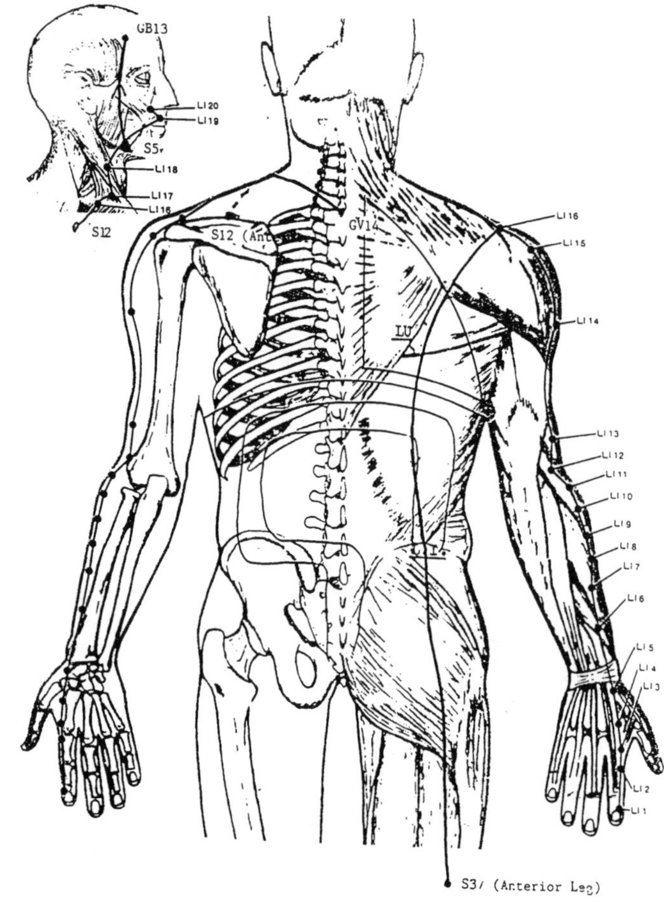

*Figure 25.3 — Large Intestine Meridian With Internal Pathways*

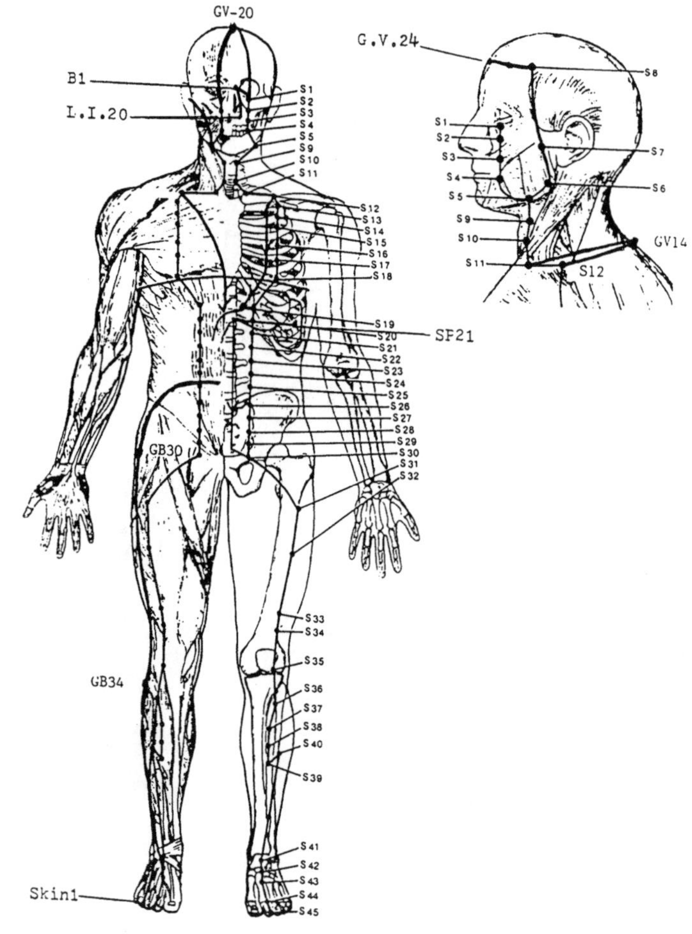

*Figure 25.4 — Stomach Meridian With Internal Pathways*

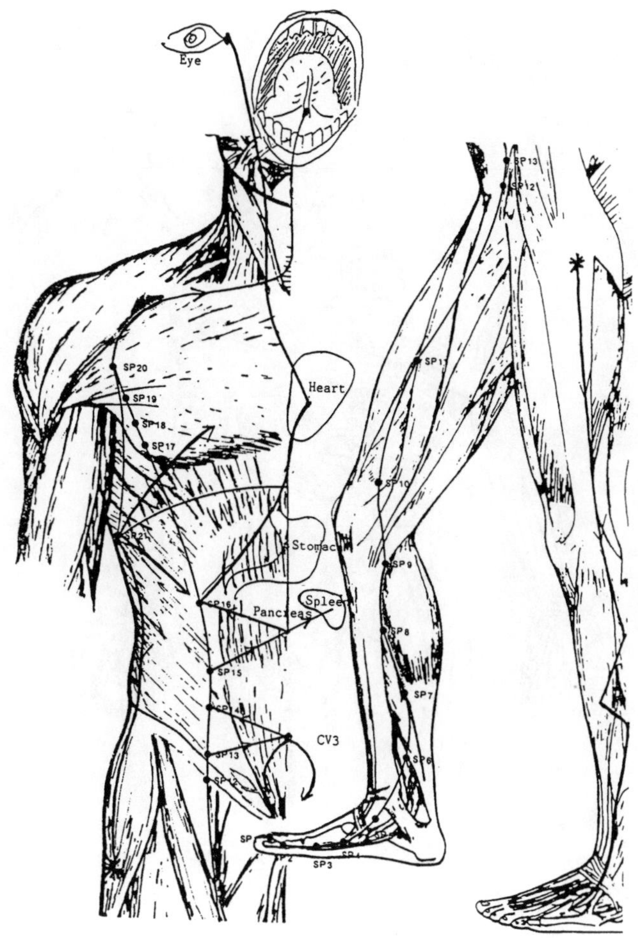


*Figure 25.5 — Spleen Meridian With Internal Pathways*

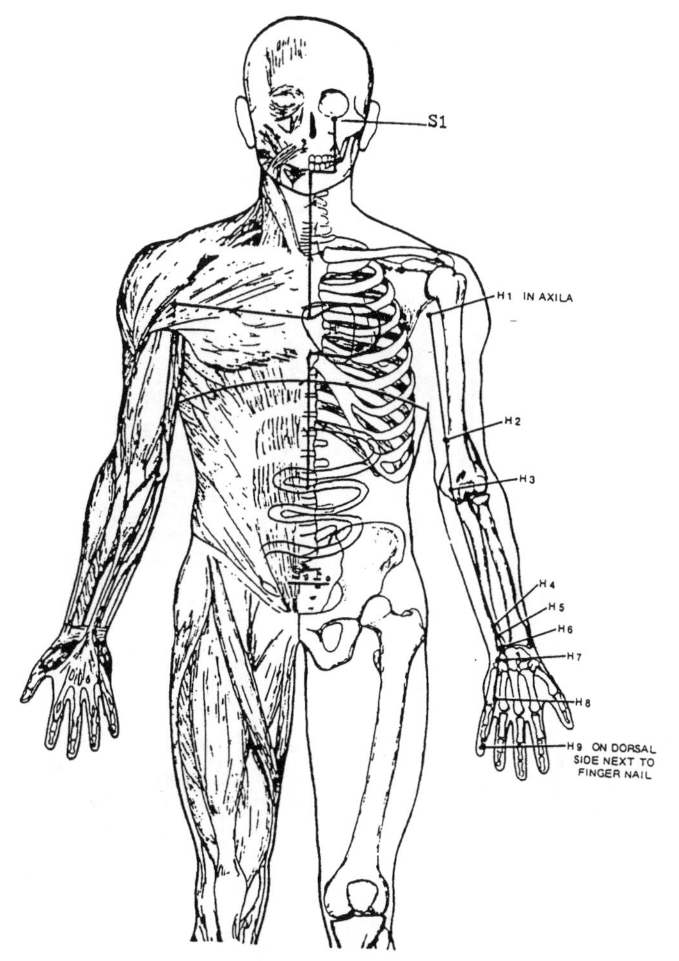


*Figure 25.6 — Heart Meridian With Internal Pathways*

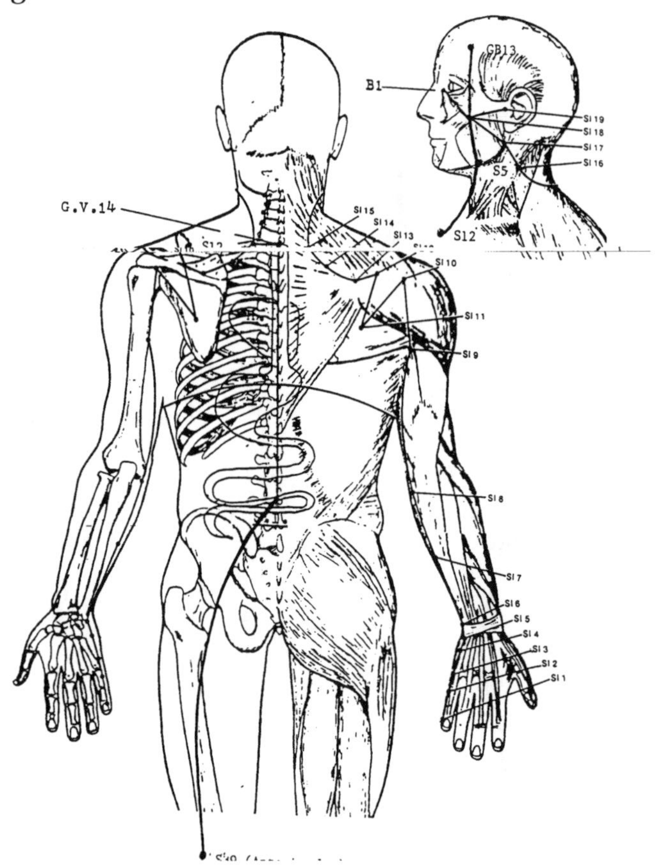

*Figure 25.7 — Small Intestine Meridian With Internal Pathways*

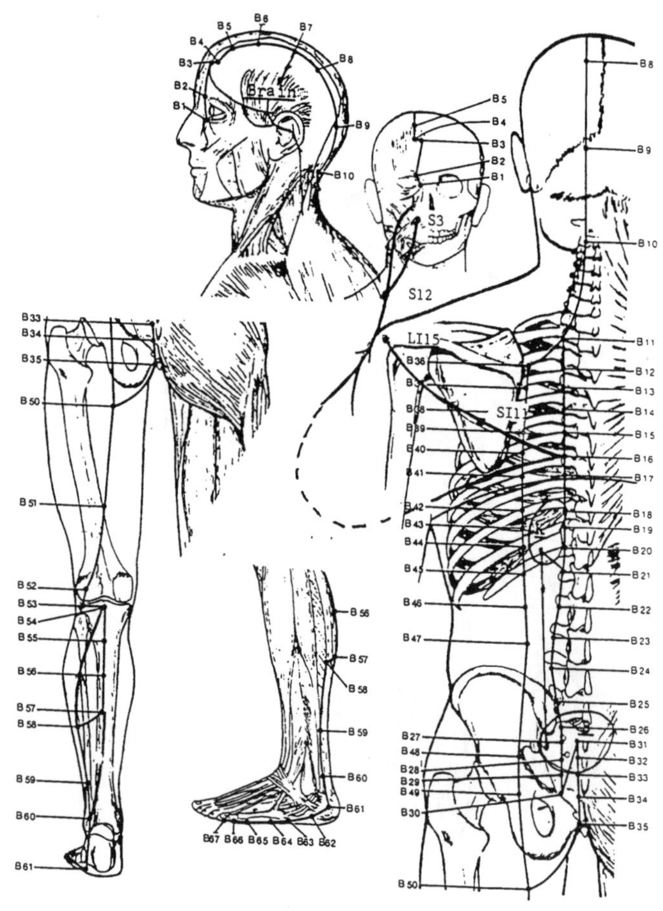

*Figure 25.8 — Bladder Meridian With Internal Pathways*

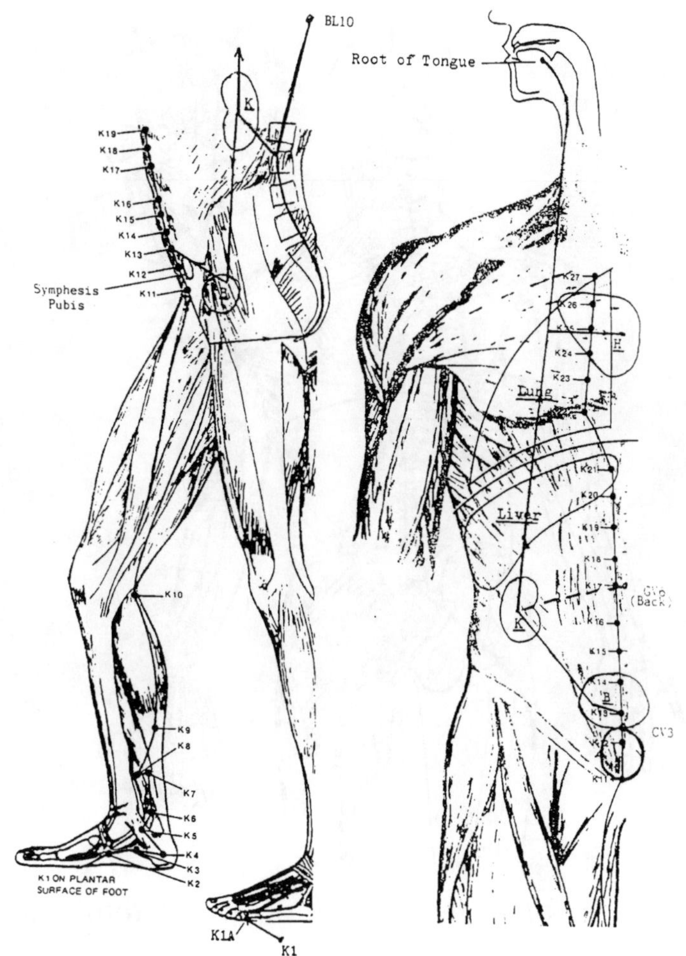

*Figure 25.9 — Kidney Meridian With Internal Pathways*

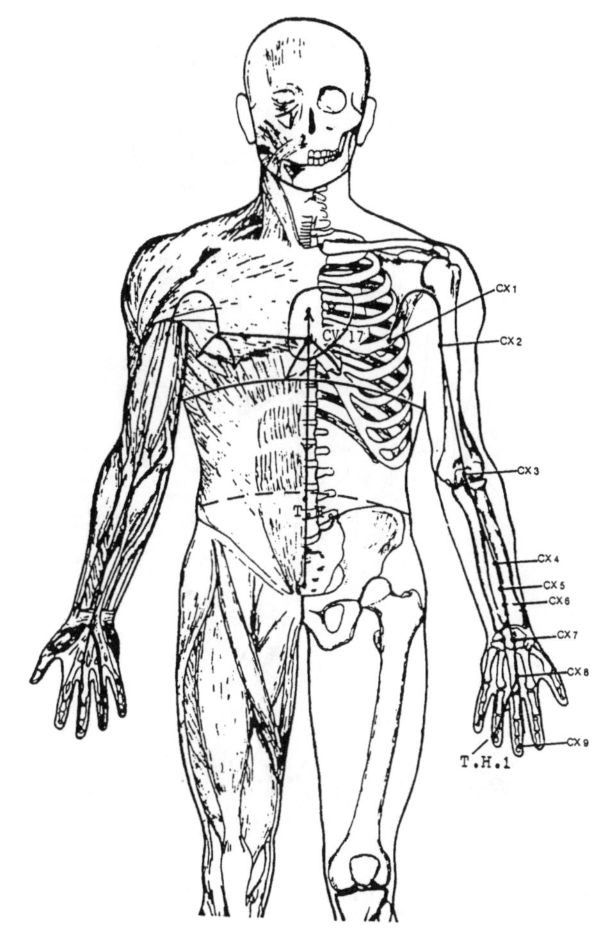

*Figure 25.10 — Circulation Sex (Pericardial) Meridian With Internal Pathways*

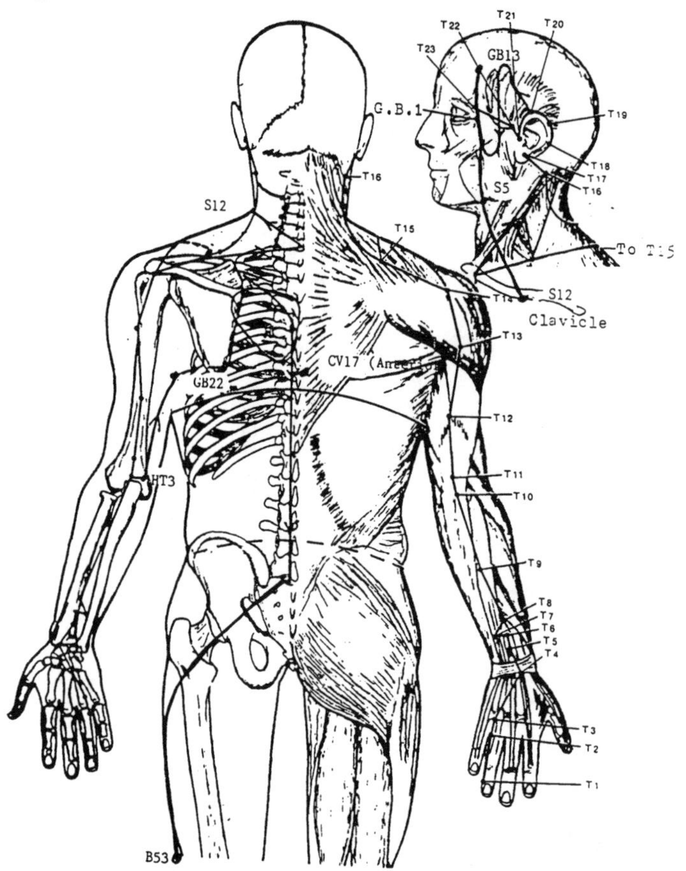

Figure 25.11 — Triple Heater Meridian With Internal Pathways

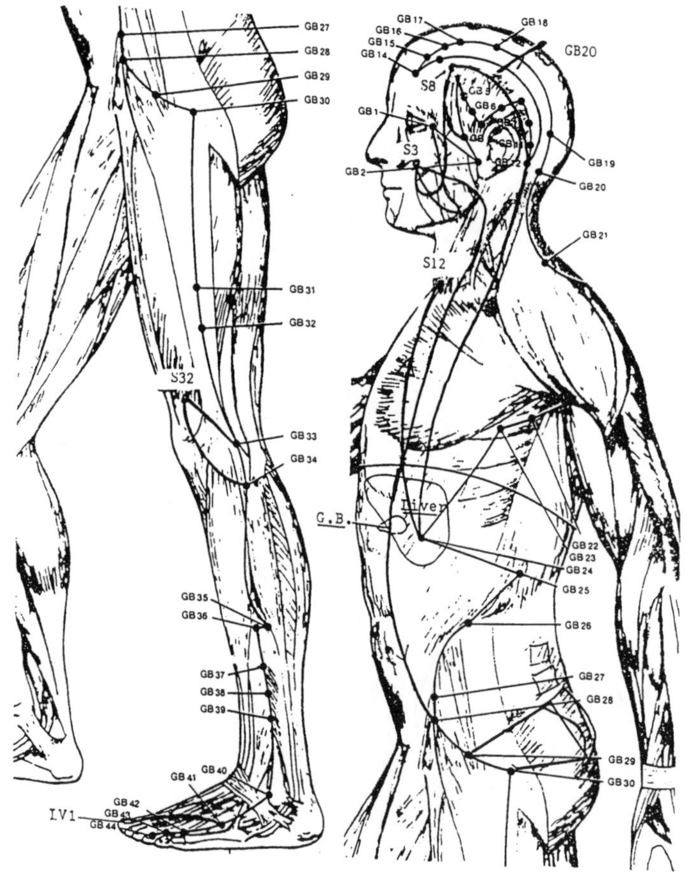

Figure 25.12 — Gall Bladder Meridian With Internal Pathways

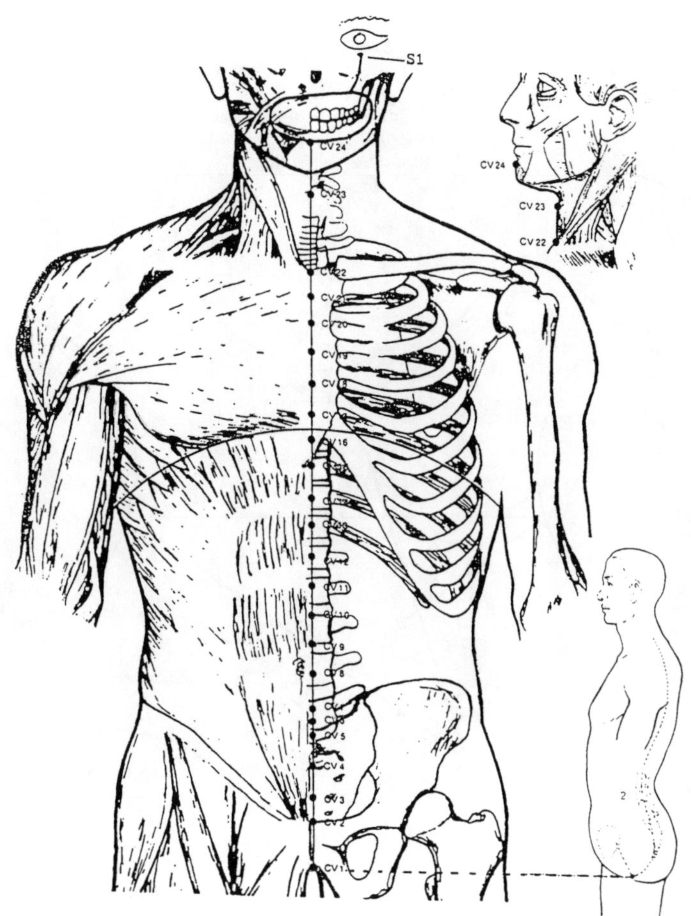

*Figure 25.13 — Conception (Meridian) Vessel With Internal Pathways*

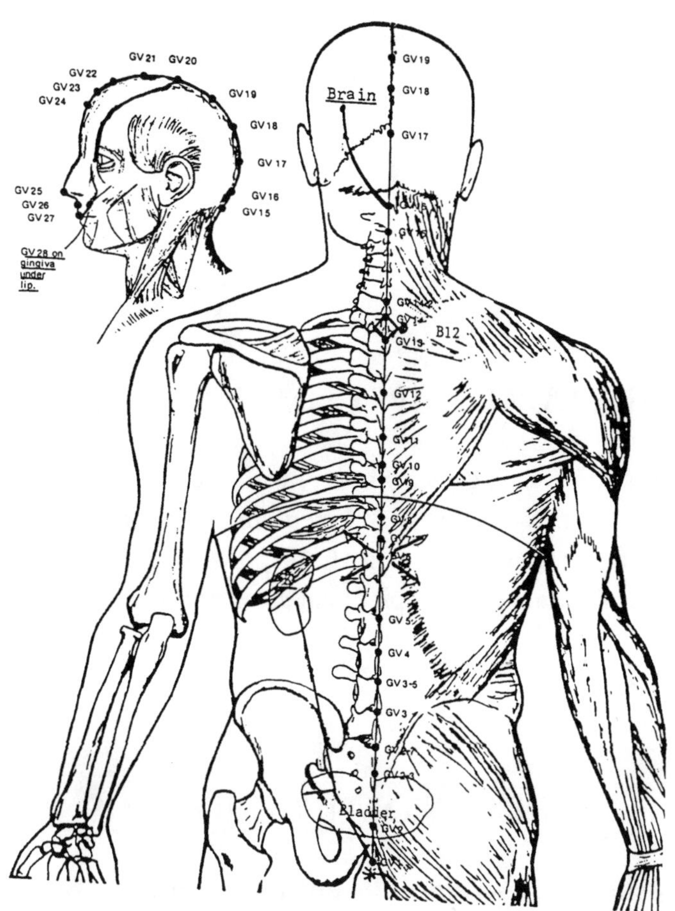



*Figure 25.14 — Governing (Meridian) Vessel With Internal Pathways*

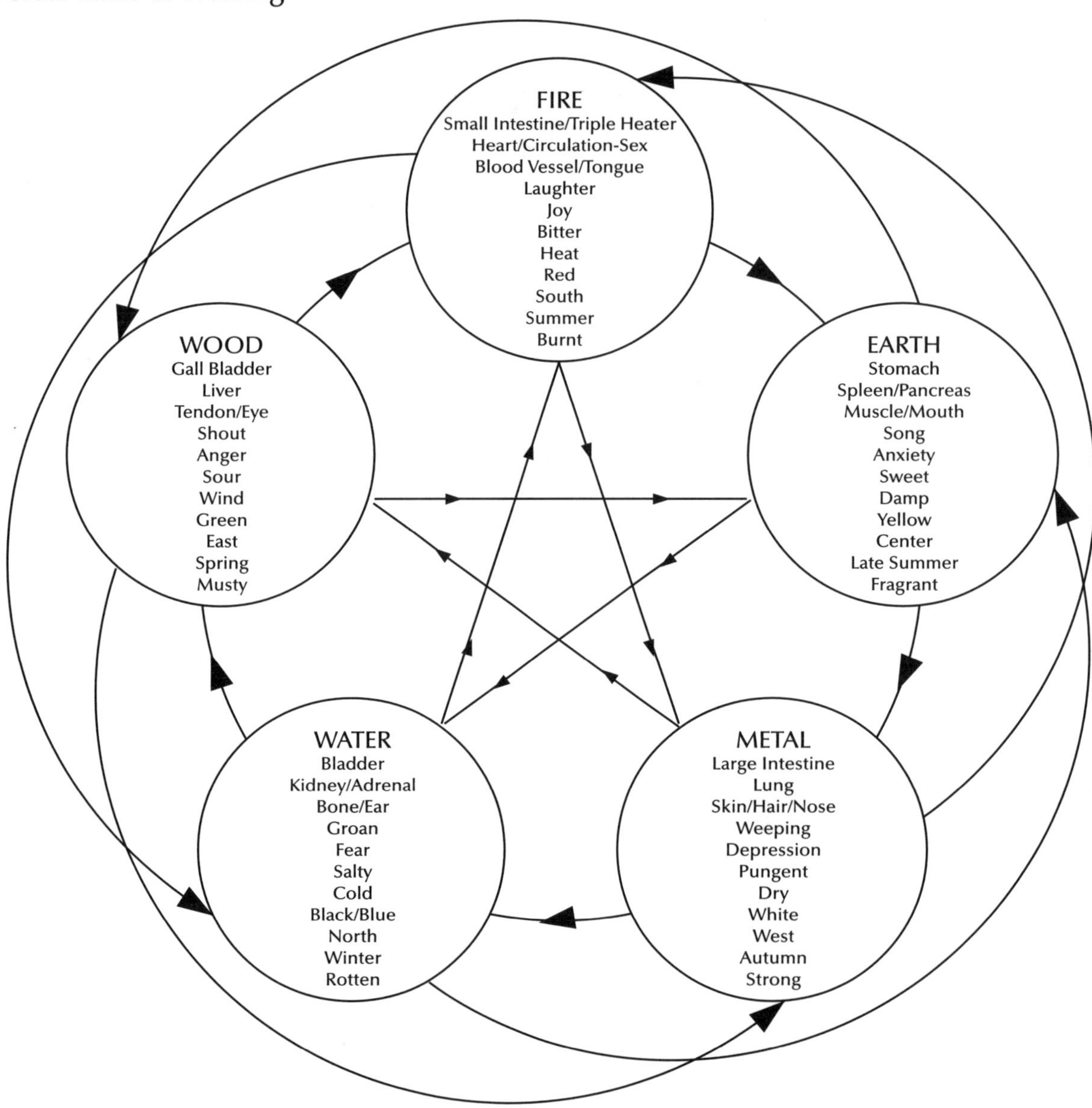



*Figure 25.15 — The 5 Phase Flow Chart*

## THE LAW OF FIVE CLIMATES (SEASONS)

A patient can exhibit internal physical, sensory and psychic response patterns that are related (usually aggravated) by the climate (season of the year). Oriental medicine teaches that these climate characteristics have been internalized by the patient and are entirely or partly responsible for his/her poor health. This concept is not entirely foreign to western medicine. For example, heat stroke and hypothermia are internalizations of climatic conditions.

## THE LAW OF FIVE EMOTIONS

**A healthy human being should experience the entire gamut of emotions as appropriate.** When an individual becomes fixated on any one emotion, it interferes with the normal functions of the being and produces dis-ease associated with the phase relating to the inappropriate emotion.

## LAW OF TONGUE DIAGNOSIS

**Changes in the texture and color, and moisture of specific geographic parts of the tongue reflect long-term dis-ease related to specific viscera.** This principle is used in much the same way as naturopaths use iridology in the west. See figure 25.16.

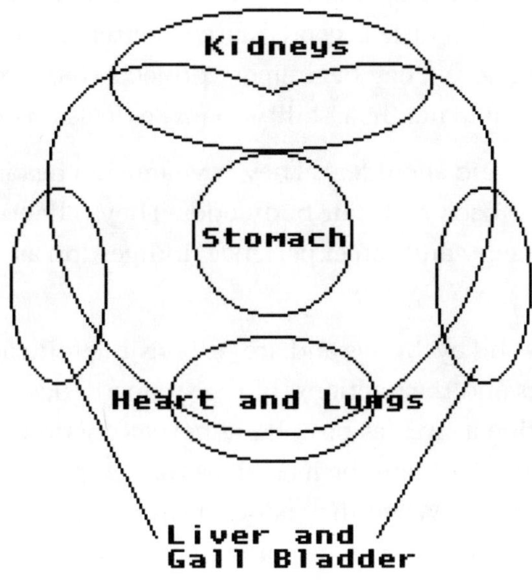


*Figure 25.16*

In oriental medicine, ch'i (qi - num, kundalini, life, innate, vital force) and blood circulate as a unit. By feeling the pulses, the movement of the blood which is initiated by and integrated with ch'i, interference with ch'i flow can be determined. The healing energy of the living being is determined by distinguishing between hot or accelerated metabolism and cold or retarded metabolism. The location of the involved organ is determined by superficial and deep pulses. The virulence of the dis-ease is determined by excess or hyperfunction and deficiency or hypofunction and the summation of Yin, cold, deficient and internal and yang, heat, excess and external. See figure 25.17.

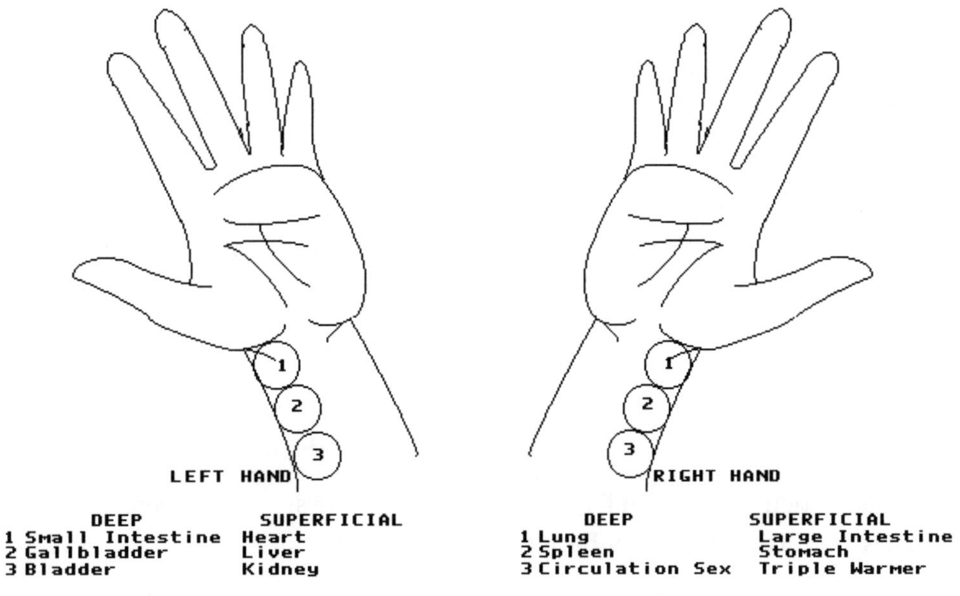


*Figure 25.17 — Location of Pulses*

# LAW OF WOOD

Individuals dominated by the Liver/Gall Bladder meridians are adaptive, cunning and fiercely independent. They are eager, innovative, reformers, revolutionizers and implementers. They wield power and influence naturally but yet are willing to comfort, break with tradition and endure hardships. They perceive sacrifice not as a loss or inconvenience but as liberation. They galvanizes others and thrive in America where ambition, achievement and single-mindedness are admired characteristics. They push themselves and others. Their mind fix is "There is only one right way, my way." If a little is good, more is better. They exhibit inconsistent moods, fatigue, nervousness, irritability and anxiety. They begin more projects than they can finish. They produce self-generated pressure and tension which impairs their ability to make decisions and their perception of reality.

They register tension in the neck and shoulders. They have tension headaches in the temples, inflamed eyes, tightness of chest, strains in the lower back and sour body odor. They rely on stimulants, sugar, fats and spices; overeat, eat on the run to generate energy and can experience  indigestion as a result. Joint and muscle pains are common as is an erratic energy level.

These meridians control the iris and eyebrows and are responsible for  cataracts, glaucoma and visual defects of the lens. They control tears and the unctions  of the sympathetic nervous system which produce arousal, excitation and powers of action as well as peripheral nerve function. They also control bile and produce dis-ease such as jaundice and hepatitis. They are the meridians that eliminate metabolic wastes, collect and direct blood and ch'i and control blood pressure. When they allow stasis of blood, it produces lumps, masses, tumors, fibroids, clots, chronic inflammations of chest, abdomen and pelvis. The wood meridians also control external genitalia and healthy sexual and reproduction functions as well as conditions such as prostatitis, epidymitis, urethritis and painful ejaculation. They also control tendons, ligaments, small muscles that move joints and nails. They represent and control the "Birth Phase" of life.

# LAWS OF FIRE

The individual dominated by the Heart/Small Intestine, Triple Heater/Circulation Sex meridians exhibit excitement, enthusiasm, enchantment and persuasiveness. This individual is a natural salesperson having a lively  sense of humor, is jovial, optimistic, generous, imaginative and articulate. They enjoy touch, love of speech, and wear their hearts on their sleeves but also have a rich inner life that is easily affected by other people. They are constantly responding to stimuli, are seductive and inspired but the power of discernment can be overloaded resulting in anxiety, confusion, and a sense of dread when overwhelmed. They can be hyperactive, nervous and may have difficulty focusing their attention. Their hands become warm and moist and they perspire freely when they are excited or busy.

They like hot spicy food, warm weather and emotional fervor and can exhibit an inability to rest, sleep and replenish their resources. Cardiac arrhythmia and cramps, with a feeling of isolation and melancholy are common in chronic cases. Friends, family and associates of these individuals may feel they are fuel for their demands and desires. At times, they can babble and have disjointed thoughts, mania, delusions, hallucinations, nightmares, and rushes of physical sensations. They become disappointed when their life does not equal their dreams and will over-indulge in foods that produce heat and dryness such as curry, sugar, alcohol, coffee, tea, chocolate and salt which in turn produce weakness. They crave ice water and cold drinks.

Their tongue is red and their mouth can have sores. They are thirsty and experience hot flashes because this meridian controls arteries and arterioles. They have complaints of the complexion, tongue, external ear and corners of the eyes.

These meridians also propel the blood, care for the spirit or the totality of the being which is the seat of moral and spiritual faculties, impart a sense of individuality and maintain awareness and alertness. Emotions of surprise, inordinate sorrow or overwhelming joy are associated with these meridians as well as conditions such as heart attacks, strokes, agitation, unrest, forgetfulness, sleep disturbances, incessant talking, disturbing dreams, aberrations of behavior, difficulty finding the right words and short- term memory loss. Shortness of breath, purpleness of the lips, fingers and nose and blood in the urine, stool or sputum are characteristic dysfunctions of these meridians as are fluids regulated of the blood and perspiration. Urethritis, cystitis, ileitis, duodenal ulcers and enteritis are also dis-eases associated with these meridians. These meridians control the "Growth Phase" of life.

## LAWS OF EARTH

The Spleen and Stomach meridians dominate individuals who value serenity and stability; they rely on positioning and leverage to influence others and they focus on extended networks of relationships. They have amiable, polite dispositions, engaging smiles, and eagerly organize other people's lives. They have a round body with solid hips and thighs.

Home functions as their center of operations and they become territorially attached to it. They have difficulty saying no and are languid, selfish, and over-protective. They resist change, anticipating that it may risk serenity and stability. They store supplies in anticipation of future need. Their life centers on pleasing others and there is little time left to fulfill personal needs, which sometimes creates an empty feeling amid a life of plenty; consequently, they eat to try to fill the emptiness. They commonly have retarded digestion and gravitate to quick fixes of starch, sugar, vitamins and concentrated food supplements.

They can be obsessive and oscillate between empty and full, indulgent and denunciatory. They are self-centered and self-depreciating, grandiose and defeated, meddling and apathetic and tend toward binging and starving. Mental concentration, recollection and reflection is slow but they adapt to endure stress without undo harm.

Their bodies extract and convert nutrients and transfer energy and mass from one site to another and into ch'i and blood, muscle strength, flesh and viscera. These meridians also control large muscles and flesh, lips, mouth and eyelids and the fluids of the lymph, saliva and digestive enzymes, lubricants of the joints and mucous membranes.

Prolapses, hemorrhage, bruising, varicosities, belching, hiccups, nausea, regurgitation, inflamed gums, diarrhea, anemia, dry skin and hair, blurry vision, pale lips and nails, vertigo, fatigue, muscle atrophy, palpitations and insomnia are all disorders of these meridians. Earth Phase is the phase of maturity.

## LAWS OF METAL

The Lung/Large Intestine meridians are the regulating centers of spirituality, standards, measurements, aesthetics, defenders of morals, principles and beauty. They control intelligence, memory, creativity, imagination, instinct, procreation through genetic coding and survival.

These individuals tend to be immaculate, impeccable, well-organized, controlled, methodical, efficient, disciplined, and need to understand how everything works. They adhere to rigid schedules, are duty bound, authoritarian, dogmatic, detached, discriminating, mechanical in response, and perfectionist. They sacrifice pleasure and spontaneity for safety and control.

These meridians control functions of the parasympathetic nervous system (inhibiting and quieting), coarse breathing and headaches, stiffness of the  chest, spine, shoulders and mental distress. The nose, sinuses, nasopharynx, bronchi, skin and mucous membranes secretions are also controlled by these meridians as are body hair and sclera of the eye.

These individuals frequently have coughing, asthma, nasal congestion, dry wrinkled skin, allergic dermatitis, hair loss, varicose veins, and are sensitive to drafts and change of temperature. They also have diminished immunity, asthma, spastic colon, constipation, lack of perspiration, dryness of skin and mucous membranes as well as sneezing, sinus congestion, and itching. The wind and sunlight aggravate them and they are sensitive to all aspects of internal and external environment. The Phase of Aging is represented by these meridians.

## LAWS OF WATER

The Water meridians are represented by individuals who are tough, self-possessed, and idiosyncratic to the point of being controversial. They are restless searchers for truth, visionary, insatiably curious and play with ideas. At the same time, they are paragons of integrity, hold to opinions even when unpopular, are stoic, unresponsive and inaccessible, negative, cynical, and suspicious.

They are not morning persons. They engage in minute self-scrutiny of how their body functions and feels, and they tend to suck the life energy out of others but do not return it. Time is their great healer but once their health fails they become fearful, suspicious, stingy, lack faith, and desire and motivation collapse. They are willing to endure the pain but not the limitations of illness.

They have large heads, large bones, and pear-shaped bodies. The ovaries, testes, brain, spinal cord, spinal column, bones, bone marrow (RBC formation) and calcification, teeth (dentition), pubic and head hair, inner ear, pupils, anus and urethra, sexual secretions, sexual impulses, sexual characteristics, ovulation, ejaculation, fertilization, gestation are controlled from these meridians. The cerebral spinal fluids, hypothalamus, pituitary and adrenal glands, tears, saliva, mucous, urine, sweat, cerebrospinal fluid, synovial fluid, plasma and semen also are regulated by these meridians. Poor health, developmental deformities, mental retardation, loss of and graying of hair, dimness of vision, loss of teeth, impotence and infertility are the results of imbalances in these meridians.

Their functioning is undermined by lack of sleep, excessive exercise, excessive sexual activity and work. These meridians also control urethral, anal, and cervix sphincters; therefore, they may have difficulty ridding themselves of toxins which congeal into tumors of the lower abdomen, reproductive organs, spinal cord and brain as well as hardening of arteries. Water phase is the phase of death and degeneration.

## LAWS OF ACUPUNCTURE

Research has documented that acupuncture points are points of decreased magnetoelectric resistance that modify the transmission of neural impulses between the spinal cord and the brain. The meridian points affect the peripheral micro circulation, rhythm and stroke volume of the heart, blood pressure, levels of circulating red and white blood cells and their production. They stimulate production of endorphins and other endogenous secretions and modify the holographic biomagnetoelectric fields of the being.

## PHYSICS OF AN ACUPUNCTURE POINT

Research has also documented that the magnetoelectric resistance at an acupuncture point is approximately 1/10th of that of the tissues where no acupuncture point is located. This phenomenon produces a window, mini-chakra or vortex. When the energy of the needle, electrical current, or laser enters or exits this vortex, it meets far less resistance and is able to be much more easily utilized by the dis-eased living being to normalize the aberrant energy pattern(s) of dis-ease. See figure 25.18.

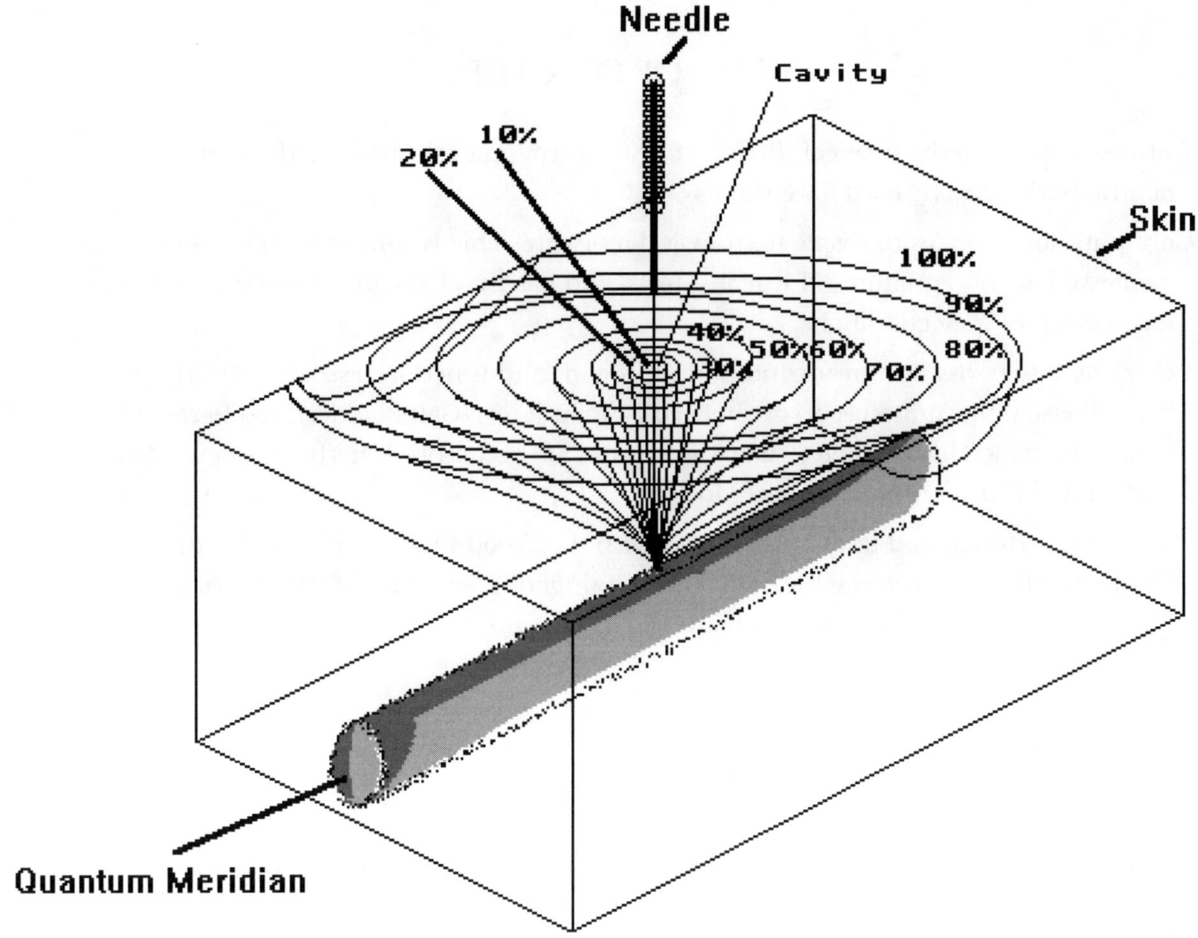



*Figure 25.18 — Decreasing Electrical Resistance At An Acupuncture Point*

## LAW OF HEALING CRISIS

An aggravation that occurs during the process of care is referred to as a "healing crisis" if, after its resolution, a patient feels and functions better than before.

## PHYTOPHARMACOLOGY LAWS

Although pharmaceuticals control symptoms, they do not resolve the pathology (i.e., antibiotics may eliminate bacteria but do not improve a person's resistance to being re-infected; diuretics rid the body of excess fluids yet do not improve renal function; aspirin controls pain without altering the course of the dis-ease.) They also produce iatrogenic side-effects such as yeast infestation following antibiotic administration, kidney damage from long-term diuretic usage, gastrointestinal ulcers and hemorrhage from excessive aspirin intake.

In phytological agents, active ingredients are formulated within the whole plant which tends to buffer adverse effects. Herbal formulas may, therefore, be formulated to antidote undesirable effects and enhance therapeutic effects.

# LAW OF QUALITIES

1. Nature - cooling herbs treat conditions of heat; warming herbs treat cold conditions; neutral herbs may be used for either.

2. Configuration - relates to shape, texture and moisture. This is similar to the western medieval Law of Signatures; if it looks, feels, and has the shape of a kidney, it is good for treating kidney conditions.

3. Color - yellow herbs best treat conditions of organs and functions associated with the Earth Phase (Spleen/Stomach); green herbs, Wood (Liver/Gall Bladder); red herbs, Fire (Small Intestine/Heart/Triple Heater/Circulation Sex) blue/black herbs, Kidney/ Bladder; white herbs,  Lung/Large Intestine.

4. Taste - a sour/fermented taste is associated with the Wood Phase, bitter/acid with the Fire Phase, fragrant/sweet with Earth Phase, pungent/spicy with Metal Phase, and salty with the Water Phase or meridian.

# LAW OF PROPERTIES

1. Dispersing - means to move and herbs in this category assist circulation, promote fluid metabolism, peristalsis, elimination and contribute to relaxation and invigoration.

2. Consolidation - means to bring functions together and it prevents the loss of normal body constituents by inhibiting excessive sweating, mucous discharge, diarrhea, hemorrhage, and urination. (These herbs are similar to astringents in naturopathic medicine.)

3. Purgative - are herbs to expel and rid the body of accumulated wastes. Herbs in this category primarily work via the lungs, nose, skin, bowels, uterus, and bladder. These include the detoxifying, anti-inflammatory, and antiphlogistic (against fever) in naturopathic medicine and those which stimulate menses, urine, sweat, phlegm, undigested food and feces.

4. Tonification - means to augment, support, replenish and strengthen. Herbs in this category have a marked effect on digestion and metabolism and increase the resistance of the patient.

# LAW OF HERBAL EFFECTS

All herbs affect ch'i, moisture and blood but not all herbs have specific effects upon specific organs.

# LAW OF FORMULAS

A herbal formula is designed to fit a particular patient just as a key is made for a specific lock. To achieve maximum results, a formula must be developed specifically for a particular patient and that patient's dis-ease at that particular point in time. As the status of the patient's health changes, the formula must also change in order to achieve maximum results. No two patients are exactly alike; two patients with the same western diagnosis may be prescribed two different herbal formulas in oriental medicine. This is referred to as the patient's constitutional formula.

1. Herbs that tone are usually complemented by herbs that disperse in order to prevent hyper-tonification.
2. Herbs that disperse are complemented by those that consolidate to prevent over-stimulation
3. Herbs that consolidate given with those that disperse prevent over-consolidation.
4. In the weak or elderly, toning without circulation will contribute to the deterioration of the patient's health.
5. An herb with a strong affinity for a particular organ system will shift the effects of all other herbs in the formula to that organ system.

# LAW OF TEA PREPARATION

Herbal formulas are generally administered in the form of teas. To prepare, simmer the herbal formula in 4 to 6 cups of water for 30 to 60 minutes in a covered glass, ceramic or stainless steel pot or until the fluid has been reduced to 1 cup. Repeat the process with the same herbal formula but using one less cup of water; combine the two and drink immediately.

# CULINARY LAWS

In the western reductionistic non-vitalistic society, food is described by its protein, calorie, mineral, vitamin and fat contents. In oriental expansionistic, vitalistic society, food is considered to be far more individualistic. **One man's meat is considered another man's poison.** For example, raw fruits and vegetables are cooling (yin), not because of refrigeration but because they promote loss of body heat and secretion of fluids. Fried, broiled, fatty and spicy foods are warming (yang) because they absorb the heat of cooking and generate body heat stimulating circulation. Yet foods in oriental medicine cannot be strictly classified as yin or yang except in their relationship to the individual's current circumstances.

## LAW OF FLAVORS

Salty - tones and concentrates

Sour - astringent and contracting

Bitter - eliminating and descending

Sweet - expanding and relaxing

Spicy - accumulating and dispersing

*Figure 25.19 — Flavors Chart*

The Spleen meridian governs all activities during digestion including that of the liver, gall bladder and pancreas. If ch'i is blocked, it follows the path of least resistance and can even reverse normal patterns and, therefore, one should never continue eating until full but should leave space in the stomach for the movement of ch'i.

# Chapter 26
# SPIRITUAL HEALING

*"Anguish of mind has driven thousands to suicide;
anguish of body, few. This proves that the health
of the mind and spirit are of far more consequence
to our happiness than the health of the body,
although both are deserving of much more
attention than either receives."*

— Colton

## IN PERSPECTIVE

From a purely academic perspective, some might balk at the idea of including spiritual (or what some would call faith) healing in this textbook. It is nevertheless a widely used quantum form of healing. In fact, it probably is the most ancient and globally dispersed form of healing, being found in some form in almost all cultures throughout history. For these reasons and others that will be discussed, it is also the most difficult to reduce to a clear and concise narrative.

## LAW OF CREDENTIALS

The credentials of healers vary from group to group. The most liberal believe that individuals qualify as healers in and of their own volition. The most conservative believe that healers are selected by the universal intelligence or governing power (God) of the universe, based upon compliance with well established criteria (laws) and that healers must specifically receive authorization and power to heal prior to undertaking their work. The former provides great opportunity for all manner of charlatans while the latter restricts the privilege to a relative few with acceptable credentials.

While both views would initially seem to have some merit, an understanding of universal laws and their application lends far greater credence to the latter. **If universal laws are not obeyed, then it is not possible that the results of abiding by those laws can be achieved.** After all, that is one of the purposes of law, to achieve consistent responses. There can be no disagreement. **Truth cannot be arrayed against truth. If such a thing were possible, all things would be in confusion.** There are those who say that spiritual healing is a "miracle" and, as such, has nothing to do with laws or that it is the suspension or overruling of laws. But is that reasonable? **What suspends a law? The only logical answer is a higher law, just as a higher court of law can overrule or suspend a lower court of law's ruling.**

# LAW OF LEVELS

This leads to yet another question. **Can a healer who is living a lower order law (is less faithful to the laws) truly heal an individual who is living a higher law (is more faithful to the laws) than the healer?** Philosophically, this can be stated, "You cannot lift and lead another unless you are standing on higher ground." The healer must also consider whether or not the patient's health actually would be caused to deteriorate due to the inferior lifestyle of the healer.

# LAW OF THOUGHTS

**Thoughts are things (anti-matter things). If they exist at the anti-matter level, there must be a balance (Yang-Yin) counterpart produced on the matter (physical) level.** Thinking about, discussing, studying and researching dis-ease (pathology) forms a template around which additional physical dis-ease is produced. Conversely, thinking about health produces a template around which greater health on the physical level is formed.

# LAW OF DEVELOPMENT

Some well-meaning but naive parents and legal guardians have adopted the philosophy that they will let their children decide about spiritual matters when they become adults. This position is as irrational as believing that children can develop into well-adjusted productive adults if they are not taught manners, or the work ethic, or respect for the laws of the land, or the value of human life and respect for property, or the need for an education until they can legally determine for themselves if they want the benefits of being an literate, self-disciplined, responsible citizen.

Statistically, there is only a remote possibility that such a totally undisciplined individual would ever begin to conform to the social standards, to develop a work ethic, to value life and property, to begin to obey civil laws, or to obtain the benefits of an education. The vast majority would be destined to live lives devoid of the understanding and benefits of this refining and enriching knowledge. **Numerous authorities find that a child who has not been taught basic concepts and skills by the age of eight will never fully master them.** It is, therefore, irrational for any well-meaning, educated parent or guardian to believe that spiritual training can be an exception to this Universal Law of Development.

Nevertheless, reductionistic thinking parents and guardians, who otherwise consider themselves to be responsible, logical individuals, turn such spiritually destitute young adults loose each year. Yet, these same parents and guardians are horrified at the thought of their wards entering the 21st Century illiterate in the use of computers because they recognize the severe handicap such lack of knowledge will place them under in being able to efficiently and successfully function in the modern world. Without spiritual training, these young adults are incapable of functioning in the in the one-half of reality that encompasses the quantum or spiritual world. Sadly, they could not be less prepared for the quantum world of the 21st Century and beyond.

# THEO-SCIENCE

The central question then becomes: How does one qualify for this "calling" or "gift' of healing which allows the bearer to suspend lower laws and thereby allow higher laws to function unrestricted and provide the healing? This has traditionally been the domain of theology but, as we are beginning to see, **this issue has proved to be the wedding of the traditional roles of science and theology.** In fact, it leads us to the point where science and theology merge into theo-science. Thus, in quantum healing, science and theology are not in conflict but are harmonious extensions of each other.

**The next question is, can universal law have numerous interpretations?** Can different individuals or groups of healers use different standards and still be in harmony with universal law? Or would it be more reasonable to expect that Universal Intelligence (God) requires all to comply with the same standard? If so, then there may be many unauthorized "healers" masquerading as the authentic article.

Certainly no purely scientific and academic discussion is capable of providing complete answers to some of the above questions. This reality was acknowledged by Selbie when he said, "When an eminent man of science declares that his chemical or biological research justifies him in saying that there is no God and there is no future for man, he is going beyond science. It may be quite true that his research does not discover for him either God or immortality. In the nature of the case, they could hardly be expected to do so. But to build upon this failure a theory of the universe  which includes these as possibilities is not a scientific position."

This is why theo-science and its answers can only be sought and found in the quantum (beyond the corporal, anti-matter) or spiritual realm of faith. (Faith being defined in the context of this chapter as an acceptance of things beyond the solid state realm.) It may take generations or even millennia before all can reach the common consensus but theo-science seems to leave one inescapable conclusion. **If spiritual healing comes from Universal Intelligence (God) then at some point ALL will need to conform to the same theocratically established standard of spiritual healing.** To do less would be to continue to prostitute science as a high and sacred calling.

In the final analysis of the concept, all forms of healing must to some degree be a form of spiritual, quantum or anti-matter healing that requires the practitioner to conform with the universal laws.

# Chapter 27

# SUFI MEDICINE

*"Allah did not create any illness without also
creating the remedy, except death (old age)."*
— Mohammed

## THE GRAND LAW

**The GRAND principle of Sufi medicine, which is inseparable from the Islamic faith, is that it is not possible to be healthy, in its fullest sense, without living a life in conformity with divine laws.** To the Sufi, the healing of the sick is considered to be the most important of all services to humanity. Central to all of the doctrines of Sufi healing are the connections between health, the heart, wholeness and holiness. Being so intertwined with the Islamic faith this makes the origins of Sufi healing about 1,400 years old.

## LAW OF SPIRITUAL DOMINANCE

There is a hierarchy in the universe and in healing, the spiritual (religious teachings) always takes precedence over and subdues and controls inordinate appetites of the material, mental and emotional planes of the individual.

## LAW OF THE NATURE OF DIS-EASE

Dis-ease is not our enemy; rather, it is a mechanism that cleanses, purifies and balances us by removing toxins on the physical, emotional, mental and spiritual planes.

## LAW OF ASSISTANCE

No herb, food or any other substance (drug) or procedure (adjustments, acupuncture, surgery, massage, fasting, etc.) can heal in and of itself; when properly selected, these therapeutics can only aid and assist the being in its own self-healing.

# LAW OF STATIONS

Each individual is at a particular station or level of personal development and what may be healing to an individual on a higher level may not work on, or even be harmful for, an individual at a lower level. The dominance of types of dis-eases experienced by an individual may be classified according to the station of development of that individual. The higher and further one rises in the evolution of self, the more one is tested. When one attains the ultimate level of unity with Allah (God) there is no longer dis-ease.

# LAW OF DIET

Worldly life is one of the stages of the journey toward Allah (God) and the body is the vehicle for this journey. It behooves the traveler, then, to maintain the body in optimum operating condition so that deviations of discomfort and malfunction do not distract him from concentrating upon the ultimate goal. **Proper diet (which includes in the Sufi sense of the word the anticipation of, the preparation of, and the consumption of foodstuffs)** is one of the primary means of ensuring the vehicle (the body) will be able to perform its assigned and proper functions.

It has been said that **the stomach is the home of dis-ease.** Therefore, if indiscretion in diet can cause dis-ease, corrections of diet can heal dis-ease. Sufi medicine teaches that, **"The most important hospital in the world is your own kitchen."**

When people enter the dining area only moments before eating, they are deprived of the extended intake of the scents and mental impressions derived from the planning and preparation of the meal which psychologically and physiologically program some of the most important digestive processes. Therefore, the diner cannot receive maximum benefit from the meal.

**The entire process of digestion must be thought of as one of heating or cooking the nutritive substances.** The Persian word "pokhta" meaning "to cook" can also be translated as "breaking down of food into its nutrient components." Speaking to this "cooking," Mohammed said, **"The main cause of dis-ease is eating one meal on top of another."** In other words, not allowing the body to finish "cooking" the first meal before requiring it to begin processing another meal or overeating.

# LAW OF FOOD CLASSIFICATION

Hot/cold -1st Degree - slight action on metabolism

2nd  "   - metabolic changes

3rd  "   - profound effect -(medicinal herbs, etc.)

4th  "   - cessation of metabolism, poisonous  herbs,

        used only in minute amounts (almost homeopathically).

*Figure 27.1 — Law Of Classification Of Foods*

## ADVICE OF THE PROPHET

**Correct religious principles and correct medical principles will always be in harmony for they are expressions of the same universal law(s).** When they are not in harmony, it is because medical science has not caught up with religious science. Given adequate time, medical science will confirm the correctness of true religious principles. A sampling of such utterances of Mohammed are as follows: "Less food, less sin" and "The stomach is the home of dis-ease and abstinence the head of every remedy."

## LAW OF OILS

It is believed that the medicinal use of each flower (plant) in healing was first made known to man by divine revelation. It is also part of Sufi teaching that **mixing these phytotherapeutic agents with alcohol destroys the essence (vital force) of the plant and renders it unsuitable for healing purposes.** In Sufi medicine, there are about 60,000 different medicinal plants or plant substances but the most frequently prescribed are the pure oils of amber, frankincense, myrrh, violet, sandalwood, musk, rose, jasmine, hina, cud (aloeswood), and jannat al-fardaws (an herbal blend).

These are most generally administered by **rubbing a small amount of the oil on the back of the right hand and rubbing it over the beard area, across the clothing on the chest and into the wrists. A second favored method is to apply a drop at a point in the concha of the ear which corresponds to Shen Wen (Ear point 102) in acupuncture.**

## LAW OF HERBAL FORMULATORY

Generally speaking, Sufi practitioners resort to modification of diet before herbal formulas are considered for use.

## LAWS OF PREPARATION

1. Formulas should be prepared in accordance with established instructions.
2. Unless the instructions specifically state "coarse powder", the herbs should be ground to a powder fine enough to pass through a sieve of 100 mesh.
3. When making decoctions (boiling in water), the container must be removed from the heat at the start of the boil and allowed to steep for 5 minutes. The decoction should then be strained and drunk warm.
4. When a formula calls for a 50 percent reduction, evaporation should be done over a medium flame.
5. If the instructions call for sugar, it must be fine, raw powder. Unfiltered honey may be used in its place.

6. If the instructions call for soaking the herbs overnight (24 hours) and there is no time, they may be soaked for three to four hours and then simmered for five to six hours. (This latter method is frequently used in winter.)

7. "Waters" are made by soaking 1 to 2 ounces of the herb(s) in 1 pint of pure for 4 to 6 hours. Strain and use.

8. When the formulatory calls for equal amounts, it is by weight or volume.

## LAWS OF STORAGE

1. Decoctions must be prepared for single immediate use.

2. Do not expose prepared remedies to direct sunlight unless that  is specifically stated in the instructions as part of the preparation.

3. Never store herbal formulas in open containers.

4. All containers should be glass that has been cleaned and dried before placing any preparations in them and they should be airtight.

## LAWS OF PRESCRIBING

1. Remedies are usually prescribed twice a day.

2. Remedies taken in the morning should be taken on an empty stomach.

3. Remedies to be taken after meals should be administered 15 minutes after eating.

4. The word "quantity" indicates that it is taken as a single dose.

5. When "vehicle" is mentioned, it is interpreted as 1 cup of milk, water, or tea.

6. When no vehicle is mentioned, the remedy should be taken with water.

## LAW OF FOUR ESSENCES

Each of the essences (akhlat, khilt - singular), or stages of digestion, is produced as food is broken down into ever smaller components of nutrition. Thus, phlegm does not necessarily have the negative connotation found in western medicine; phlegm produces the lubricating and protective discharges, digestive enzymes, saliva, etc., of the body. **Only abnormal digestion produces the excessive and abnormal phlegm associated with this word in western medicine.** The four essences are:

Blood - hot and moist

Phlegm - cold and moist

Bilious - hot and dry

Atrabilious - cold and dry

## LAW OF FASTING

Fasting is the oldest form of natural healing but if applied incorrectly can result in severe disorders and even death. **Fasting is the epitome of a natural way of life.** Abstinence strengthens self-control, forbearance, sacrifice, and morality and heightens awareness of Allah (God).

## RULES OF FASTING

1. The intent of the fast must be stated.

2. The period of rest (fasting) must extend from sunrise to sunset.

3. During the fast, total abstinence from the following is required: food, drink (including water), smoking or consumption of tobacco, sexual intercourse and all forms of negativity, backbiting, fighting, cursing, arguing and similar behavior.

4. Willful ejaculation and vomiting must be avoided.

5. Pregnant, menstruating or lactating women, the seriously ill, the aged, children under 12 years of age, and the insane are exempted. Designated fast days must be made up by menstruating women. Children may fast for part of a day.

6. One should be as charitable as possible during a fast.

7. One should read and recite the Holy Qur'an (scriptures) as much as possible.

8. **True fasting is not achieved until a perfect health and spiritual blessings are experienced.**

9. The fast is broken after sunset with a date or glass of water and a modest meal.

## LAW OF HEALING CRISES

Healing crises occur by nosebleeds, involuntary vomiting, diarrhea, perspiration and excessive urination. These are events that western medicine labels as illness or dis-ease and tries to prevent. Synthetic chemical drugs immediately put an end to these healing actions. (This is much the same as the cleansing concept in naturopathy.)

## LAW OF POSTURES (SALAT)

In western culture, the word posture denotes a stance or an exercise  but to the Islamic faithful, it denotes something far different. It is an indispensable **spiritual practice leading to Allah (God).** It is performed at five distinct times during the day; before and extending to sunrise, at noon, when the sun is at a 45-degree inclination to the horizon, when the sun sinks below the horizon, and approximately one hour and twenty minutes after sunset. **The procedure includes thoughts, spoken words and physical actions.** Because of their deep religious significance and out of respect for Islamic beliefs, the teaching of the precise doctrines, postures, utterances and thoughts is best left to a member in good standing and in authority within the faith.

The belief is that if one is noble enough to give up selfish desires and serve humanity solely for the sake of pleasing Allah (God), the reward, after passing through the trial, is total and unrestricted health, protection, grace, enlightenment and favor of Allah (God).

# LAW OF BREATHING

Breathing also holds great significance within Sufi healing not only with regard to healing. To the Sufi, it probably appears to be one of the most neglected aspects of physiological healing in the western world. Within Sufi philosophy (theology), breathing has four distinct functions:

1 It is the means by which life is bestowed by Allah (God).

2 It is the means by which divine attributes are conveyed to mankind.

3 It is  responsible for creating the balance and harmony of the living being.

4 It carries the life-supporting elements from the exterior of the living body to the interior and transforms them into life-sustaining physiological functions.

Breathing, in the Sufi sense of the word, is not synonymous with oxygen. **It is the complete package of the above four concepts which controls the negative entropic (-S/T) functions of the living being producing increasing levels of order, organization, intelligence and spirituality.**

But breathing in the Sufi concept goes still further. It is accompanied by specific recitations (chants or prayers may be a more meaningful term for westerners) designed to move the patient closer to the Deity by cleansing, purifying and spiritualizing the individual.

# PRIMARY CONSIDERATIONS

For the Sufi, four things are considered in the cure of dis-ease:

1 Phytotherapeutics and diet;

2 Restriction of certain substances such as pork and alcohol and also lusts;

3 Practicing of postures [salat] and breathing; and

4 Praying.

Of these, **prayer is considered the most superior form of medicine.**

# Chapter 28
# THE SCOPE OF HEALING ARTS AND AGENTS

*"Man has always fought fiercely*
*to preserve his ignorance."*
— Robert Quillen

## CONFUSION

Scope of healing agents and scope of practice are frequently confused and considered as synonymous within the medico-legal realm. Nothing could be further from scientific fact.

## SCOPE OF PRACTICE

Scope of practice is an illogical and unscientific artificial legal classification. It has been created to protect "turfs" from other practitioners. While this may serve the legal profession and legislators well, it does immeasurable harm to the sick and suffering and to the progress of the healing arts in general. For example, a chronic dental abscess can produce a liver problem but the dentist, who would be the most likely practitioner to identify the connection, cannot legally treat the liver problem. Or a chiropractor may become aware of Pott's Disease (tuberculosis of the spine) but legally cannot care for that condition because of the scope of practice restrictions in some jurisdictions. Or a naturopath who identifies the need for an episiotomy during childbirth is legally prevented from performing this procedure by the medical practices act.

The point is that it is scientifically impossible to dissect the parts and functions in a bio-dynamic living being and send them to specialists as we do with auto parts. The carburetor goes to one individual's work bench, the starter motor to another, the pistons to yet another location to be ground and then these parts are reassembled into a functional whole. The concept of specialists is completely foreign to all forms of medicine except allopathy. In the vast majority of the world's healing arts, one cannot be a scientific healer of a part of a bio-dynamically whole being. Therefore, specialists and/or licenses for healing the separate parts of the body is illogical. Chiropractors cannot scientifically  be restricted to the spine, nor dentists to the mouth, optometrists to the eyes, podiatrists to the feet, neurologists to the nerves, cardiologists to the heart, etc.

# SCOPE OF AGENTS

The scope of healing agents also teaches the same vital lesson. A drug, a phytotherapeutic agent, an adjustment, a psychological evaluation, a surgery, massage, acupuncture or hypnosis affects far more than just angina, or the kidney, the spine, the psyche, the arthritic hip, spasms of muscles, the organ after which the meridian is named, the subconscious and so on. **Every agent of care must be evaluated for its total effect upon the living being.** Ignorance of this fact is the major cause of iatrogenic dis-ease. **There is no form of health care that does not, to a greater or lesser degree, affect every aspect of the total living being.** To believe otherwise is to be out of touch with the reality of our inseparably interconnected universe.

# UNIVERSAL LAWS

The basic principle of this text is that the various forms of health care are for all practical purposes utilizing the same principles of healing by different names and from different perspectives.

# THE LEGAL STANDARD

In our legal system, truth is established by the testimony of two or more witnesses, never upon the testimony of a single witness. The testimony is even more desirable and certain when these corroborating witnesses have never  had interaction with each other. Such a standard has been established in this text.

To illustrate, African Medicine arose in cultures different from all others and in most cases without a written language from the dawn of time until the present. The Ayurvedic system of healing originated at approximately 2,000 B.C. on the Sanskrit-speaking and writing Indian sub-continent. Chiropractic was formulated in the English-speaking American mid-west in 1895 A.D. Homeopathy originated in the late 1790s A.D. in the Germanic-speaking portion of Europe and Native American and Oceanic Medicine was born in the western hemisphere among peoples who spoke hundreds, if not thousands, of different and often unrelated languages from antiquity to modern times and who either lacked a written language or wrote in hieroglyphics. Oriental  Medicine emerged in the Chinese-speaking and Kanji-writing portion of Asia and Sufi Medicine in the Arabic-speaking and writing Middle East in 400 A.D. Yet, as our text has documented, to an amazing extent these systems all have the same basic principles.

This is in spite of widely-dispersed time frames, a variety of cultures, diverse and totally unrelated forms of spoken and written languages, and  geographic dispersion under circumstances when transportation and communications over the vast distances involved were non-existent or primitive at best. Therefore, we have been able to establish precisely the legally acceptable criteria that we set forth earlier in this chapter. **The laws of healing are indeed universal in their nature even though their application may vary.**

# BOOK IV
# SENIOR TEXT

# INTRODUCTION TO THE SENIOR TEXT

*"O God, give us serenity to accept
what cannot be changed, courage to change what
should be changed and wisdom to distinguish
the one from the other."*

— Reinhold Niebuhr

## THE LIGHT AT THE END OF THE TUNNEL

You are now within reach of the goal that you have sacrificed so much to achieve. If you have mastered the universal laws of healing contained in this text, you have been forever changed. What more, then, could there possibly be to deal with? Herein lies another essential truth. Truth always leads to more truth. It is a grand and eternal round. We will never arrive at a point where we can rest on our laurels. To do so would be to slide backwards and lose what we have. It would make a mockery our entire effort to this point.

As you near the end of your formally outlined educational curriculum, you deserve a well-earned rest. But be wary of resting too long for it can become a degenerating habit. In reality, your true education as a healer is just beginning. As you begin working with actual patients rather than learning from textbook assumptions and ideal classroom situations, you will find that many of the procedures that were supposed to work simply don't. And things that you have been told don't work, in certain situations do.

As a progressive healer, you will likely become frustrated when you find that many of your professional organizations are far behind in their understanding of the true potential of your profession. Many seem frozen with fear. Members seem to prefer the mediocrity of marginal acceptance and status quo to advancing the principles of true health care. You will likely find that you have little in common with less progressive colleagues since they quite simply cannot comprehend what you are talking because they lack a functional understanding of the universal laws of healing. It is well said, "The higher, the fewer." You, as a progressive, vitalistic, quantum practitioner are about to learn firsthand the significance of that statement in your personal and professional life.

Rather than allowing any shuns from your fellow practitioners to

discourage you, be thankful that you have the knowledge to lead your profession and educate  as many as are willing to listen. As for the rest, hope that some day they will be willing to bring their minds and lives into compliance with universal law but don't wait around for them. If Columbus had waited for everyone to be ready for the exploration of the western ocean, many of us would still, 500 years later, be sitting on the docks in Spain.

Be valiant to yourself, to truth, and to trying to understand your place in the grand scheme of things. This is the ultimate benchmark of greatness. Each of you must now decide if that is what you want and are ready to pay the price for it.

# Chapter 29
# WHAT DOES THE FUTURE HOLD?

*"To come forth into the light of things,*
*let nature be your teacher."*

— Wadsworth

## FREE LICENSE

The future provides a freedom not enjoyed in the previous chapters of this text have not enjoyed. In discussing the past, one needs to be certain that the data is consistent with history. In the discussion of present practices, the text must correlate with current knowledge. But the future is free for pure speculation and the discussion of healing need not be bound by facts; indeed, this would be counterproductive. The mind must not only be free but encouraged to fantasize. Such freedom frequently proves to be a major and frightening challenge to the disciplined scientific mind. Scientists are so accustomed to having their minds conform to parameters of factual restraints that they tend to feel naked and vulnerable outside of that familiar framework. Yet it is this very training that must be, temporarily, abandoned if scientists are also to be philosophers.

## WHAT IS PHILOSOPHY

First, however, it is necessary to clearly understand the purpose of philosophy. Philosophy is an attempt, a guess, or a hypothesis to explain something about which we have inadequate or no knowledge. As we develop our data base and begin to apply the knowledge in a consistent clinical manner, philosophy progresses to the art form. When we can apply this knowledge consistently time after time, we have entered the realm of science. Therefore, science and philosophy are the polar opposites of each other. Universal Laws dictate that **more of one means less of the other.** To teach precisely the same philosophy as the Nei-jing, Punarvasu Atreya, Hippocrates, Lindlahr, Palmer or Hahnemann is to admit that there has been no progress made toward science. Thus, as our science develops we must develop new philosophical questions and new answers for those questions.

## THE SAGES

Does this mean that we do not revere the sages? Exactly the opposite is true. We revere and try to emulate their most sterling quality, the pioneer spirit that led them to philosophize in the first place. This is what allowed them to advance with such giant strides beyond their contemporaries, to be of even greater service to humanity and to become immortal in the annals of healing.

## STAR TREK

The theme of the Star Trek televison series is to "boldly go where no one has gone before." This is the true purpose of philosophy, to boldly explore new possibilities, regardless of how abstract they may seem to be.

## THE LAW OF PRIME

Quantum (energy) force is the medium through which healing takes place. If there is a force, then logic dictates there must be a generator of that force. That is a universal unchangeable law. Within chiropractic, this generating entity is called "Universal Intelligence"; in homeopathy, "Vital Force"; in oriental medicine, "Ch'i". In theology, it is referred to as "God". In pure science, it is labeled "The Prime". Regardless of what they  call it, all of the above disciplines attest to its existence. It would therefore seem reasonable that in the future, healing will be forced to become more and more associated with, to understand and to model this prime entity. This undoubtedly is why in so-called "primitive" cultures healing is so closely equated with deity. In reality, these so-called "primitive" cultures, and forms of healing may be far more "scientific" from a quantum perspective than solid state western forms of health care.

## SCIENCE OF THE FUTURE?

Should this be true, in the final analysis, the ability to be a great healer may center around how we conform not only to the irrevocable prime laws in our professional practice but even more importantly, in our private lives. As horrifying as it may sound to the old school philosopher, scientist or academician, it is conceivable that theology could be the ultimate science of the future.

## EXTREMES OF HEALING PHILOSOPHY

In an effort to assist our scientifically trained and restricted minds become more flexible and comfortable in the unrestrained world of philosophy, let us postulate the ultimate example. If we stretch our philosophy to the very outer limits of our imaginations, what might be some of the characteristics and results of such an ultimate healing science? Such an exercise will make less radical philosophical concepts seem well within the range of practical possibilities. This approach is critical because, to borrow a phrase, "Without vision, my people perish." To state it yet another way, "If it is imaginable, it is attainable." Maybe not in our lifetimes, or even a hundred lifetimes, but sometime, somewhere, in the vast expanse of our existence as a race, it is achievable.

Healing could conceivably progress to the point where solid state forms, and even our current solid state research methods, could be totally outdated by energy applications if our technology were focused on the quantum energetic nature of individuals. This could provide us with the tools to make the quantum leap from where we are to where we can go.

The development of some type of full body quantum energy scanner is moving closer and closer to becoming a reality. Just as thermograph reads and interprets the infrared signature of the body, and just as the SQID (pronounced Squid) can read the magnetic field of an object, so too could a scanning system capable of detecting the rest of the energy spectrum being produced by a living person be developed.

We would have to take the time and trouble to learn what the various energy signatures from the body mean. This could only be done by clinically correlating and verifying thousands of cases. Just as thermograph can be highly accurate in finding a Peripheral Nerve Entrapment Syndrome, so could scanning equipment be programmed to recognize cancer, MS, or even a common cold in any of its stages or manifestations.

## THE QUANTUM FIELD SCANNER

The forward thinking individual would recognize the monumental nature of this task. It would indeed take years of work and huge numbers of dollars to accomplish. The outcome, though, would be worthwhile. Inappropriate or unnecessary testing (blood, colon scopes, MRIs, CT scans) would be eliminated. Doctors would not be ordering tests from a sincere fear of missing something or from a greedy desire to make more money. Considering how rampant fear and greed are in the medicine today, the "investment" in a whole quantum field diagnostic scanning system would be returned within a relatively few years.

Primary efforts would be put into developing accurate diagnoses. This would please the 200,000 patients who would otherwise die each year due to unnecessary surgery as well as those millions suffering from iatrogenic dis-ease. At this stage, the treatment modalities would be conventional medical, chiropractic, ayurvedic, acupuncture, homeopathy or naturopathic techniques. As revolutionary as the whole quantum field scanning equipment would be to patient care, it would significantly impact treatment. Since fewer than 20 percent of all medical modalities have proven to be effective, treatment regimens could be rendered that would improve the patient's quantum field energies with the knowledge that this improvement will show up in the physical body eventually.

Think of how streamlined each profession would become. We could shed those techniques, concepts, teachings and dogma that have plagued us and we could focus on what works! We could disallow all the other unsuccessful or partially successful approaches; they would go the route of the germ theory and of bleeding patients to get rid of the "bad humors" in their bodies. Think of all the tonsils, gall bladders and uteruses that will be saved. We will finally learn that we cannot make a person whole by removing his/her vital parts.

## TRUE HEALTH

With these two revolutionary approaches in place, patients will get well and stay well. Society can change its standards to emphasize maintaining  individual health instead of treatment of dis-ease. No longer will the illogical practice of babies being fed soy-based formulas fortified with only 10 or 15 vitamins and minerals be continued while our pets are given food that contains 40 to 50 nutrient supplements. Prenatal formulas won't come from pharmaceutical houses looking for future business; society will insure that we do what works because anything less will be failure and perhaps even a crime. Prenatal care will be designed to maximize the genetic potential of each individual.

Birth defects will not occur and the average IQ of the general population will rise steadily until everyone functions at the level we now consider "genius". We could measure the effects of food, additives, chemicals, TV programming, music, lighting, medications, religion, nutrition, adjustments, acupuncture, phytotherapeutic agents, and many other variables on the quantum energy economy. Why would we choose to use anything that did not improve us or raise us to new levels? This is all within our grasp!

## QUANTUM FIELD HEALTH CARE

Eventually, we will be able to improve all of our care methods. Instead of trying to affect the quantum level indirectly by treating the physical body, we will learn to access it directly. Diagnosis and treatment could be done in one facility. With the ever-increasing speed of computers, millions of pieces of data could be obtained, matched with thousands of known dis-ease patterns and corrected with modalities allowing the quantum field to be balanced within moments.

## ANTI-VIRAL PROGRAMS

Consider the anti-viral program used to debug a computer. Imagine running an anti-viral program on a patient's quantum energy field and neutralizing mononucleosis, herpes, and other conditions. Initially, patients probably would need to do this fairly frequently, perhaps monthly, but as greater levels of health permeated all individuals and all levels of society, they might only need the care once or twice a year.

We would be able to eliminate the "heroic" measures used in allopathic medicine to save lives. Gone would be surgery except for accidents and traumas; no radiation or chemotherapy would be needed. There would not be a need for root canals or restorative dentistry since we'll have a race of healthy people. Specialists would be retrained to become Quantum Physicians (QPs) and could start to truly help patients at every level of each patient's total being.

It is obvious, then, that all the "hidden agendas" of huge companies, governments, cartels, monopolies and other established groups would not be able to continue manipulating the world's population for gain because we would be able to monitor the short- and long-term effects of virtually everything including the effects upon our quantum energy levels.

Taking this one step further, imagine how efficiently we could "test" a potential therapy. While in a quantum field scanner, the practitioner could administer a new therapy, see what patterns manifest, develop a match for the disrupted energy pattern in the computer and the testing would be complete. We would know when to use what therapy, for what duration, exactly when to change it, when to discontinue it and when to pronounce the patient truly well.

## THE FINAL STEP

The final stage will be to outgrow the need for this technology. Healers would be trained to do the same thing for us intuitively while returning the emphasis and responsibility for health and proper living to the individual. Until then, the dynamic adjustment, the specific acupuncture treatment, the correct homeopathic or phytotherapeutic agent will be necessary but temporary crutches to be used until healing reaches the higher planes of understanding by applying the quantum laws of healing.

Once trained a practitioner could visualize the energy template of Lycopodium, Kali Carbonicum, Hypericum or any other remedy and project the healing energy pattern into the patient's being. A quantum chiropractor could  visualize the total holographic QPNIMT subluxation complex and conceptualize an adjustment returning the complex to its normal juxtaposition and proper QPNIMT function.

Or an acupuncturist could envision energy being adjusted at the indicated acupuncture point to correct the imbalance.

For the sake of discussion, if such healers could be developed, they would have to be of the caliber and nature of the prime itself. Is such a transformation possible? "Yes" seems to be the tenet of religion while "No" seems to be the answer of solid state science. "Likely" is the quantum science answer.

## INCORRECT APPROACH

If the above points are theoretically correct, then almost all current solid state research is counterproductive. All disciplines within complementary healing seem to be presently scrambling to "prove" themselves according to the solid state "research principles" of reductionism. Yet, the issues we are discussing are quantum in nature. One cannot become the leading authority on apples by studying oranges. **If quantum healing is indeed the future of healing, then the greater portion of future research must be oriented toward the quantum components of healing.**

Assuming, again for the sake of discussion, that the above is correct, then the healers of the future will also have to guard this energy from being drained or interfered with by adverse influences **for without the non-corporal or energy component, the quantum healer is helpless.** This no doubt will require significant changes in the life style of many, if not all, healers to insure that they remain in tune with the prime force.

Additionally, this may mean that therapies such as Counseling, Hypnosis, Ch'i (Qi) Gong, Heliotherapy, Radionics, Chromotherapy, as well as some others, may be purer quantum forms of healing and, thereby, may supersede the cruder physical forms.

## UNBELIEVABLE

Granted, these concepts seem to border on the impossible. But what would our ancestors from the middle ages have thought of central heating, running water, bathrooms, air conditioning, airplanes, super tankers, railroads, freeways, computers, atomic energy, electricity, plastics, radios, telephones, synthetic fabrics, organ transplants, men walking on the moon, X-rays, ICBM missiles, radar, infra-red night vision, lasers, microwaves, homeopathic remedies, life support systems, test tube babies or cloning? The only thing that makes our projection of futuristic philosophy fantastic is that we do not yet understand the technology necessary to make it commonplace.

## PHILOSOPHER OR HISTORIAN?

Philosophy is intended to be the leading edge of our professions, not the shackles that hold us in place. **Philosophy's true destiny is to lead us to new goals and unexplored visions.** Philosophy is the one dome under which the scientifically trained are allowed and encouraged to abandon scientific restraints and proofs. To simply teach what our professional progenitors philosophized about is in reality to be a historian and not a philosopher at all.

Obviously, this approach is critical for those who have never been exposed to basic principles. But to be teaching the same principles at the post-graduate level is to admit that nothing new has been conceived and that no progress has been made.

# DANGER

On the other hand, there is also a major pitfall in philosophy. The ancient Greeks became so fond of conceiving and debating new ways of thinking that no one wanted to work. This proved to be a major factor in their downfall. As D. D. Palmer said, "Too much or too little is dis-ease." Philosophy for philosophy's sake is not the goal. **The goal is the advancement of the human race.** Therefore, the goal of philosophy is to move closer and closer to ultimate truths. In order to achieve this, it is necessary to abandon any and all untruths and modify partial truths. **It can, therefore, be said that one of philosophy's purposes it to keep us a little off balance, humble, teachable, and open-minded. A philosophy that is too comfortable is ancient history and not philosophy at all.**

# Chapter 30
# THE ECLECTIC REALITY OF HEALTH CARE

*"Nature knows no trifling; she is always sincere,*
*always serious, always stern; she is always in*
*the right, and the errors and mistakes*
*are invariably ours."*

— Goethe

## ALL IS CONSTANT, ALL IS CHANGE?

There is an old adage that says the only things you can count on are death, taxes and change. The conflict between man's longing for a constant world and the reality that the world is in constant change is as old as the race. The Egyptians, the Chinese, and Ayurvedics, by 2,000 B.C., were discussing this principle. By 500 B.C., the Greeks debated it in attempts to explain God, spirit (non-corporal or anti-matter), matter and the human condition: either all was one (constant) or all was change.

Today, quantum mechanics and physics accepts the premise that the universe is in constant flux, expanding and changing moment by moment. Yet, there is structure and order to this constant change. Each moment of flux is in direct proportion to the moment prior to it and the response is always the most desirable one. This observation leads to the conclusion that universal intelligence/prime does not allow for random change but, rather, requires order. Therefore, everything that exists in our fluxing universe is required to react to these changes. This response is the universal principle known as: adaptation. **For anything to continue to survive, it must adapt.**

The problem is, can we adapt fast enough to survive in our modern polluted world? In Figure 30.1 R. L Wysong, B.S., D.V.M., illustrates we that our organisms have adjusted to a natural unpolluted environment for a time frame which is 16.5 million times longer than the sudden deluge of demands being made on it in today's polluting society. The current mode of sickness care which refuses to address the miasma, diathesis, phase, dosha of dis-ease cannot accomplish such a dramatic task. Only by dealing with the basic miasma, diathesis, dosha, phase (genetic) weakness can we allow the Innate Intelligence to successfully make such dramatic adaptations is such a short time frame. To do less is to allow the human race to commit genocide.

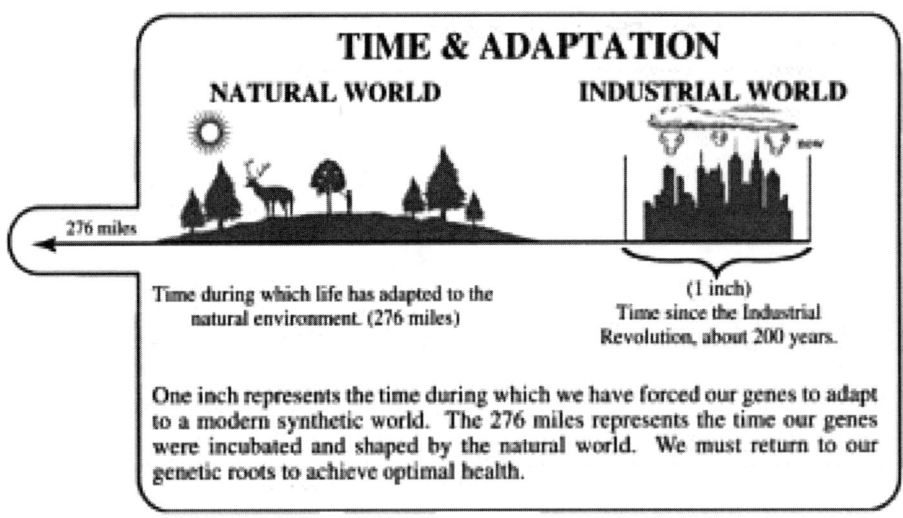


*Figure 30.1 — Pollution, Time And Adaptation*

## THE UNIVERSAL LAW

R. W. Stevenson, D.C., Ph.C., in writing of this universal principle, said "Adaptation is a continuous process. . . It is never constant and unvarying as are other universal laws. Adaptation is a universal principle - the only one of its kind. It is the principle of change; unlimited; everywhere present; embracing a wide range of subjects, used for or among all; unrestricted in application, adapting to all." He continues, "Adaptation is the intellectual ability that an organism possesses of responding to all forces which come to it, whether Innate or Universal. All organisms have the benefit of Intellectual Adaptation. If they did not, they could not be alive. . . ." Since change is a universal law, all things must conform to it including our thinking or philosophy,;if not, our professions are dying.

## LAW OF PHYSIS

Physis (Greek for "nature" or "natural balance") is the root from which the word "physician" is derived. Remove man and the universal laws of physis (nature) will return the planet to its pristine state. Remove the interference in dis-ease and it does the same for the individual.

**Thus the duty of the physician, as discussed in the Freshman text, is to restore health rapidly, gently, permanently (by establishing physis or the self-healing mechanism); to remove and destroy the whole dis-ease in the shortest, surest, least harmful way, according to clearly defined and comprehendible principles (laws).** But to stop here is to leave the job only half done!

**Once physis is achieved the healer must cease being the physician (facilitator) and become the doctor (Latin for teacher). To continue to unwisely facilitate would produce dis-ease. The patient must now be taught a life style conducive to maintaining physis. Not to do so would be to allow the patient to become dis-eased once again.**

# QUANTUM VECTORS

Dozens of articles and texts have been published on quantum non-neural communications in the living being but many of our professions have failed to make provisions for it within our philosophies. Einstein said, **"It is possible there exist human emanations that are still unknown to us. . . . The knowledge about man is still in its infancy."** We used to believe if we knew one thing and then another, then we knew two things, because one and one are two. We are now discovering that we must learn more about the "and". In western reductionistic medicine, we believe if we know pathology and anatomy, then we know healing. We are now discovering that we must learn more about the subtle num, kundalini, innate, vital, ch'i, life and universal forces, the "and".

W. Tiller, Ph.D., of Stanford University's Material Sciences and Engineering Department, states, **"By subtle fields of energies. . . . I do not mean weak fields or energies. . . .The subtle fields are normally only very weakly coupled to our physical fields so we generally see only small effects. However, under a favorable set of circumstances, they can be strongly coupled and then massive effects are possible."** (Such as changes in health.)

Tiller continues "Future technologies in this area will reveal energy content and utilization of such fields that are many orders of magnitude larger than that due to any of our presently known physical fields." Again, "Subtle energies are real energies that are not directly observable because they function at the level of. . . negative energy. . . . They can be converted to observable in our present human condition only via an intermediate transducer. Today these transducers are primarily living systems. . . . One known potential, the magnetic vector potential, appears to play the role of 'bridge' between the subtle, unobservable energies and physically observable energies associated with electric and magnetic fields."

We are familiar with biological vectors but few comprehend the mathematical vector, "A complex entity representative of a directed magnitude, as of a force or velocity, and represented by a system of equal and parallel segments." In chronic dis-ease vectors have a compounding effect. See Figure 30.2.

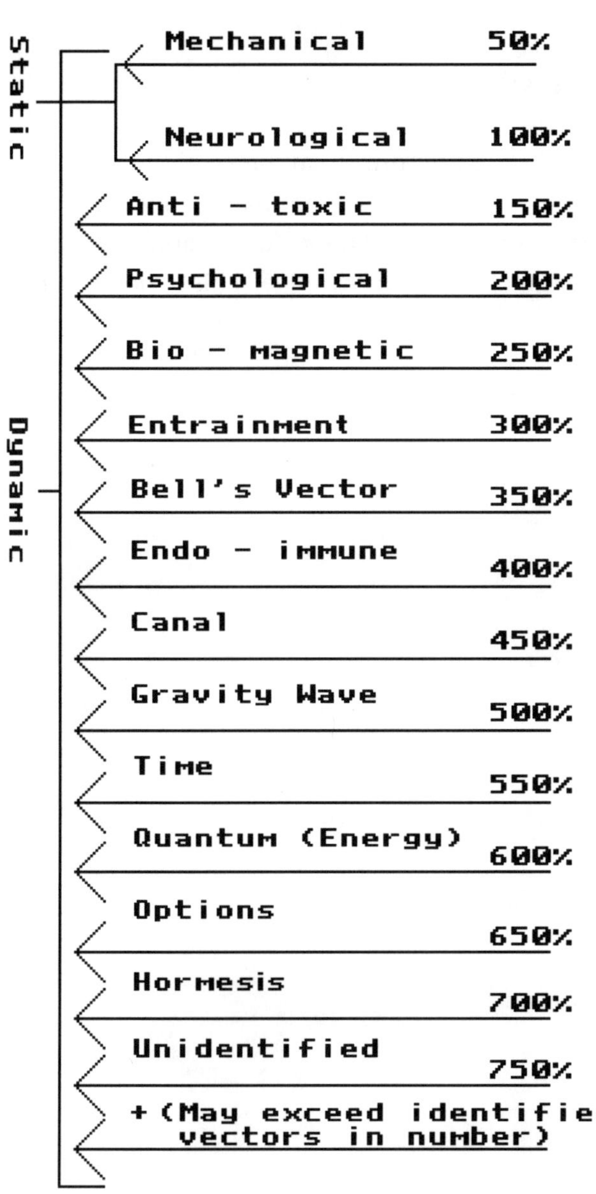


*Figure 30.2*

Allopathic medicine is the only medical system which has ever existed that does not have a vitalistic, expansionistic approach to illness and health and does not contain any concept of biological energy.

D. D. Palmer also discussed this, **"We are surrounded with an aura; that we pass from our bodies a subtle, invisible substance known as magnetism; that this emanation may be either repellent or attractive. . . heat, magnetism, odor and no doubt other unseen forces emanate from our bodies in all directions. . . .There is an emanation from us, not magical or miraculous, but subtle, invisible substance, capable of perception..."** H. Lindlahr, M.D., adds, ". . .The  physical body should be looked upon as something which is part of a much larger whole. . . the physical body is subject to the influence of energies which are brought to bear on it and flow into it both from these other bodies and from outside."

# DUALITY OF REALITY

Science of the 19th and early 20th Centuries was based upon the erroneous Newtonian assumption that everything could be explained in mechano-chemical terms. This remains a pillar of non-vitalistic, reductionistic medicine and has tainted the quantum healing arts too. This is troubling because the basic premise of all natural healing arts, that living entities have the innate ability to heal themselves, is quantum in nature.

# THE QUANTUM LEAP

More has been learned about the num, kundalini, vital, innate, ch'i, life, universal forces of life in the past twenty years than in all previous history; unfortunately, the natural healing arts are not major contributors to this learning. As we study the works of Oriental, Sufi, Ayurvedic, Chiropractic, Native American, Naturopathic, and African healing, we find in all this num, kundalini, vital, innate, ch'i, life knowledge. This is not surprising for all true healers must draw from the universal source.

# Chapter 31
# FROM SICKNESS TO HEALTH

*"The superior doctor prevents illness;*
*the mediocre doctor cures imminent illness;*
*the inferior doctor treats illness."*
— Chinese Proverb

## RETRACING

Retracing was one of those subjects alluded to during our formal professional educations but evaded when the students addressed specific questions to the faculties regarding it. I have since come to understand this was because few, if any, of the faculty members actually understand this critical vitalistic principle. What we do not understand ourselves, we cannot teach to others.

What follows in this chapter is a refined and updated version of principles that have been published by numerous authors over the last several hundred years. They are not modified in the sense that they were incorrect in their original conclusions but, rather, clarified and further refined in order to be of more practical value. Such graphic representation cannot possibly depict every conceivable situation that could arise and, as we come to understand more and more of the quantum components of healing, the graphs will likely need further revision in order to more accurately represent what is actually taking place within the living bio-dynamic being as it heals itself.

## PARAMETERS

In order to clearly comprehend the graphs, we must visualize them as a cylinder that has been cut horizontally at the D (death) line and flattened out. See figure 31.1. The closer we move toward the H (health) line on the vertical axis, the healthier we are. The D, death line, or point of maximum dis-ease, being the polar opposite of health, is the point at which the organism can no longer sustain life. Thus, if we render excessive care, it becomes iatrogenic causing the patient to return to dis-ease. For example, an iron deficiency (Yin - too little) produces anemia, but an excess of iron (Yang - too much) is toxic.

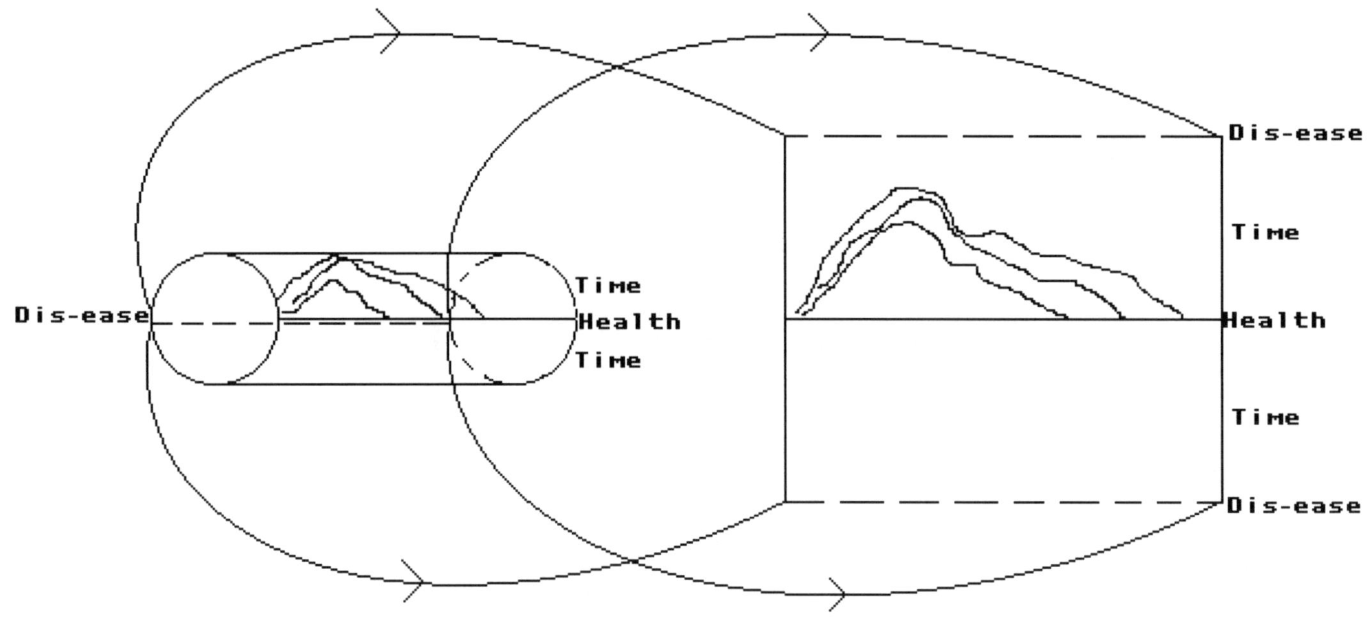


*Figure 31.1 — Origin of Retracing Graphs*

The horizontal axis equates with the passage of time since care was initiated. This is, however, not a fixed factor for the following reasons:

1 **Different therapies work at different rates of speed; some take longer than others but they all tend to follow the same general healing pattern.**

2 **Time is related to the degree of vitality of the patient's recuperative powers.** If an elderly grandmother and her six-year-old grandchild each have the same dis-ease, the child will heal far faster, as a general rule, than the grandmother. **The critical factor is for the healer to clearly comprehend what an adequate time factor is in each individual case.**

3 **The living being is bio-dynamic, meaning that it fluctuates constantly within acceptable limits. Evaluating a patient on the basis of a fixed time frame can result in false conclusions.** For example, a hectic schedule for several days, a lack of sleep, poor eating, and high levels of stress can result in an energy level deterioration which retards healing but which has little or nothing to do with the appropriateness of the care being rendered. In such instances, a longer time frame is necessary in order to arrive at a true picture of the patient's innate recuperative powers.

It should also be clearly understood that specific factors such as sexual desires, appetite, body temperature, etc. can be tracked on these graphs. The sexual desire is the mechanism used to pass num, kundalini, innate, vital, ch'i, life force on to future generations. If a person with no sexual interests experiences increasing sexual desires during illness, it can be a valid indication that healing is taking place. Other examples that could be graphed are the status of the auto-immune and central nervous systems and the acupuncture meridians involved.

The lines representing the various factors being graphed are represented as constantly undulating. This depicts the fact that the living being, in sickness and in health, constantly fluctuates through a state of dynamic homeostasis. **Such routine fluctuations cannot and must not be considered as accurate overall indicators of the success or failure of a particular mode of care. Only the overall pattern can be utilized with consistent clinical success.**

## SECOND LAW OF MOTION

In physics, the Second Law Of Motion states: A body at rest tends to remain at rest, a body in motion tends to remain in motion in a straight line unless acted upon by another force not parallel to its course or opposed to it. When we say a case retraces in the reverse order of its original development we are talking about the textbook ideal. Search as you may, you will likely not find the ideal but what you will find are case after case that approaches the ideal. In reality, there are forces interacting with retracing that will cause minor variances, just as in the Second Law Of Motion, but the inborn intelligence of the living being is able, in short order, to compensate and return to its predetermined course of regaining health.

There is no guarantee, given the ever-changing environmental conditions, accidents, emotional upheavals, dietary and sleep indiscretions and other influences, that the same combination of circumstances will continue to exist that existed when the case was first evaluated. Hence, no exact mathematical reversal of the steps is consistently possible. Cases must constantly be re-evaluated and the care being rendered adjusted to present circumstances in order to avoid depletion of the num, kundalini, innate, vital, ch'i, vital force.

Lastly, healing requires energy. The body also requires energy to run its normal daily functions. If there is not enough energy to do both, the innate wisdom of the being will temporarily turn off the healing process and the healing line(s) on the graph will flux away from the H line.

It is also necessary to understand that the portion of the graph above the H line can be a mirror image reflecting the area below the H line. Nothing has changed. Moving closer to the H line still represents a movement toward health and movement away from the H line, a movement toward dis-ease.

## WHY BOTHER?

Some may ask why bother with these graphs when access to laboratory facilities, X-rays, EKGs, EEGs, MRIs, CTs is available. First, if these are your thoughts, then you have totally missed the "Big Idea" of this entire text. Secondly, many complementary practitioners are denied use of the above-mentioned facilities because of professional bigotry, prejudice and discrimination. Third, such knowledge will serve you well in emergency situations, house calls, after-hours appointments, and other non-routine situations.

The following provides an example of how such knowledge will stand the healer in good stead. A patient is delirious, running a 104F degree fever, has diarrhea, wakes frequently and has a chronic candida infection of the intestinal tract with an elevated white blood count. Within twenty minutes of care being administered, the patient is lucid, the fever has dropped a degree- and-a-half and the patient then falls into a deep sleep. There has not been time for the white blood count to change so a laboratory test at this point would essentially be worthless. But if the practitioner understands Hering's Law and what each graph is illustrating, he can be confident that the care has already triggered the patient's self-healing mechanisms.

The following graphs are examples of the patient's response to treatment.

# RESPONSE 1

## IDEAL RESPONSE TO CARE

GRAPH:

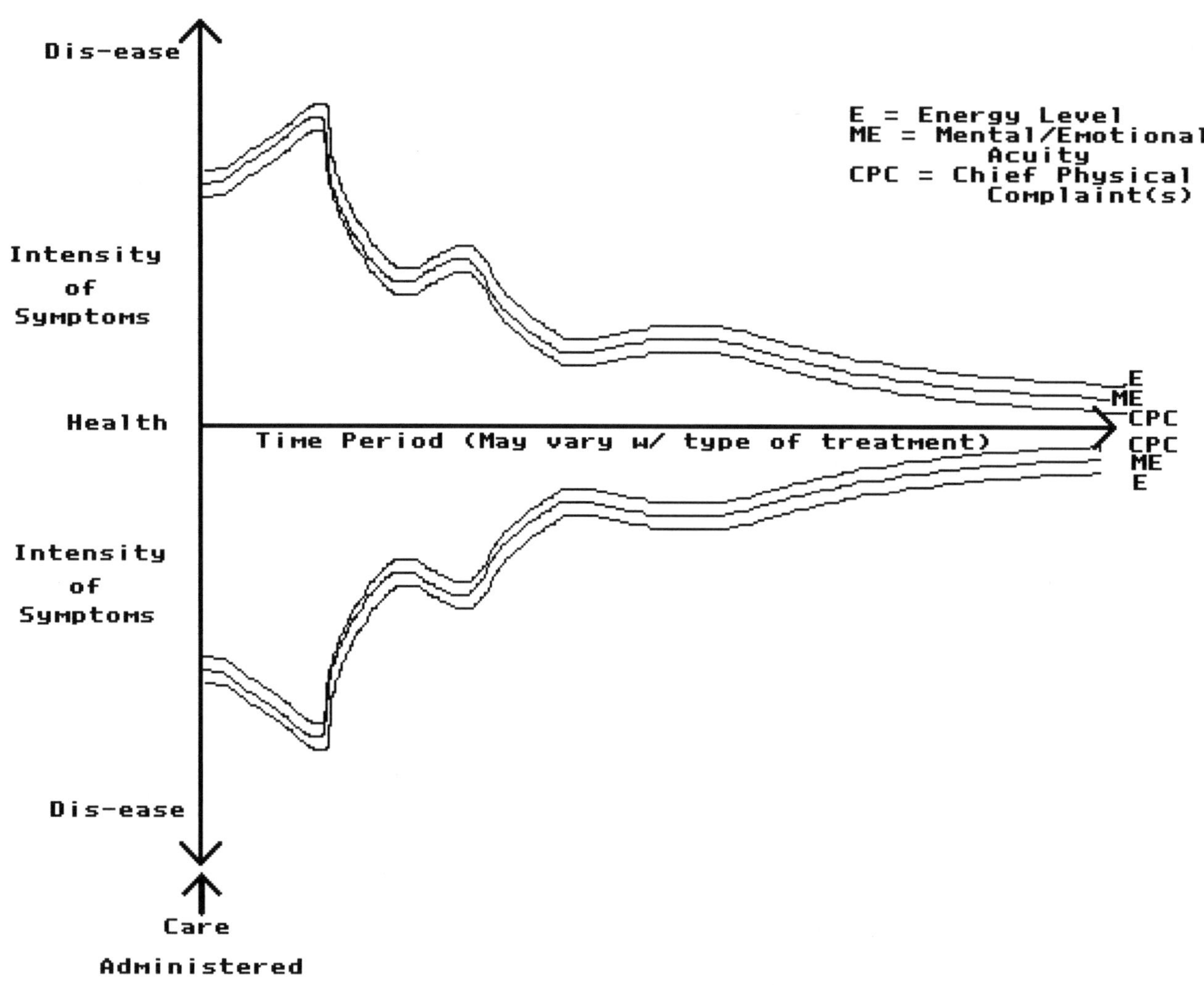


*Figure 31.2*

PATIENT COMMENTS: "I feel much better!"

TECHNICAL COMMENTS: There was a temporary aggravation indicating that the body's defense mechanism had been activated. **The dis-ease is primarily focused at the functional (nervous system) level with very little or no other organic or tissue pathology.** The effect of this correctly chosen and administered care is long lasting, meaning that it may be months or possibly even years before care might again be necessary.

Note that the lower half of the graph represents the mirror image of the upper half. This relationship is true of all of the graphs in this chapter but in order to keep the subsequent graphs as uncluttered as possible, the lower portion will be deleted. The student should ,however, keep in mind the lower configuration at all times.

PROGNOSIS: **The case has been handled correctly and the patient is in the self-healing mode.** Any additional care could be counter-productive causing the individual to become sick again.

# RESPONSE 2

## IDEAL

GRAPH:

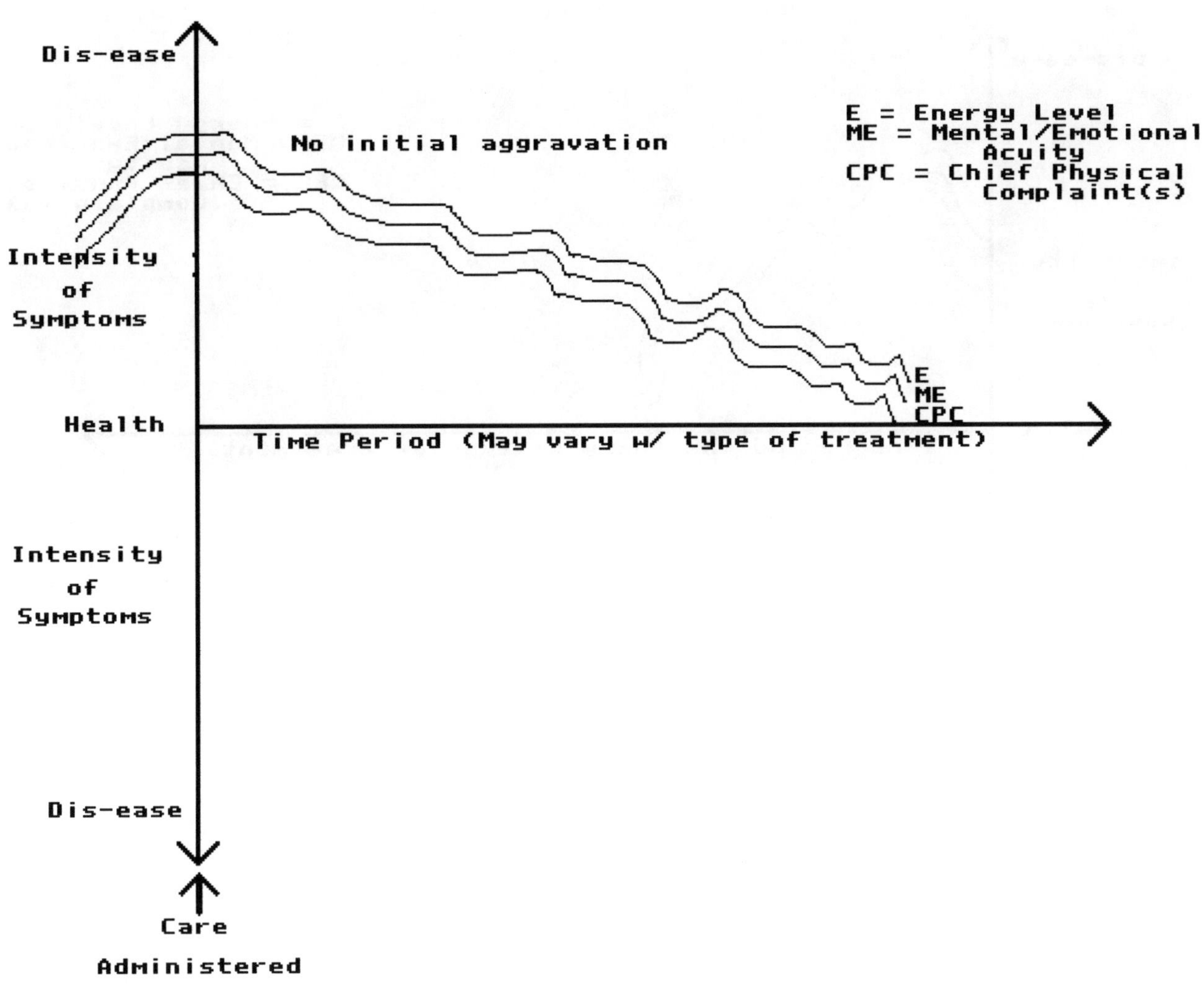


*Figure 31.3*

See Figure 31.4

PATIENT COMMENTS: "It's like a miracle."

TECHNICAL COMMENTS: The care rendered is perfectly matched to the patient's needs. The patient's symptoms were already aggravated to the maximum degree possible prior to the administration of care (as represented by the lines to the left of the vertical intensity line on the graph); thus, the defense mechanism was already at its highest levels of function and no aggravation of symptoms was necessary. **The dis-ease is primarily of a nervous dysfunction and there is little or no organic or other tissue pathology. This response is therefore highly desirable and is most commonly observed in the care of acute conditions.**

PROGNOSIS: **The outlook is excellent. It is wise to wait a long time (months or even years) before rendering any additional care. Should excessive care be rendered, the response will likely follow the pattern illustrated on the bottom half of the Response 1 graph.** Remember "Too much or too little is dis-ease."

# RESPONSE 3

## WAS BETTER, NOW WORSE

GRAPH:

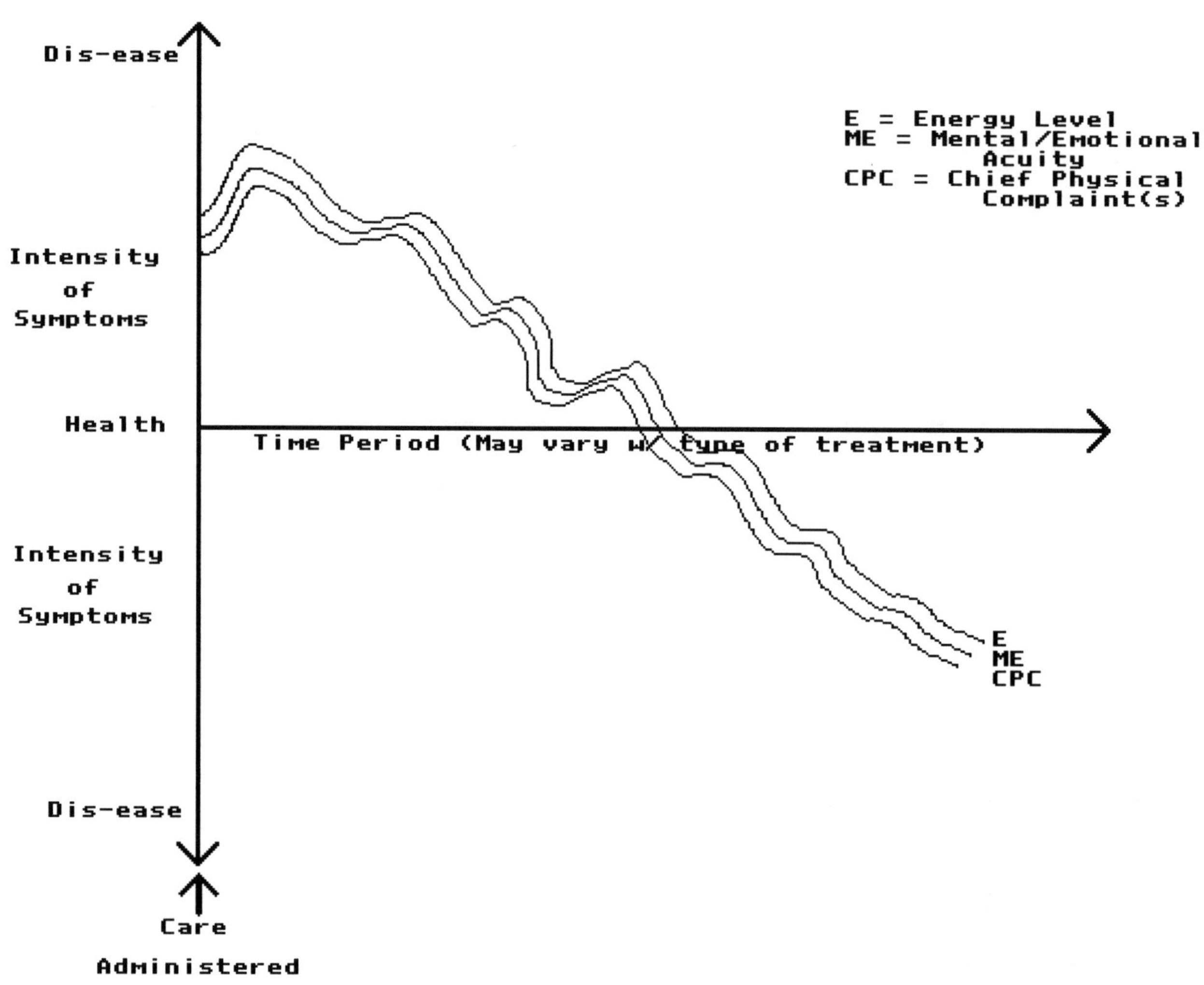


*Figure 31.4*

PATIENT COMMENTS: "I was feeling great but something went wrong. I feel just like I did when we started."

TECHNICAL COMMENTS: **The most common mistake is not knowing when to discontinue therapy. The initial response was textbook perfect but excessive therapy caused the patient to pass through health and back into dis-ease.** This mistake facilitated the dis-ease process and made it harder to resolve the original problem. If un-warranted therapy continues to be administered, the patient's dis-ease will eventually develop into an incurable condition.

This adverse response is possible in all of the following graphs. The notation "See Figure 31.4" on the lower portion of each graph is a reminder of this ever-present danger.

PROGNOSIS: Poor, if the therapy is continued; good, if therapy is discontinued at the appropriate time.

# RESPONSE 4

## MINOR SYMPTOMS SHOW NO RESPONSE

GRAPH:

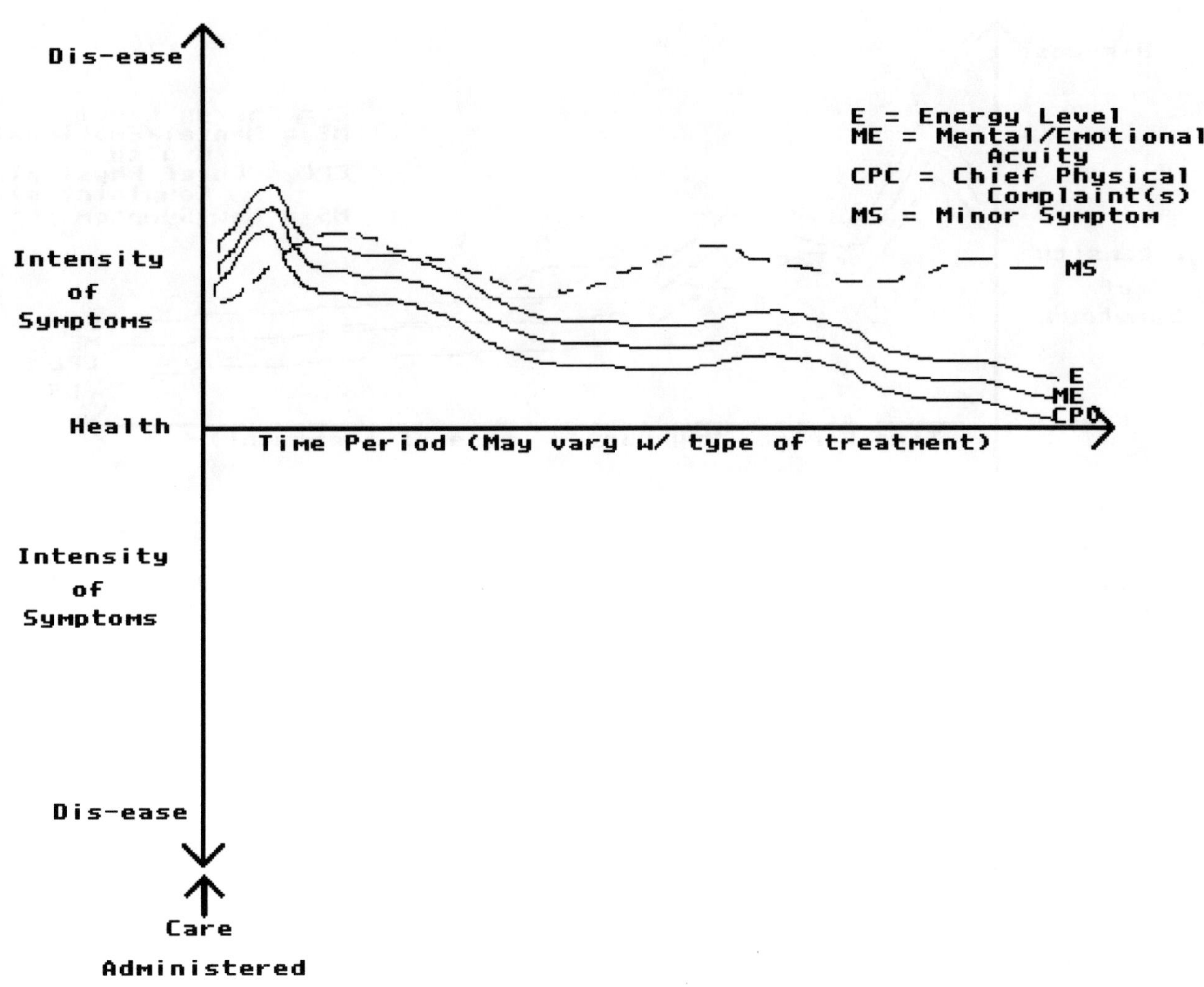


*Figure 31.5*

See Figure 31.4

PATIENT COMMENTS: "I definitely feel better but I still have a few minor problems."

TECHNICAL COMMENTS: The healing process has been activated by the care rendered. The body must be allowed to continue healing without interruption. **Perfectionism at this point will cause far more harm than good.** Rendering additional therapy will result in a Figure 31.4 response pattern developing. If minor symptoms remain for a long period of time (months), consider rendering care for those symptoms based upon their total picture at that time. As a general rule, such minor symptoms will slowly disappear.

PROGNOSIS: Very good. The healer has done his/her work successfully and **no additional care is needed** in the vast majority of cases with this response.

# RESPONSE 5

## IATROGENIC SYMPTOM CREATED

GRAPH:

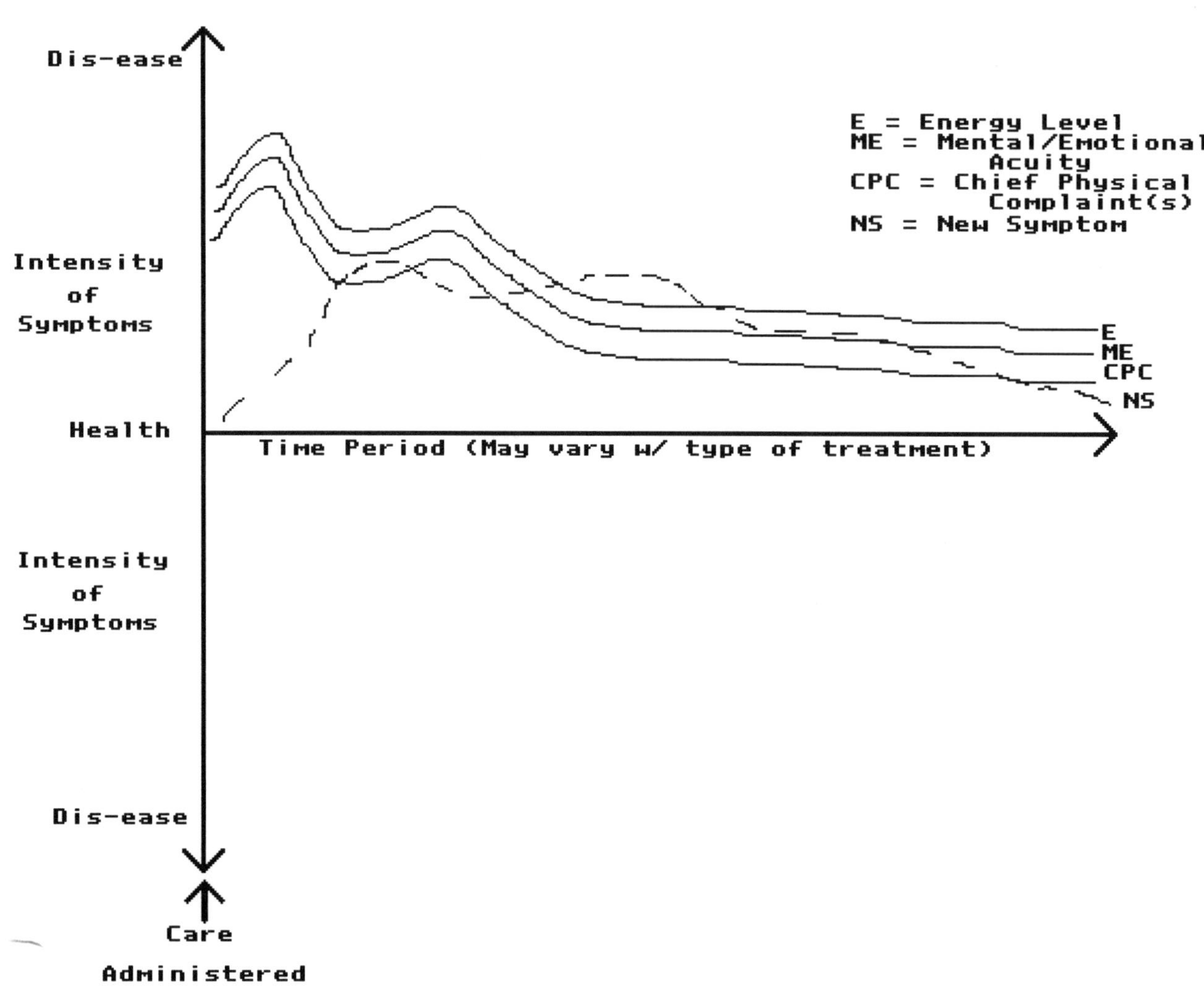


*Figure 31.6*

See Figure 31.4

PATIENT COMMENTS: "I definitely feel better but I have a new problem that I never had before."

TECHNICAL COMMENTS: This situation is commonly encountered. The healing process has been initiated. **The new symptom is consistent with correctly chosen and administered care.** The case is responding well and rendering unwarranted care would be a serious mistake and would run the risk of obliterating the progress of the case to date. **The new symptom will disappear in a few days or weeks if the healer and patient wait.** Unwarranted continuation of care at this point will cause the patient to respond in the manner represented in the Figure 31.4 graph.

PROGNOSIS: The care is correct and the patient will fully recover.

# RESPONSE 6

## MAJOR SYMPTOM IMPROVING, FEEL LIKE OLD SELF

GRAPH:

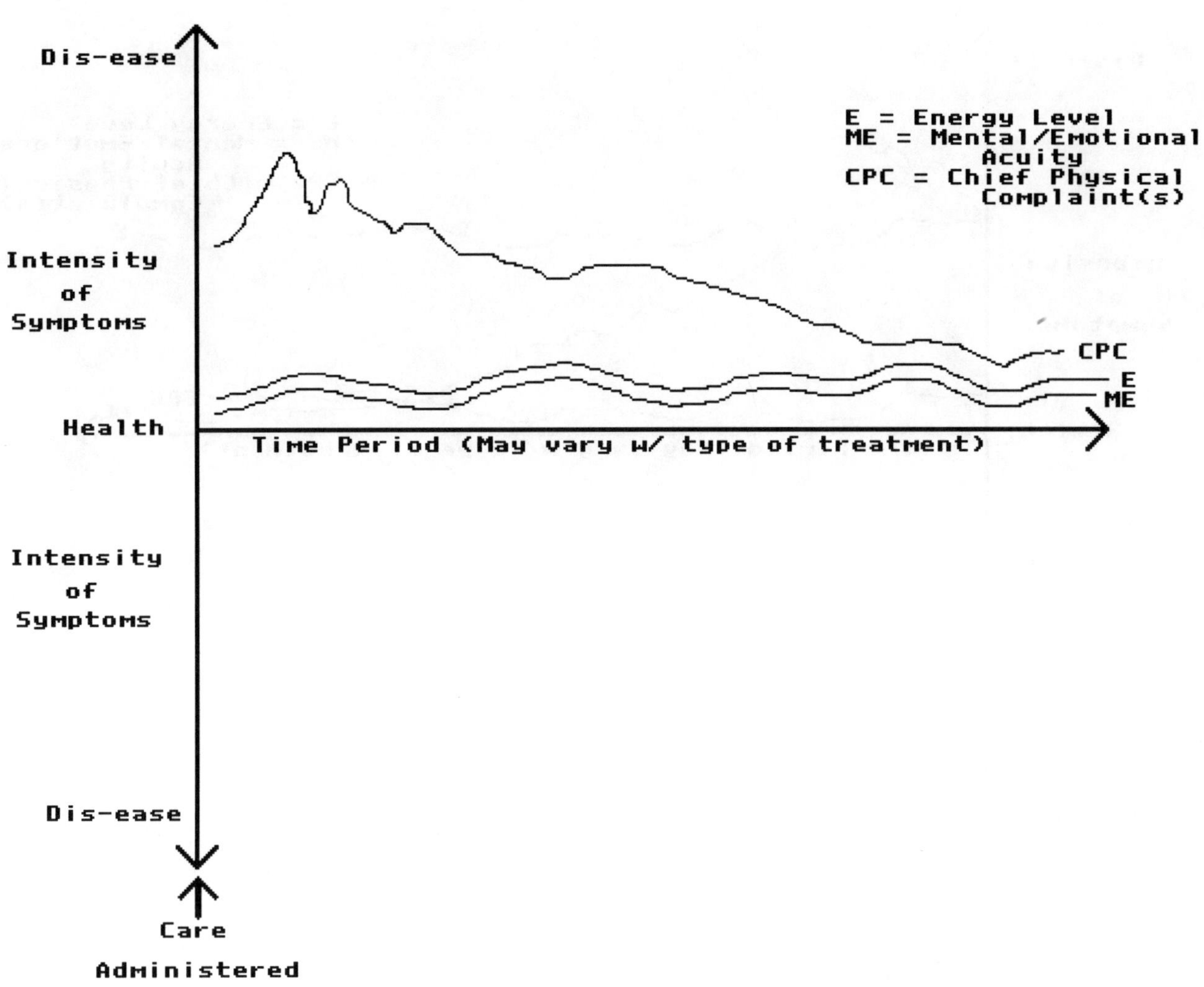


*Figure 31.7*

See Figure 31.4

PATIENT COMMENTS: "I am just like my old self."

TECHNICAL COMMENTS: **This pattern indicates that there were no adverse changes in the energy or emotional states.** This usually is a problem of relatively short duration and it has not had time to affect the deeper mental/emotional and energy levels of the patient's total being.

PROGNOSIS: Excellent. **Wait patiently.**

# RESPONSE 7

## MAJOR SYMPTOM IMPROVED, BUT STILL DON'T FEEL LIKE OLD SELF

GRAPH:

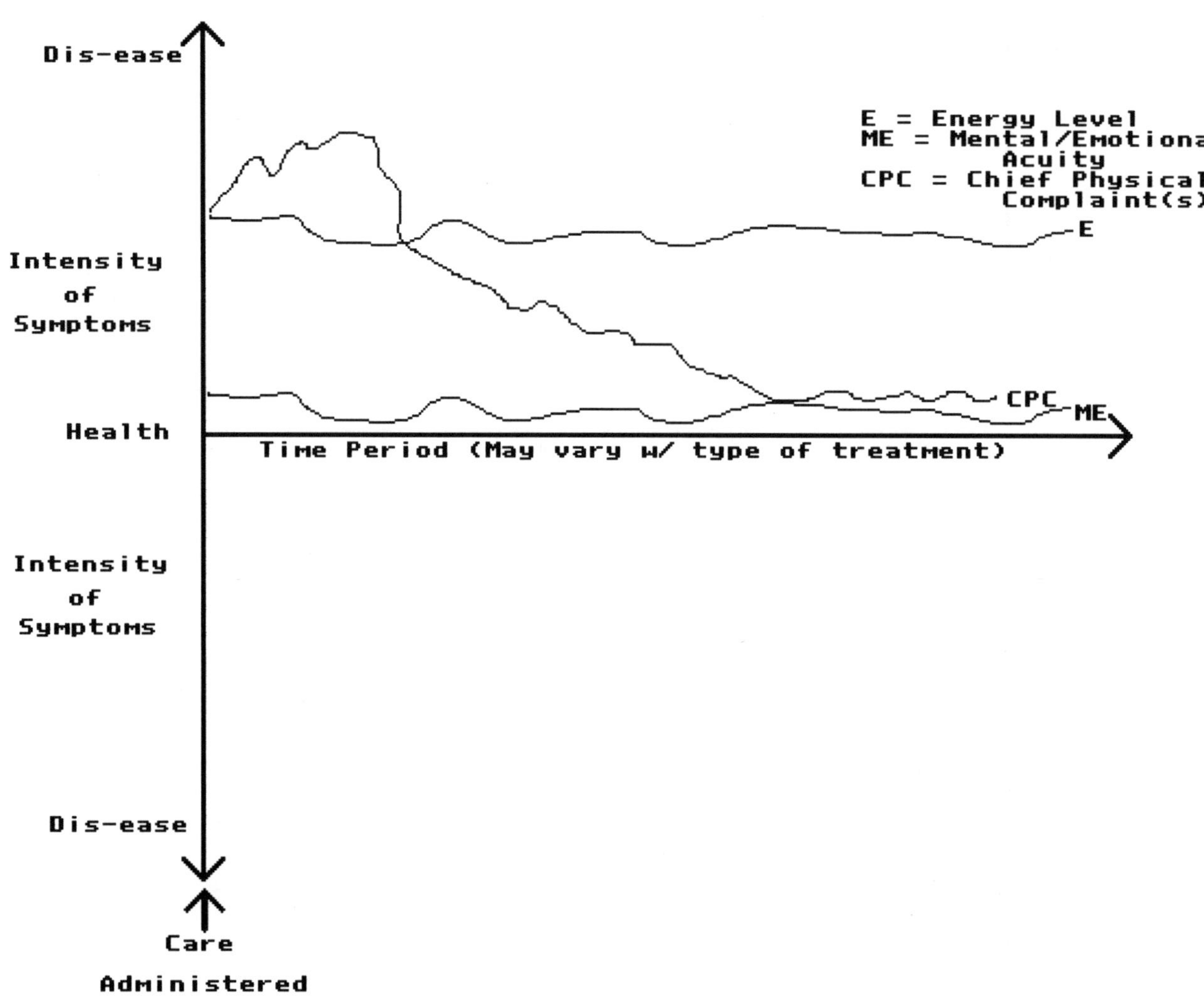


*Figure 31.8*

See Figure 31.4

PATIENT COMMENTS: "I definitely am better but still I don't feel like I used to."

TECHNICAL COMMENTS: **In very elderly patients and patients with their vital force badly depleted (i.e., AIDS patients), it is possible that the process of aging and/or the devastation of the dis-ease may never again, or may only very slowly, allow the patients to return to their former levels of energy.**

PROGNOSIS: Fair. The case may require extensive and closely monitored nursing, proper nutrition, and elimination of toxins, to aid the vital life force to increase its influence.

# RESPONSE 8

## ENERGY, MENTAL/EMOTIONAL SLOWLY WORSENING

GRAPH:

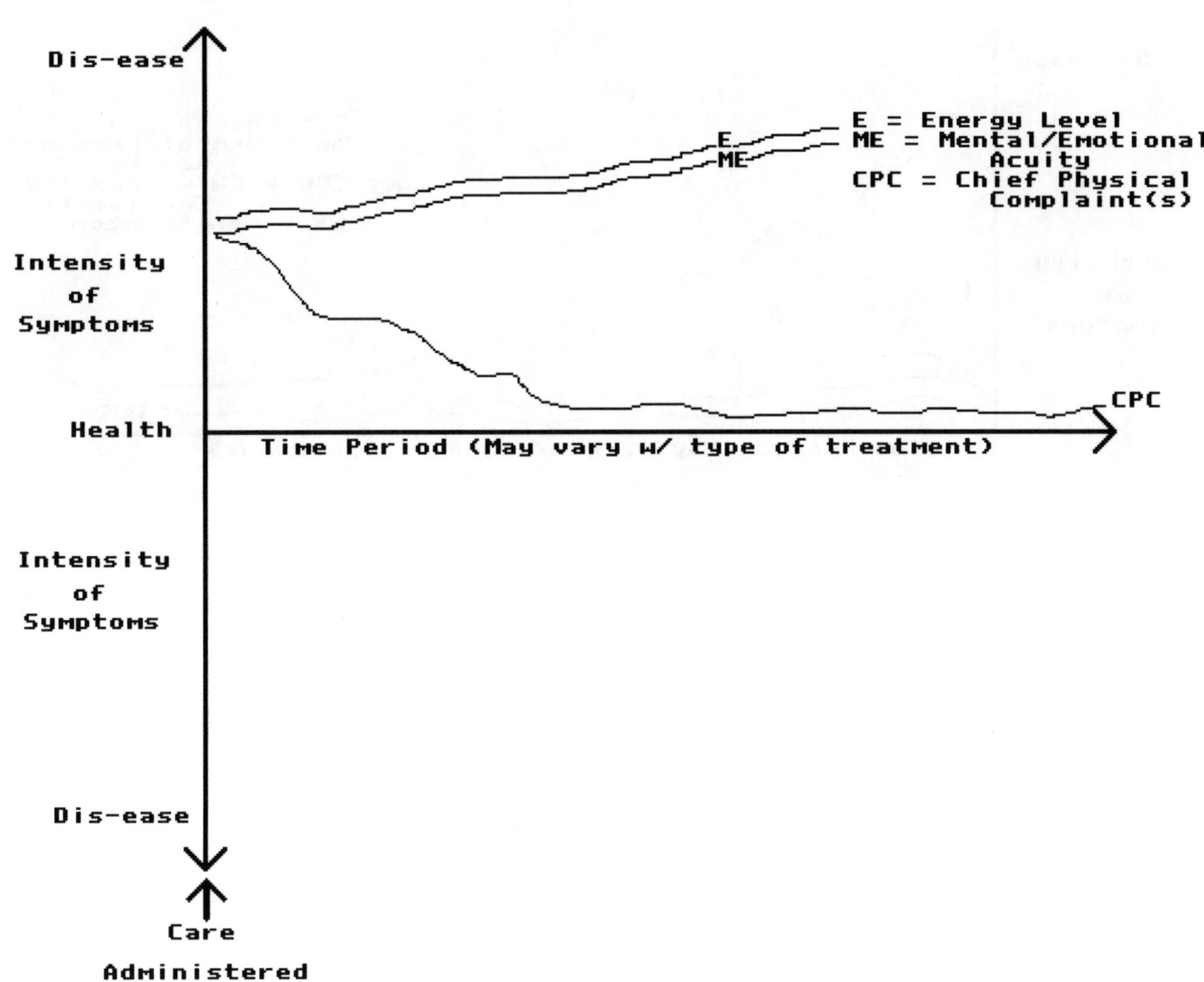


*Figure 31.9*

See Figure 31.4

PATIENT COMMENTS: "I'm some better but I still feel like I have a long way to go."

TECHNICAL COMMENTS: The chief physical component is much improved but without any initial aggravation while the energy and mental-emotional components continue to slowly worsen. **This is very likely a layered case in which the therapy has helped to expose the rest of the miasmatic, diathesis, dosha, phase picture of the dis-ease.** Such cases can be very much like peeling an onion. When each layer of symptoms is removed there is another layer hidden underneath.

PROGNOSIS: Not favorable. There is likely a better therapy that can be administered. **The case needs to be completely re-evaluated from a miasmatic, diathesis, dosha, phase perspective.**

# RESPONSE 9

## OLD PROBLEM BETTER, NEW ONE REPLACED IT

GRAPH:

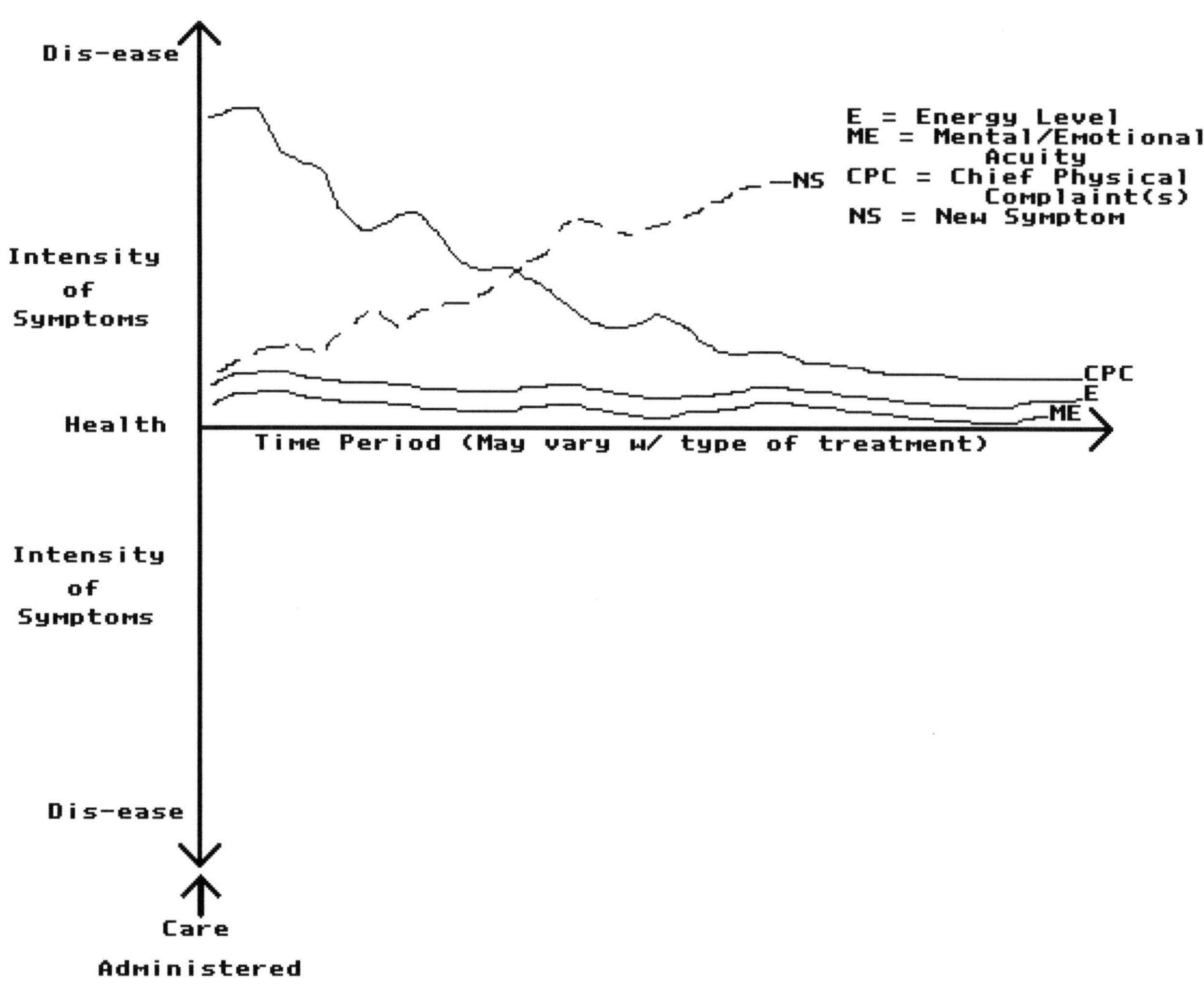


*Figure 31.10*

See Figure 31.4

PATIENT COMMENTS: "I've got a new problem now."

TECHNICAL COMMENTS: The therapy is close but not resonant with the patient's true need. **Re-evaluate the case for a more eclectic approach.** If a better choice is not evident, wait until one becomes apparent. By administering inappropriate therapy, the practitioner may further disturb the case and make it more difficult to select the correct therapy. **This is a layered case and appears to be developing a complete miasmatic, diathesis, dosha, phase picture of the case.**

PROGNOSIS: Not favorable if the developing miasmatic, diathesis, dosha, phase picture is not considered.

# RESPONSE 10

## OLD PROBLEM IMPROVING, INTENSE NEW PROBLEM

GRAPH:

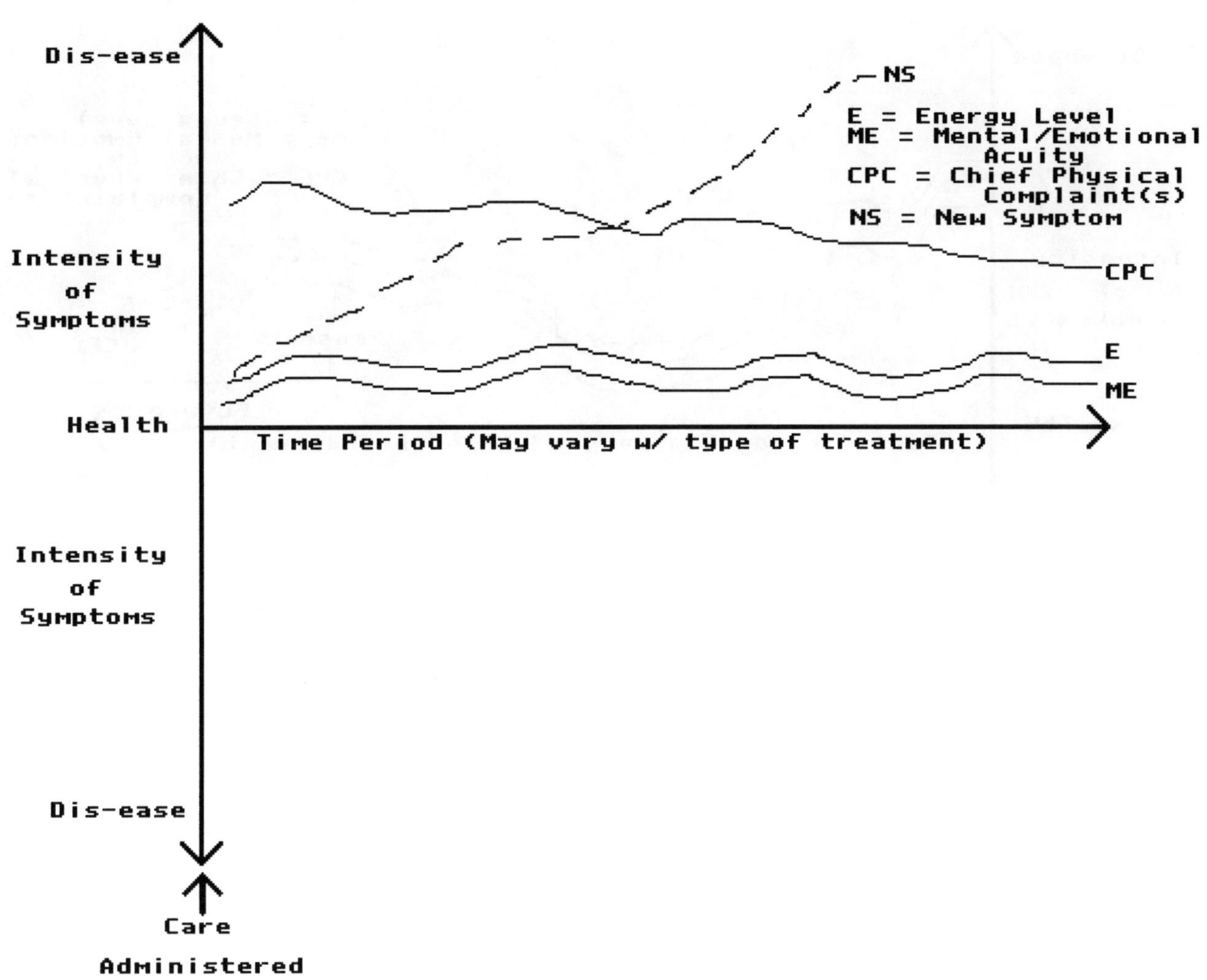


*Figure 31.11*

See Figure 31.4

PATIENT COMMENTS: "I've got a major new problem that is just killing me."

TECHNICAL COMMENTS: The new dis-ease symptom(s) is (are) more dramatic than the old condition being treated. **The complete miasmatic, diathesis, dosha, phase picture is developing very nicely.** This pattern can also be seen when the patient discontinues the use of drugs which were suppressing, but not curing, a particular symptom or symptoms of the full dis-ease picture.

PROGNOSIS: Good, with an appropriate change of therapy. Poor, if the practitioner tries to continue the original program of care.

# RESPONSE 11

## GETTING WORSE AGAIN

GRAPH:

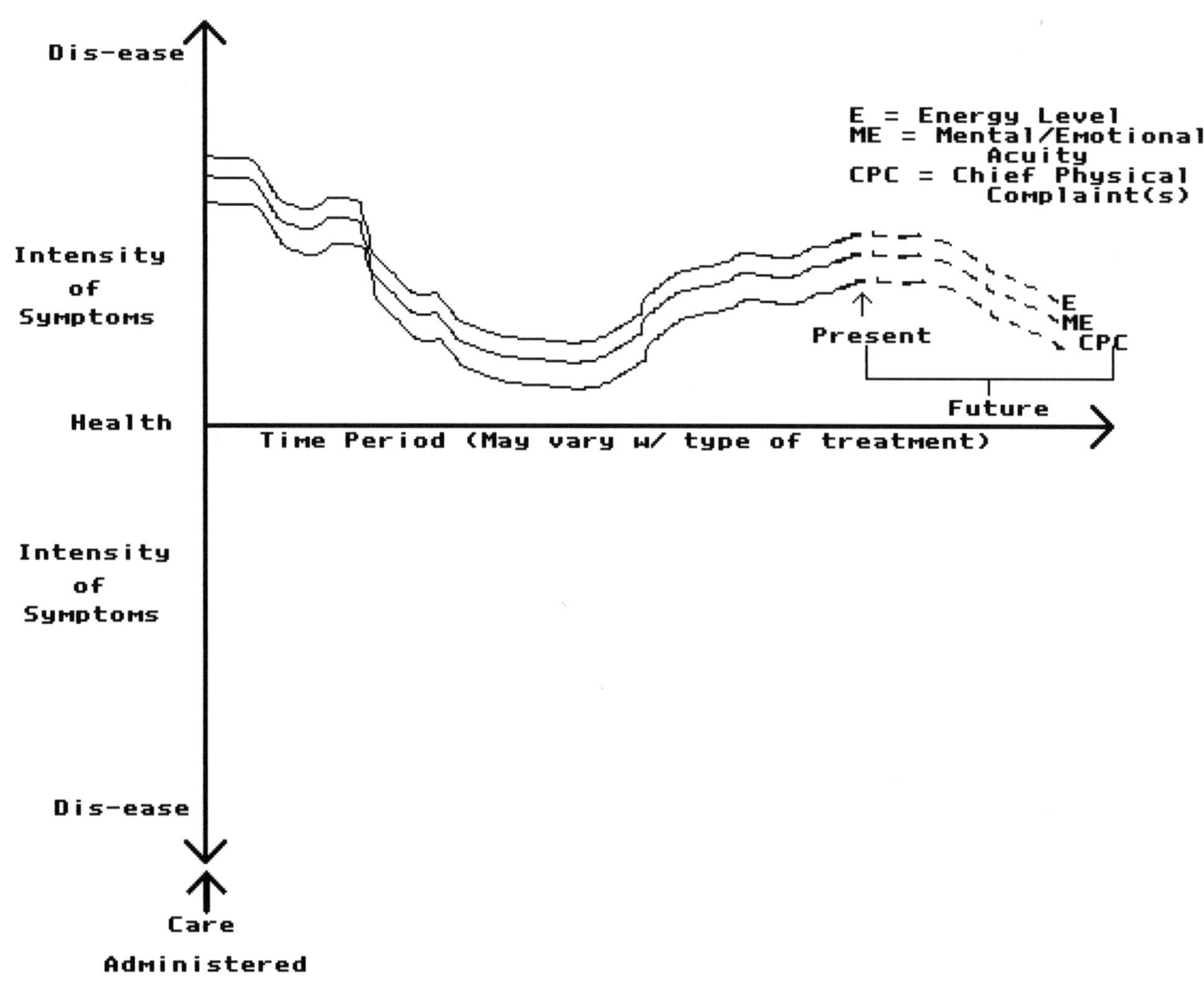



*Figure 31.12*

See Figure 31.4

PATIENT COMMENTS: "I was much better but now I am getting worse again."

TECHNICAL COMMENTS: The patient has experienced such a dramatic response to therapy that he feels discouraged when he back-slides even a little bit. **It must be carefully determined if the present symptoms are precisely the same as the original symptoms.** Frequently, in this type of response, the miasmatic, diathesis, dosha, phase basis of the disease has also been ignored. There is no definite aggravation of symptoms, only amelioration. The patient wants another treatment but to provide this will definitely disturb the progress of the case to date. If the patient cannot be convinced to wait, the practitioner should administer placebo care.

PROGNOSIS: **Wait. It is extremely likely that the healer has successfully completed the work and the innate healing power of the patient will in short order again activate the healing processes.**

## RESPONSE 12

## BACK TO WHERE STARTED

GRAPH:

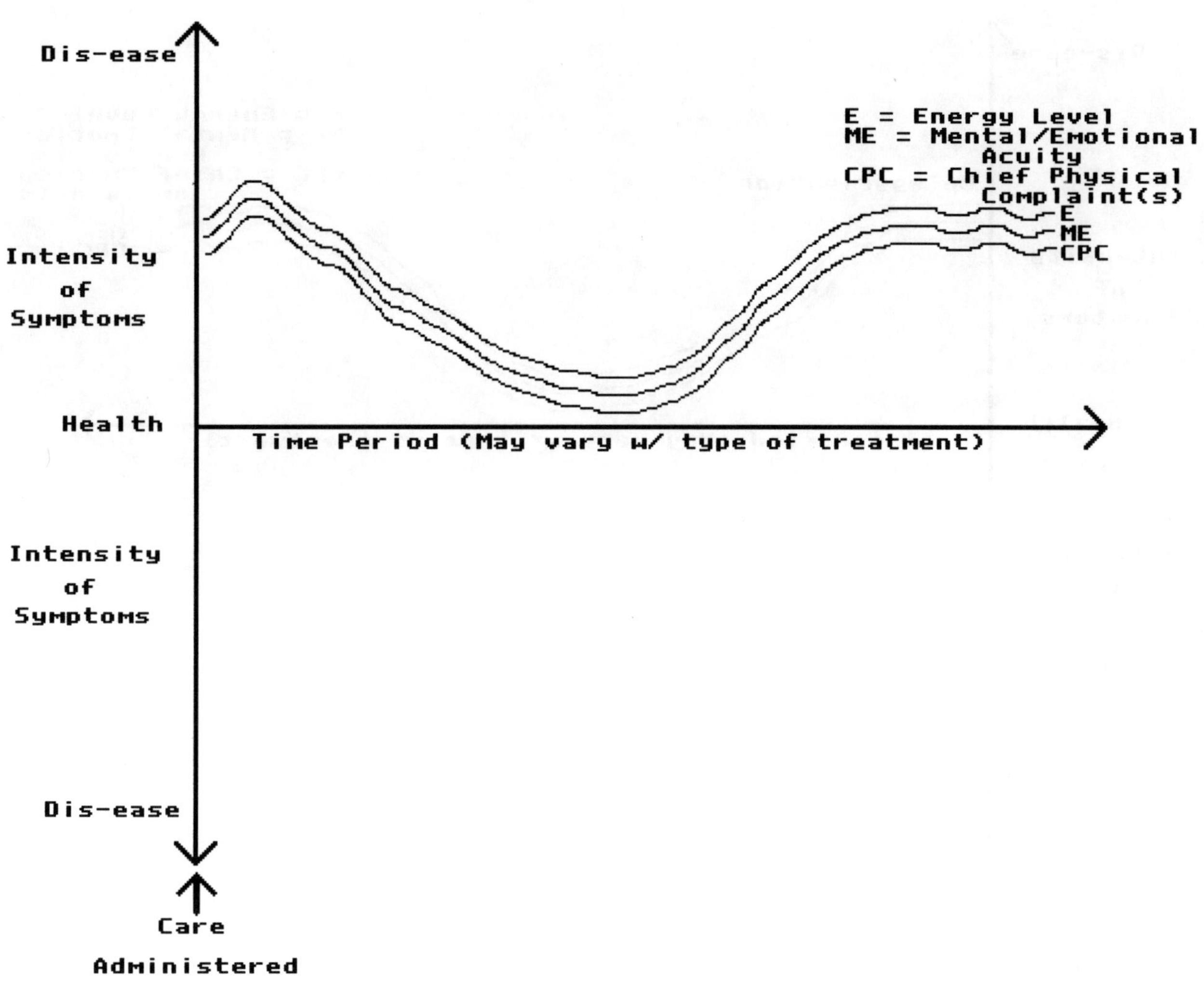



*Figure 31.13*

See Figure 31.4

PATIENT COMMENTS: "I'm back to where I started. Are you really going to be able to help me?"

TECHNICAL COMMENTS: Definite short-term aggravation followed by marked amelioration and then a full relapse. The therapy was correct but was not maintained. **Re-evaluate to determine why. The most common reason is that the miasmatic, diathesis, dosha, phase aspect of the case has been ignored. Another reason is that the num, kundalini, innate, ch'i, vital or life force is weak and unable to sustain the healing.** The vitality of the force must be nursed to the point where it is stronger through good nutrition, massage, rest, Ch'i (Qi) Gong, and other such treatments. If the picture is exactly the same as when the case was originally taken, re-prescribe the same therapy but administer it more intensely. **If something has negated the therapy, find out what it is and eliminate it. If some of the symptoms are different from the first time, the therapy must be changed.**

PROGNOSIS: Good, if the above instructions are faithfully followed.

# RESPONSE 13

## WAS BETTER, NOW THE SAME

GRAPH:

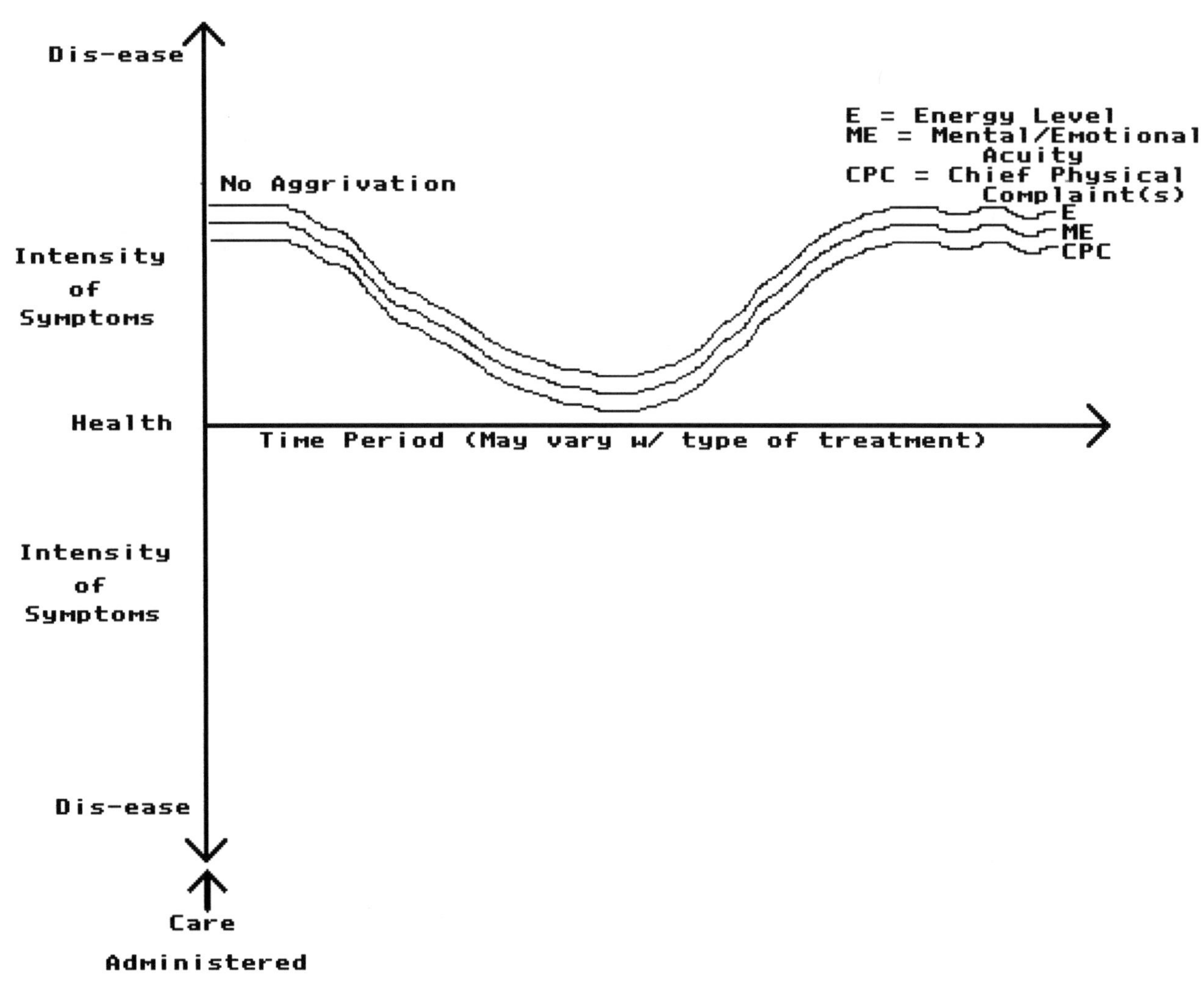


*Figure 31.14*

See Figure 31.4

PATIENT COMMENTS: "I was better, but now I'm back where I started."

TECHNICAL COMMENTS: **Amelioration without aggravation and then full relapse.** This can indicate an incurable condition but more likely the **need is for a different therapy** to match more closely the total needs of this patient. **If the best indicated therapy is continually changing from visit to visit, the possibility of an incurable case may need to be considered.** The patient may also be doing something that interferes and negates the properly selected therapy. **In the rare event that it is an incurable case, the periods of amelioration will get shorter and shorter even with appropriate care.**

PROGNOSIS: **Guarded, unless the correct therapy can be arrived at.** May have to settle for temporary amelioration if the case is incurable.

# RESPONSE 14

## BETTER, NOW MUCH WORSE

GRAPH:

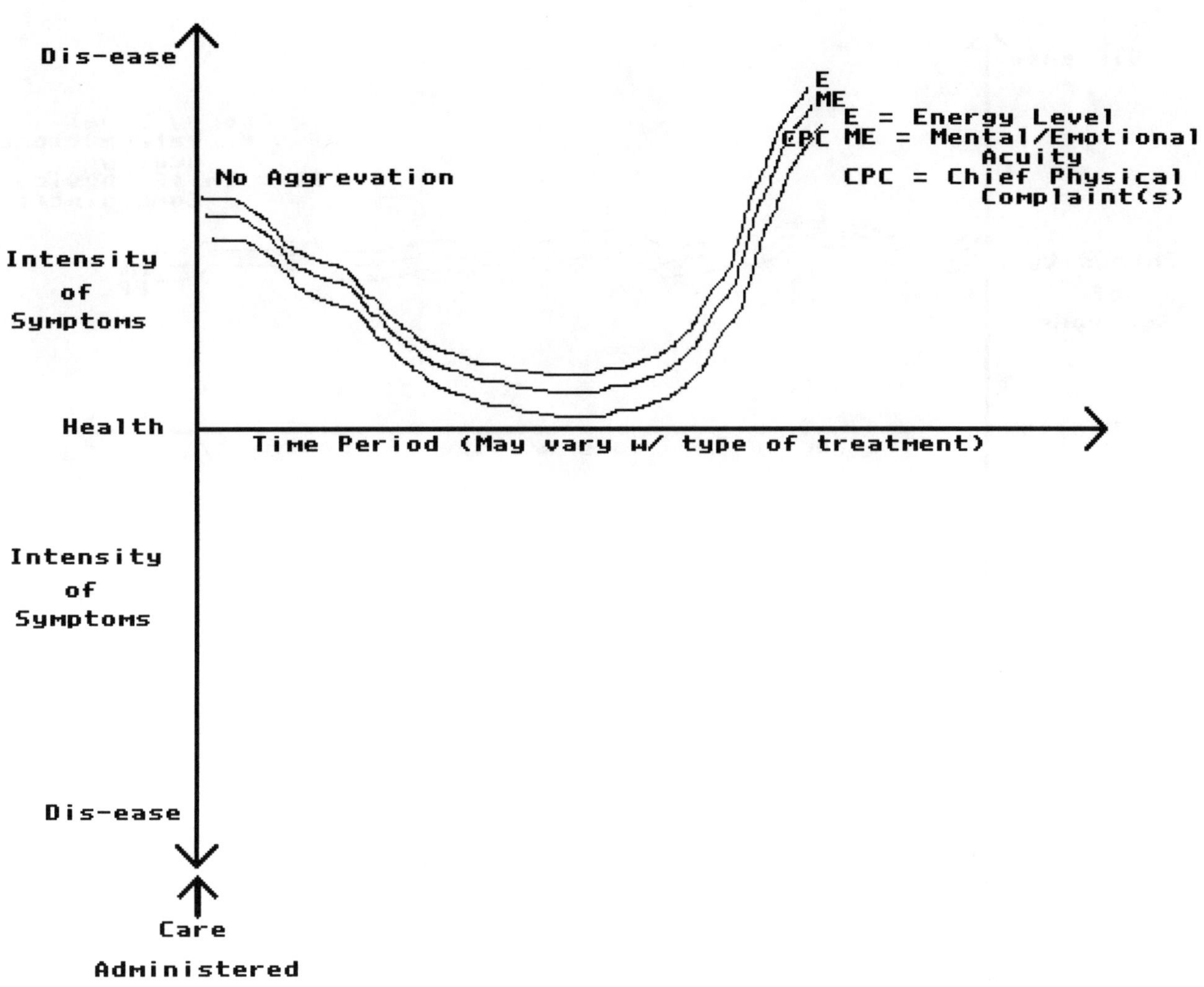



*Figure 31.15*

See Figure 31.4

PATIENT COMMENTS: "I was cured and now I am much worse."

TECHNICAL COMMENTS: Amelioration without initial aggravation followed by intensification of symptoms. **The miasmatic, diathesis, dosha, phase aspect of the case has been disregarded. The case must be re-evaluated in light of miasmas, diathesis, dosha, phases or care will be palliative only. The healing force is very weak and needs to be built up with nutrition, massage, rest, Ch'i (Qi) Gong, and other means.**

If this oversight is not rectified therapy will need to be changed frequently and such care will provide relief for shorter and shorter periods of time. Many practitioners unfamiliar with miasmas, diathesis, dosha, phase pictures would consider this case incurable. **It is incurable ONLY because they do not know how to successfully evaluate it.**

PROGNOSIS: GUARDED. There likely has been extensive damage done to the tissues and their functions. **Full recovery may take years.**

# RESPONSE 15

## NO RESPONSE, OPEN PATIENT

GRAPH:

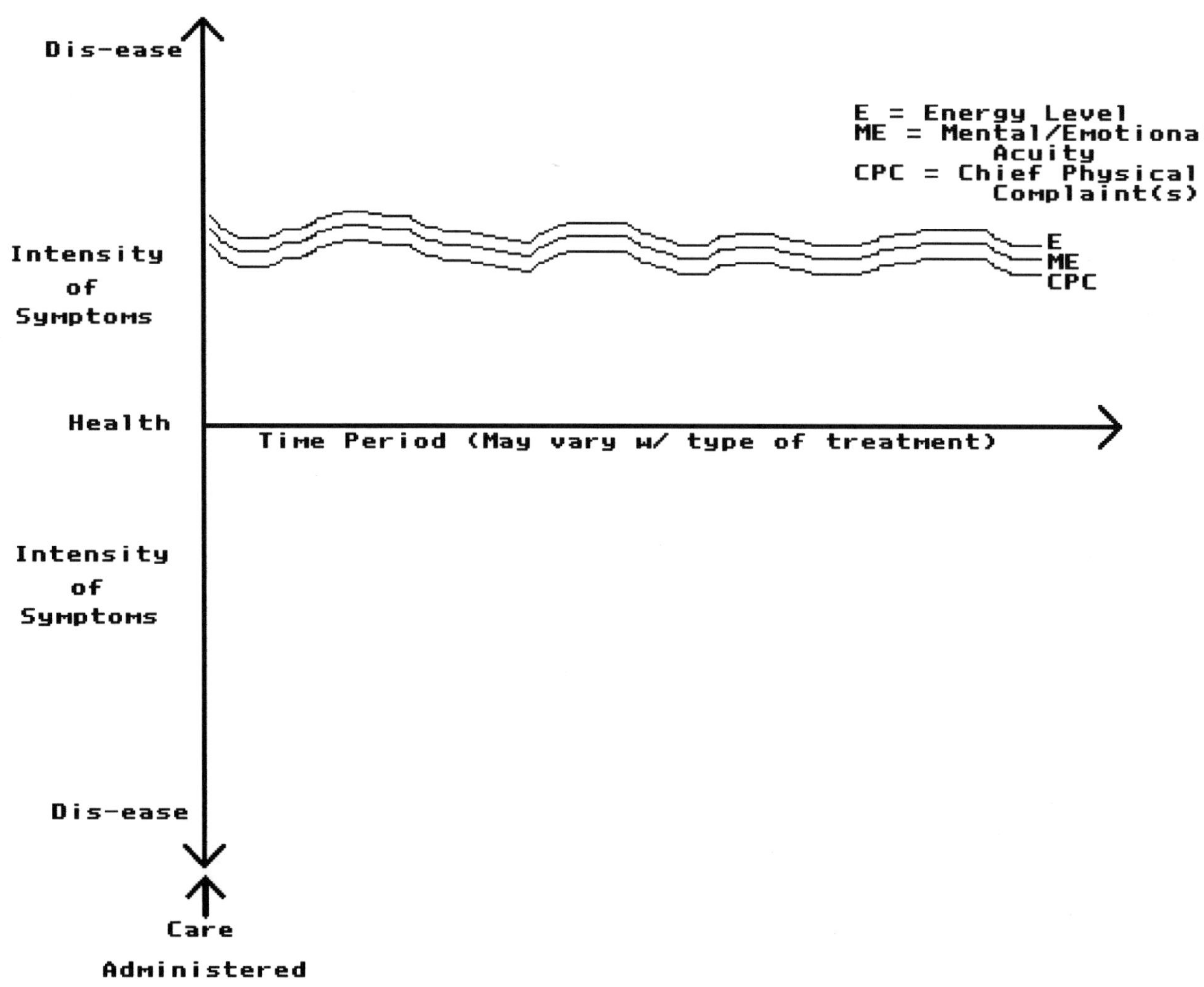


*Figure 31.16*

See Figure 31.4

PATIENT COMMENTS: "There is no change. Do you really think that you will be able to help me?"

TECHNICAL COMMENTS: The care rendered is not correct for the case. **The case must be completely re-evaluated** in order to find an appropriate mode of therapy.

PROGNOSIS: Very poor, if the re-evaluation of the case is not done; good if the case is re-evaluated and the proper therapy in found.

# RESPONSE 16

## NO RESPONSE, CLOSED PATIENT

GRAPH:

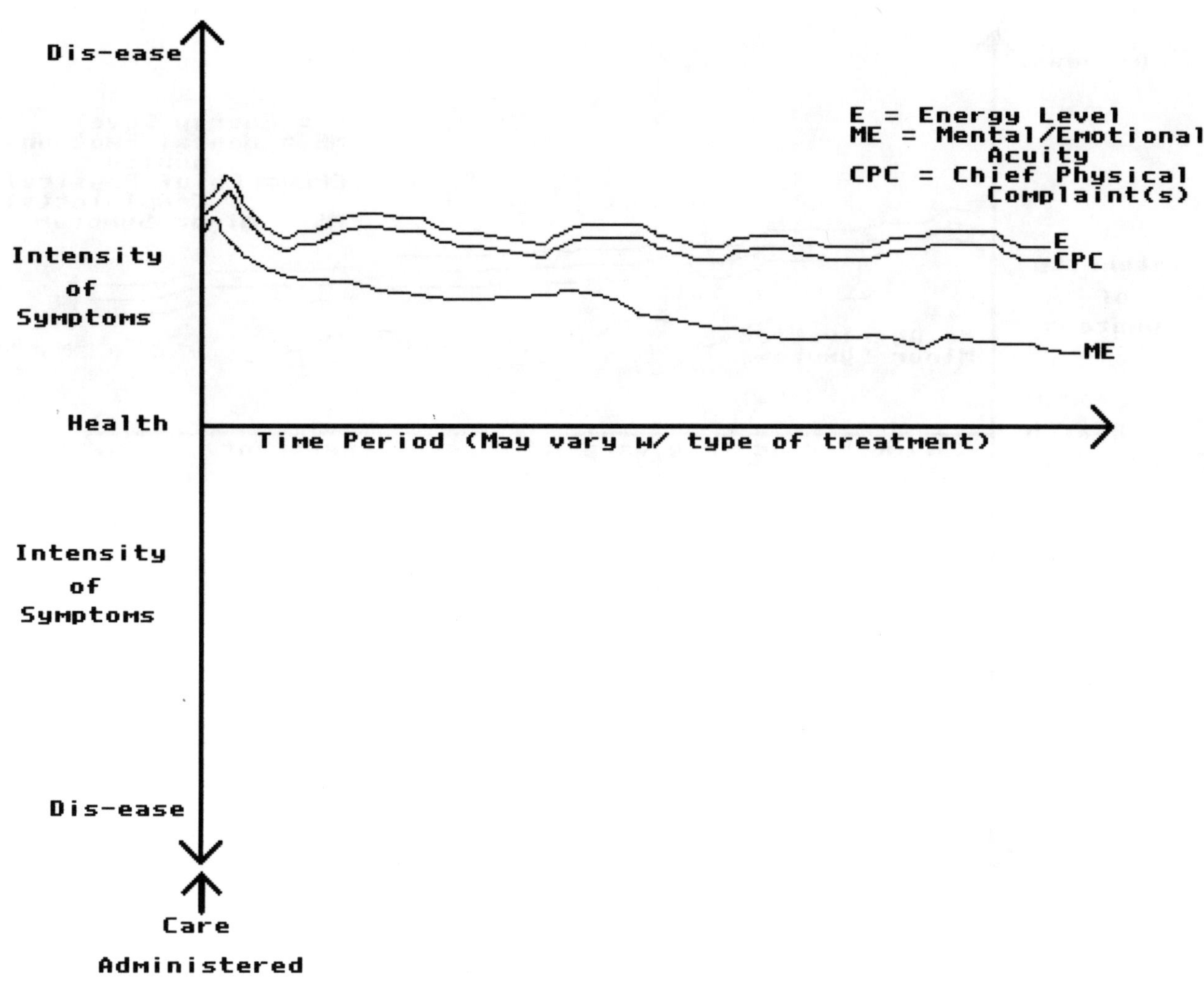


*Figure 31.17*

See Figure 31.4

PATIENT COMMENTS: "I'm the same."

TECHNICAL COMMENTS: This is the intellectualizing patient. **They have trained themselves to suppress their emotions, thoughts and expressions and to rationalize.** Such individuals tend to explain away things; so responses that are true healing are not recognized or reported because the patient attributes them to other influences such as: "Well I gave up eating meat." or "I changed my perfume so that's is why my allergies are so much better." or "I modified my exercise program so naturally I have improved."

**Closed patients are generally unimpressed by short-term change even when the change is quite dramatic. Such patients tend to withhold what to them is considered "unimportant" information. In reality, this withheld information is vital. Therefore, even small concessions have great significance to the alert healer.**

PROGNOSIS: The therapy is beginning to act on the most critical levels and patience is vital. **Wait.** To retreat could cause the progress to be stopped or even reversed as shown by Figure 31.4.

# RESPONSE 17

## MINOR RESPONSE ONLY, CLOSED PATIENT

GRAPH:

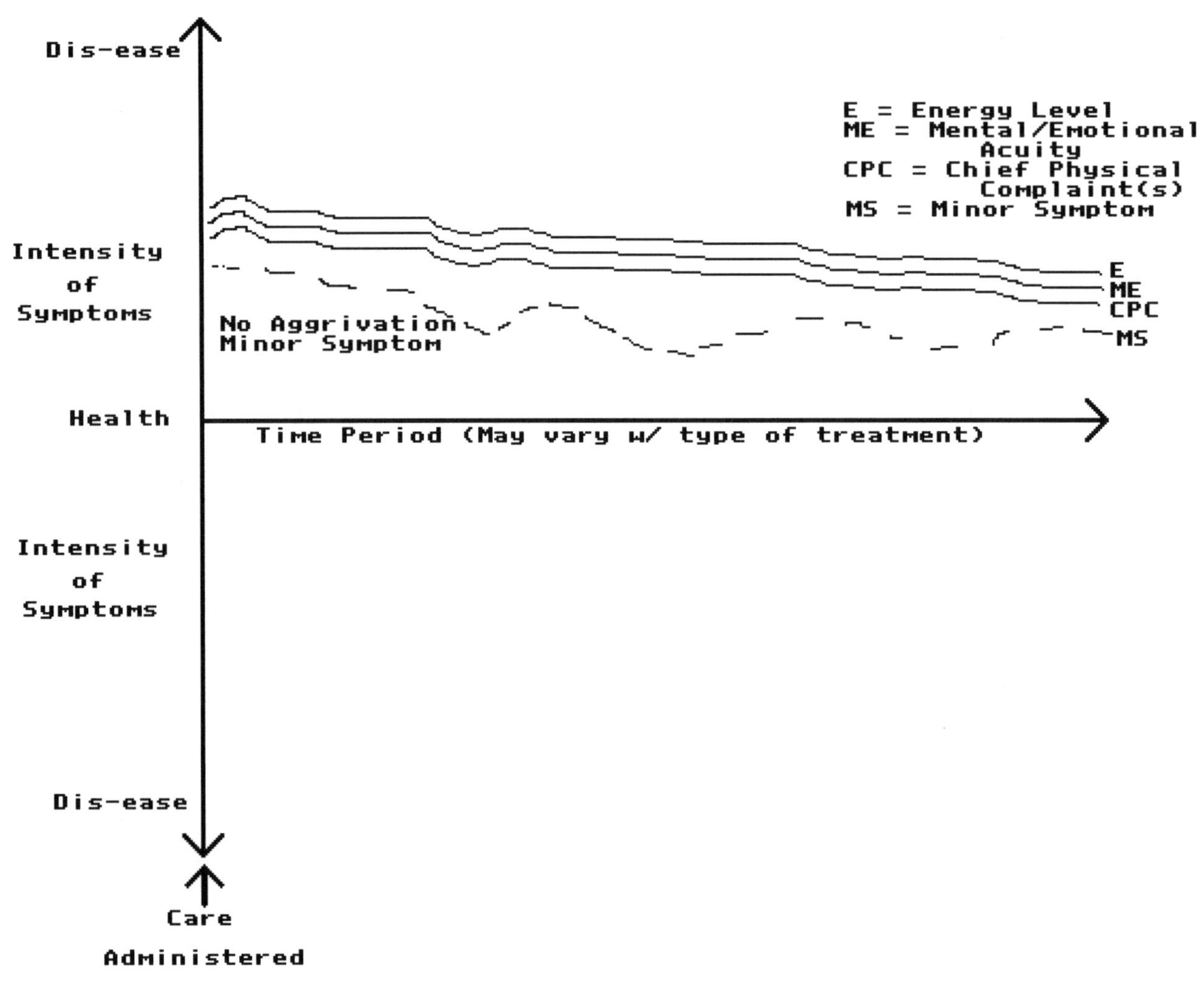


*Figure 31.18*

See Figure 31.4

PATIENT COMMENTS: "I'm the same."

TECHNICAL COMMENTS: **The therapeutic results are questionable.** This could be nothing more than a random fluctuation in bio-dynamic homeostasis or it could be the beginning of the cure. A third possibility is that the therapy is correct but has not been able to reach the deeper levels of the patient's being, in which case a more aggressive use of the therapy in question might be considered.

PROGNOSIS: **Wait. If there is no further improvement or relapse, the therapy should be changed. If slow improvements continue, allow the cure to develop without further therapy as long as the slow improvement continues.**

# RESPONSE 18

## MINOR RESPONSE ONLY, OPEN PATIENT

GRAPH:

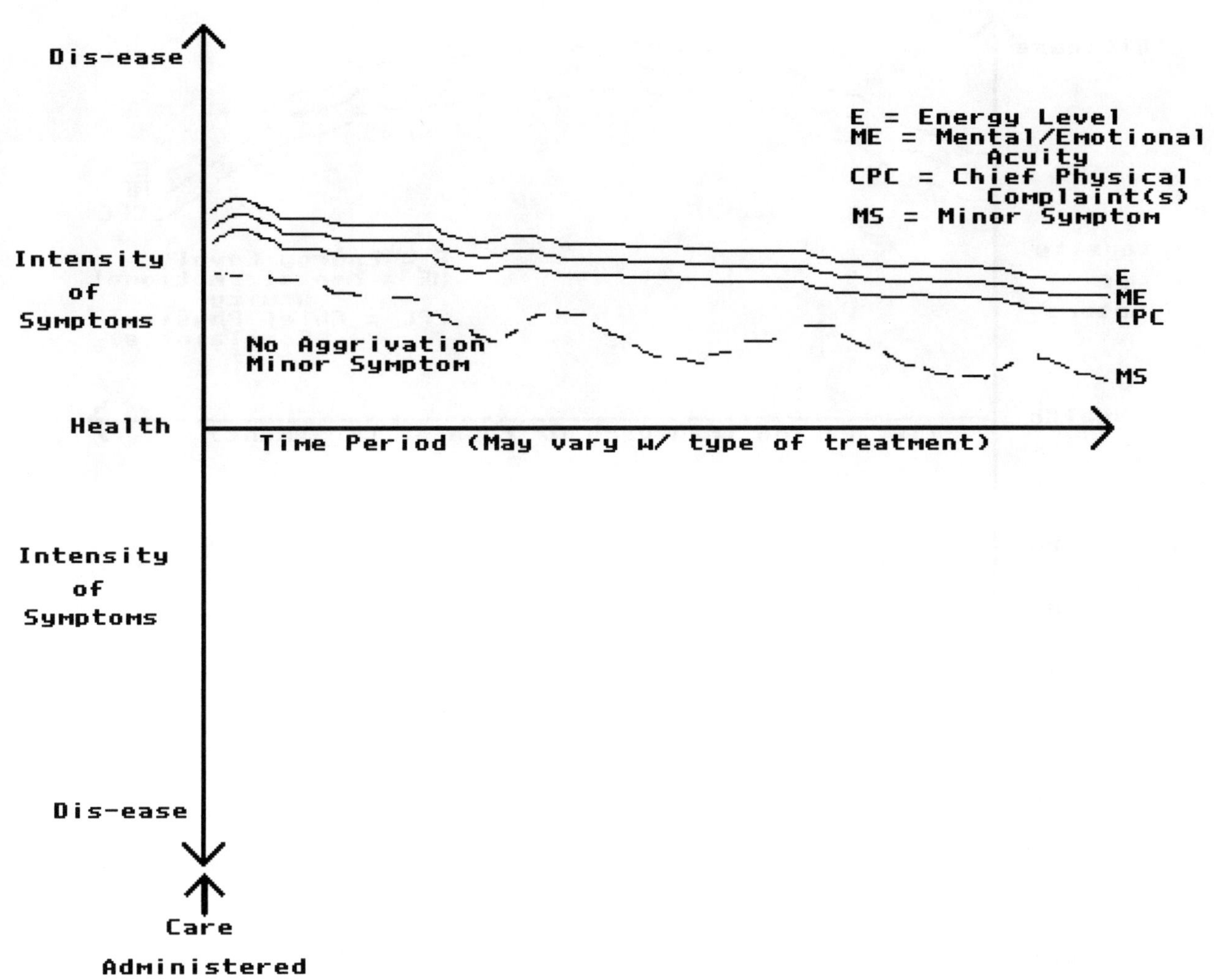


*Figure 31.19*

See Figure 31.4

PATIENT COMMENTS: "I'm the same generally but I do have a few minor improvements."

TECHNICAL COMMENTS: An open patient likes to please and will go to great extremes to find something that is improving in order to make the practitioner feel good. The practitioner must not be swayed by this patient.

PROGNOSIS: **The therapy was totally incorrect and the case must be re- evaluated for a better choice.**

## RESPONSE 19

## AGGRAVATION OF ALL SYMPTOMS

GRAPH:

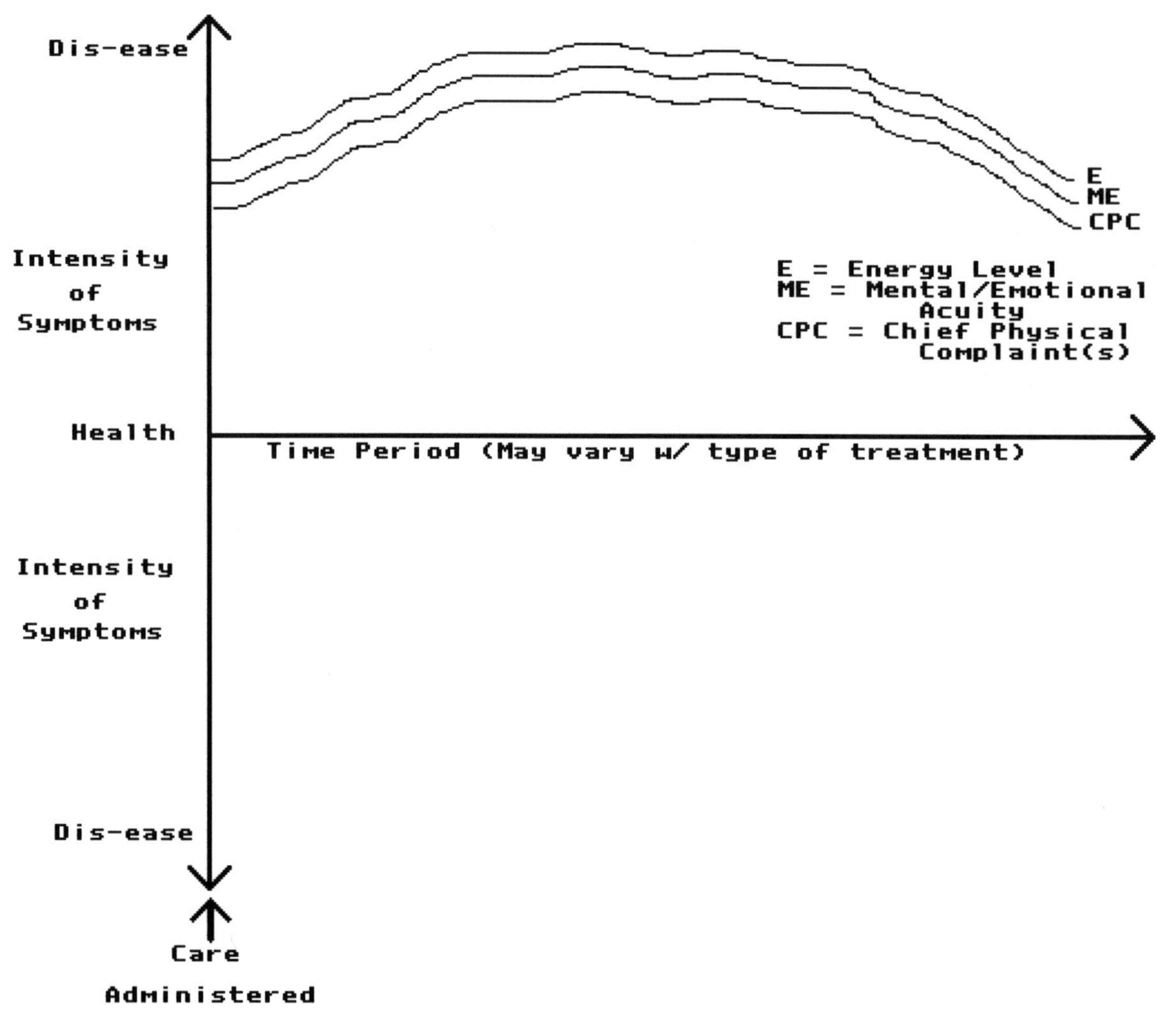


*Figure 31.20*

See Figure 31.4

PATIENT COMMENTS: "EVERYTHING has been worse."

TECHNICAL COMMENTS: **It is very typical for patients in this scenario to disregard the recent improvements. Such a pattern is indicative of a patient who has deep long-standing pathology and is frequently very discouraged and wants to influence the practitioner to do something more dramatic in order to get "quicker" results.**

PROGNOSIS: **The therapy is extremely well suited to the needs of the case and the healing process has just now begun. Great patience must be exhibited in order not to disturb the healing. Wait.** Do not continue care. Such interferences will cause the case to follow the response in Figure 31.4. Placebo therapy may be necessary in order to buy time for the healing process to work.

# RESPONSE 20

## CONTINUING AGGRAVATION OF ALL SYMPTOMS

GRAPH:

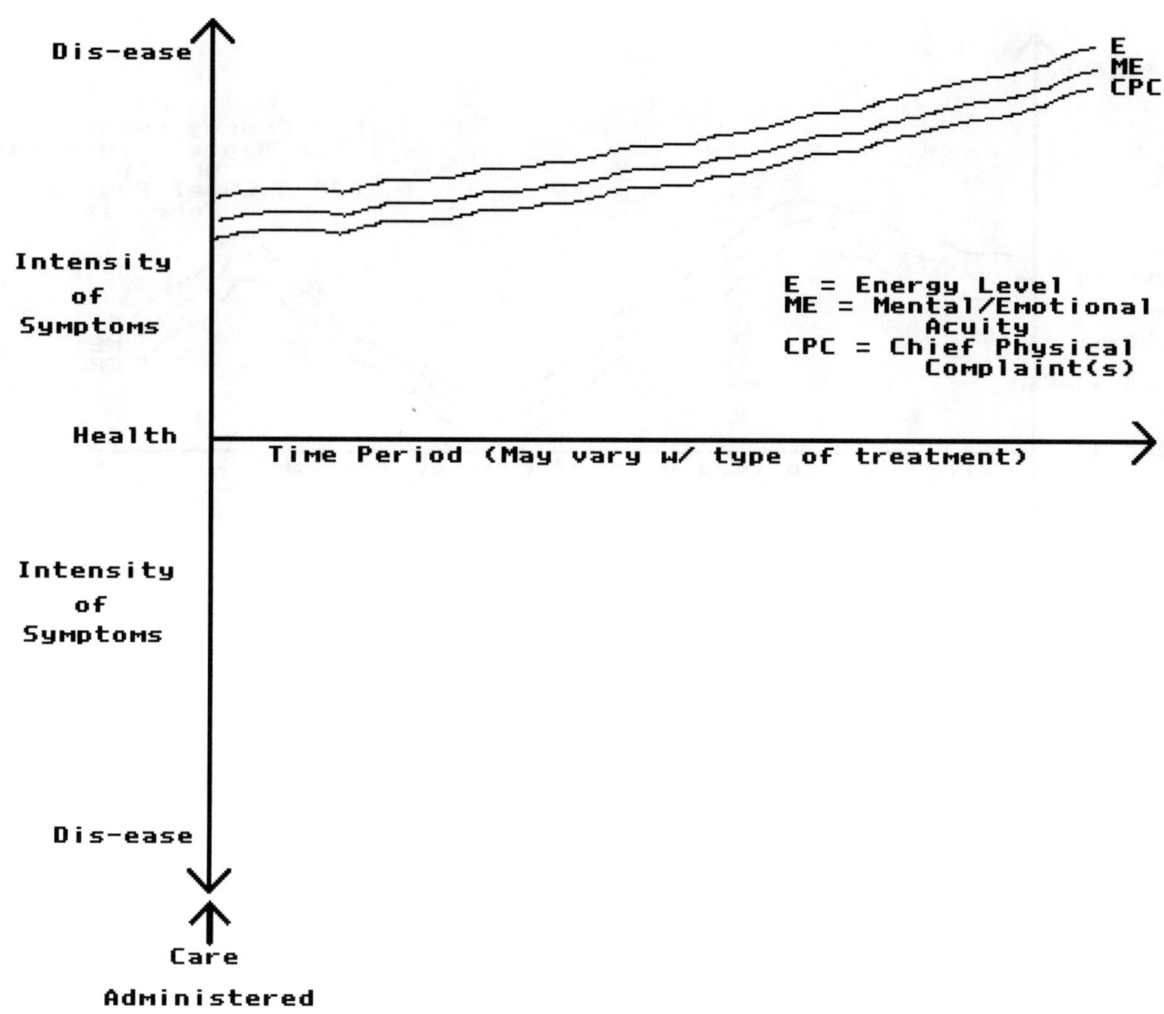


*Figure 31.21*

See Figure 31.4

PATIENT COMMENTS: "I am definitely worse in every way."

TECHNICAL COMMENTS: This pattern is seen when pharmaceutical drugs, pain killers, acupuncture, chiropractic adjustments, and other therapies have been used for symptomatic relief only have been discontinued when the therapy is determined to be inappropriate. **The case must be re-evaluated as therapy is totally incorrect.** This is the least desirable of all responses. If no palliative therapy withdrawal is involved, it means that the case is deteriorating. The best possible therapy must be instituted immediately and frequent re-evaluations will be necessary. If the therapy of choice is the same as the original, then a more aggressive form of this therapy must be administered.

**It is not unusual in such cases for a few symptoms to provide clues as to what the next appropriate therapy will be but do not rush into it. It is critical to allow healing time. Pushing too hard can cause the case to deteriorate further.**

PROGNOSIS: An optimistic prognosis can be made if the case is handled properly but disaster can result if handled improperly.

# RESPONSE 21

## AGGRAVATION, AMELIORATION, AGGRAVATION

GRAPH:

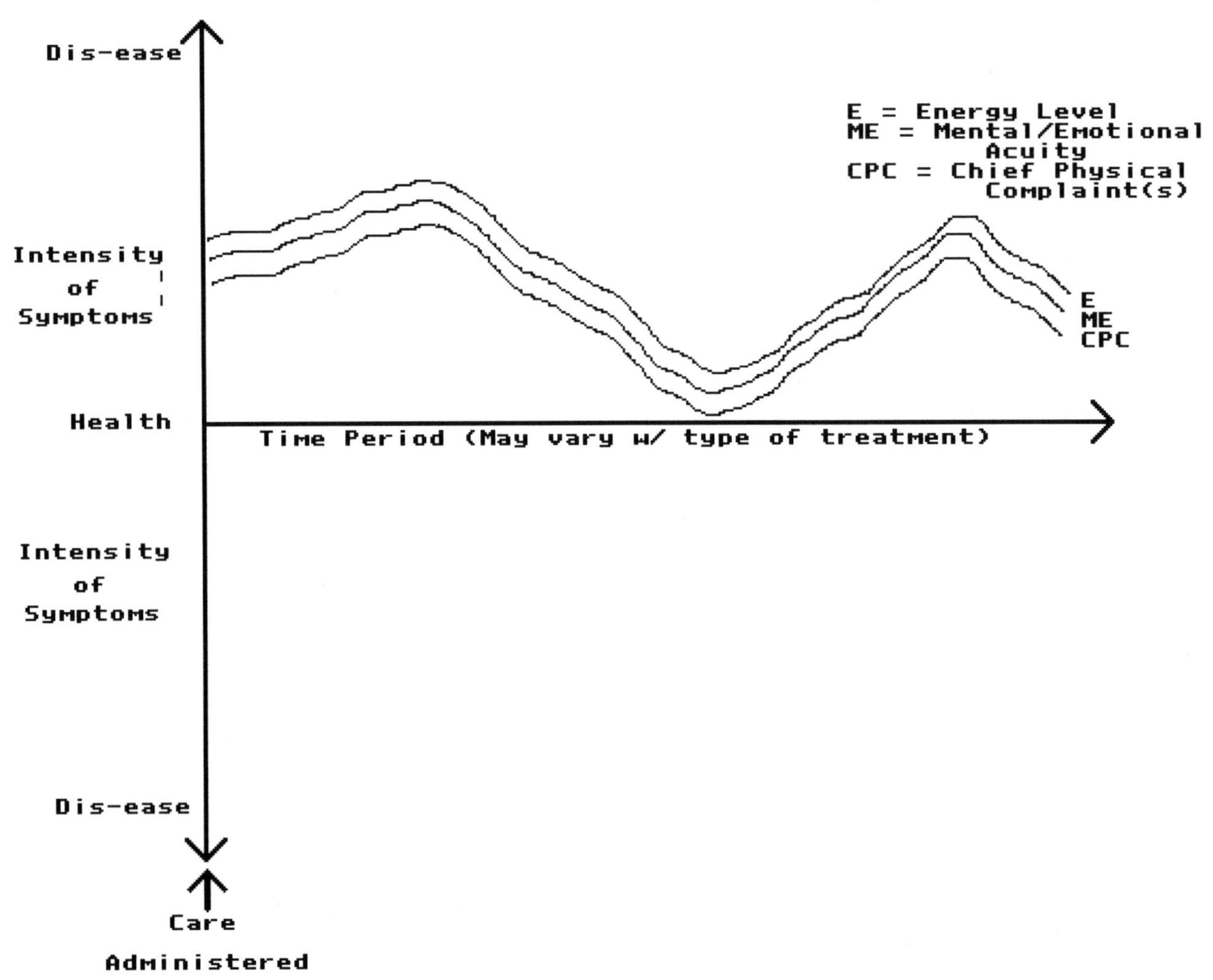



*Figure 31.22*

See Figure 31.4

PATIENT COMMENTS: "I've been worse again except for the last few days."

TECHNICAL COMMENTS: **There are severe pathological changes in the tissues. The defense mechanism is very weak but not yet non-functional. Virtually every choice in therapy must be exactly correct if progress is to be achieved. This pattern often indicates the correct therapy must be slightly modified in relation to potency, frequency or intensity.** Cases such as this have had frequent changes in indicated therapy. What worked last time may not work the next time. Ideally, such cases should have around-the-clock nursing care. Less commonly used therapies and/or procedures are frequently the ones that produce the best results.

PROGNOSIS: Nearly incurable case; prognosis **fair, if the above instructions are followed.**

# RESPONSE 22

## CHIEF PHYSICAL COMPLAINT WORSE

GRAPH:

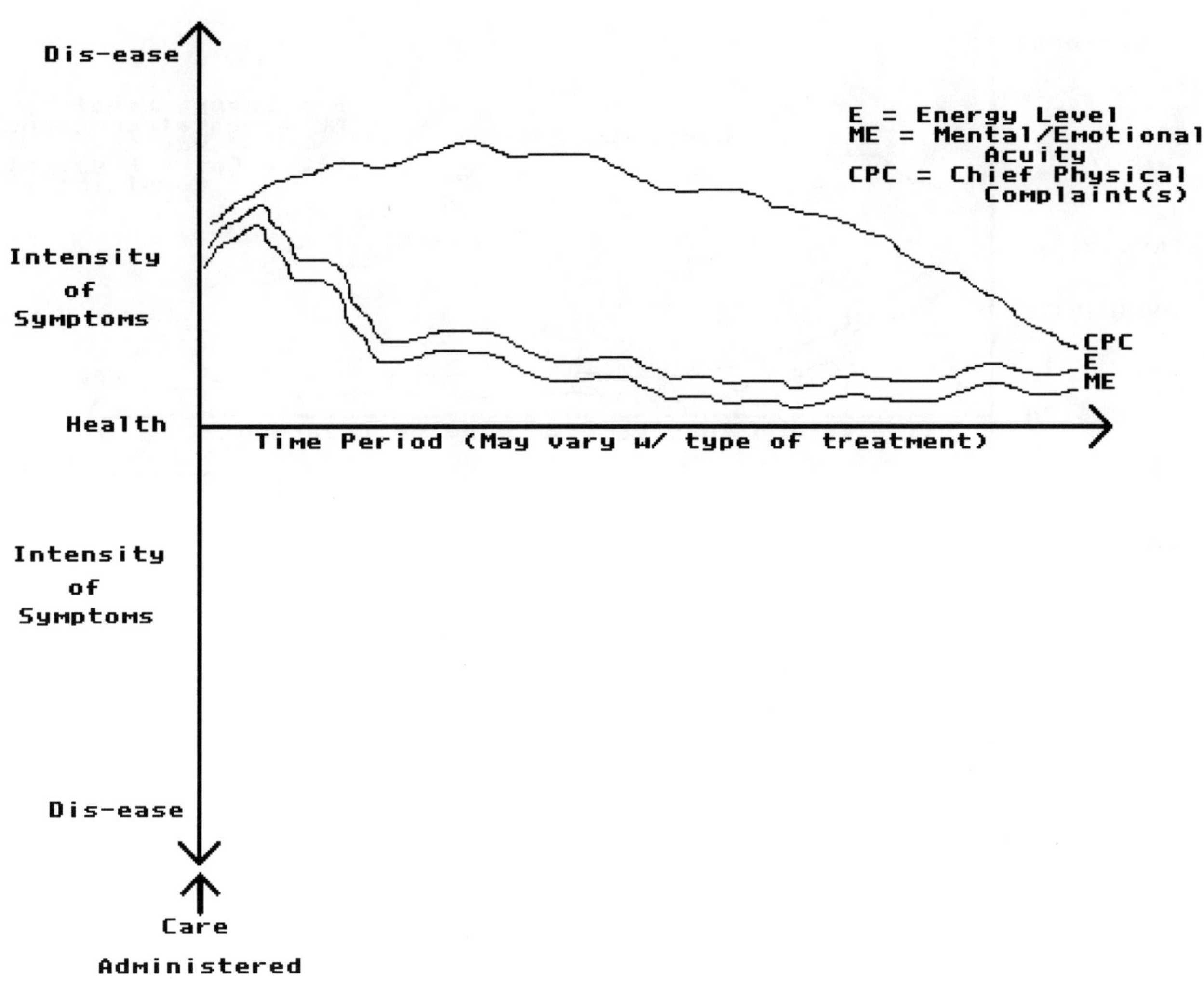


*Figure 31.23*

See Figure 31.4

PATIENT COMMENT: "I've been worse the whole time."

TECHNICAL COMMENTS: The chief physical complaint is aggravated but the energy level and mental/emotional states are slowly improving. **Since the physical suffering is worse, the patient is not normally aware of the fact that he has made improvements on the more critical levels of his being.** This situation is most frequently encountered in patients who were using pharmaceutical drugs, acupuncture, chiropractic adjustments, or phytotherapeutic agents to mask the pain symptoms and have now discontinued their use. This is the classic example of Hering's Law at work. The practitioner has already done his/her job.

PROGNOSIS: **Good. The therapy is correct. Wait and allow the body to continue the healing process.**

# RESPONSE 23

## MENTAL/EMOTIONAL WORSE, OTHERS MUCH IMPROVED

GRAPH:

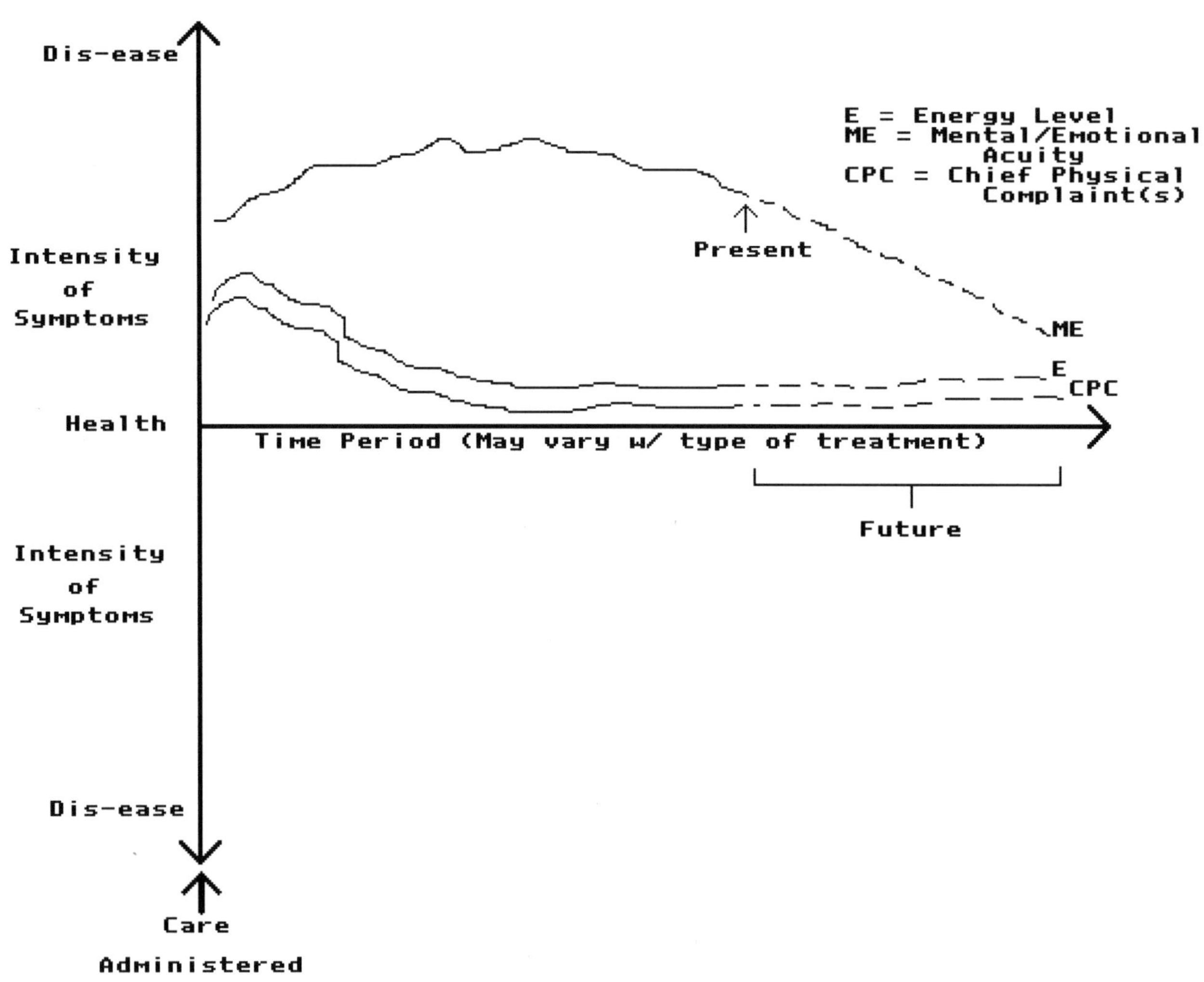


*Figure 31.24*

See Figure 31.4

PATIENT COMMENTS: "I'm steadily getting worse."

TECHNICAL COMMENTS: **Cases with mental/emotional disturbances tend to have such aggravations during the healing process. This is especially true when the patient is in counseling and is working his way through old issues which have been suppressed to the sub-conscious level.** The patient may be convinced that nothing is improving, that he is getting worse, and the will frequently press the practitioner to have "something done". Placebo therapy may be necessary to tide the patient over until the healing process is completed. Do not get in a hurry to repeat the therapy because the current therapy is still working.

**In severe cases, patients with a suicidal history may require 24-hour-a- day monitoring until the critical aggravation of the mental/emotional aspect of the case begins to show amelioration.**

PROGNOSIS: Excellent if the above directions are followed.

# RESPONSE 24

## DEFINITELY MORE ENERGY BUT HURTING AGAIN

GRAPH:

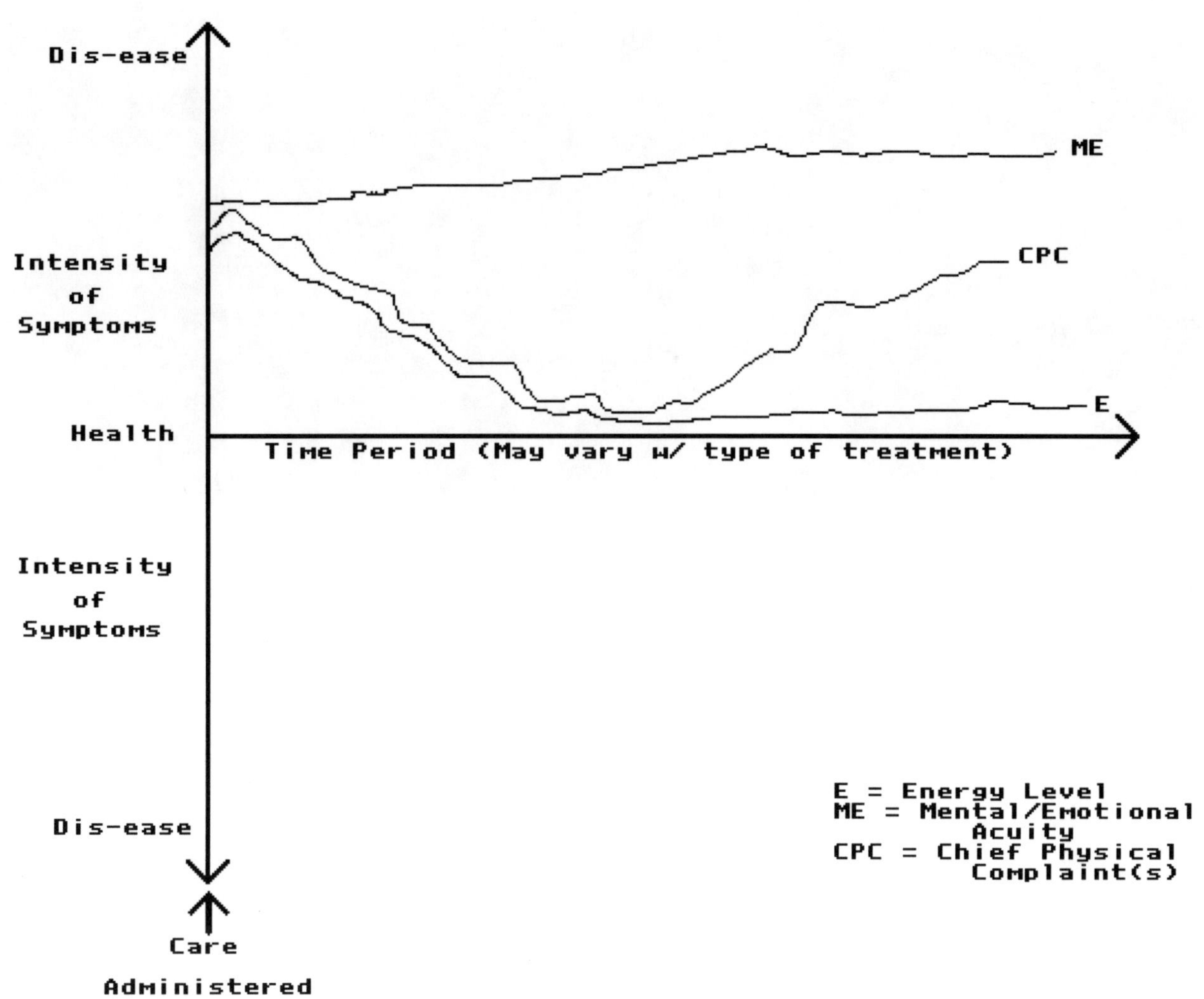


*Figure 31.25*

See Figure 31.4

PATIENT COMMENT: "I don't know what is going on."

TECHNICAL COMMENTS: These are very mixed indications and it is therefore difficult to determine with any degree of accuracy the outcome of the case at this point in time. **Waiting for further developments is the only prudent choice. If the chief physical complaints again ameliorate, it is likely the case will be resolved by the current therapy. If the chief physical complaints continue to worsen, the case will have to be re-evaluated for a more appropriate therapy.**

PROGNOSIS: Questionable

# Chapter 32
# THE IMMUNIZATION QUANDARY

*"The United States is recognized to be the most*
*over-medicated, most over-operated on and most*
*over-inoculated country in the world. We impose*
*our life-saving drugs and technologies, intended for*
*serious ailments, on minor, even trivial illness —*
*illnesses that are self-limiting and that, except for*
*symptomatic relief, do better without interference*
*from the physician. Americans think of health as*
*something that can be bought, rather than a*
*state to be sought through an accommodation*
*to the norms of nature."*

— Hurbert Ratner, M.D.
University Of California
24 February 1963

## EPIDEMICS

Epidemics have been defined as, "A widespread outbreak of an infectious dis-ease simultaneously affecting a large number of people." This is inadequate, however, as historically epidemics have varied from one time to the next time; each outbreak  may be totally different from the preceding or subsequent ones, even though it may be diagnosed as the same dis-ease. It is also well known that the symptoms characterizing each epidemic depend on various factors; climate, prevailing weather conditions, hosts, malnutrition, pestilence, war, pollution, sanitation, educational level of the populace, personal life style, religious and cultural beliefs, affluence, level of technology, politics, individual and/or group genetics, general levels of individual and/or group health, time of the year, age, race, frequency of natural and/or artificial immunization, virulence, psychological conditioning, genetic engineering, the age during  which it occurs, the portion of the globe affected, ease of transportation, beliefs, and a myriad of other factors.

## HISTORICAL PERSPECTIVE

Of all the pestilences that have swept the earth, the Bubonic Plague seems to have been the most devastating; in some instances, it killed up to 80 percent of the population. The question must be asked, why did the other 20 percent survive? They lived in the same houses, ate the same food, breathed the same air, drank the same water, came in contact with the bodily excretions of the ill, slept in the same beds, and even made love to those who perished. Was theirs the luck of the draw? Did they offer the right sacrifices to the right gods and thereby secure divine favor? Or are there other reasons, sound scientific reasons, why this 20 percent remained dis-ease free? If so, can these same principles be applied to the general population to prevent such scourges in the future? **If microbes are the cause of dis-ease, these healthy individuals should also have had the microbes infesting them and producing the dis-ease.** We know it was not because the peasants who survived in the year 1054 did so because they went to their local doctor and paid to be "immunized" with a vaccine from a pharmaceutical company. When we start evaluating the issue by strict scientific standards we find that the stock answers we have been handed in the name of "medical science" show numerous and very serious flaws.

## SMALLPOX

Historically, smallpox has existed in Europe, Asia and Africa for over a thousand years and has been documented to exist in three forms, the Veriola Minor (or Alastrim), Veriola Major (by far the most virulent form) and Veriola Vaccinae (or Cowpox - the mildest form). About of any one of these protects, at least temporarily, from the other two. This observation made by Edward Jenner, M.D., was the basis for smallpox immunization. Interestingly, history documents that until the late 1700s, smallpox was a relatively minor dis-ease with most cases reported among older children and adults, but then its pattern dramatically changed and it became the major cause of mortality among the very young, its victims being found primarily in the rapidly growing slums of the cities.

But Jenner was not the first to vaccinate; 600 years earlier in the 11th Century, Chinese and Ayurvedic physicians were using the dried scales of the smallpox lesion which were ground into a fine powder and blown into the nostrils of the patient.

## THE QUESTION

But does the immunization concept actually work? In the United Kingdom, vaccinations were made compulsory in 1853. Records show that at the time about 1,000 deaths per year occurred from smallpox. In the epidemic of 1871, 23,062 deaths occurred in an immunized English population. In 1887, Sheffield, England, recorded a 97 percent immunization rate. Yet, among its 20,000 residents, there were 7,101 cases of smallpox recorded resulting in 648 deaths.

In 1928, a Dr. Garrow wrote in the *British Medical Journal*, "The fatality rate among the vaccinated was five times that of the unvaccinated." In 1946, compulsory smallpox vaccination ended in the United Kingdom. The total deaths from vaccination recorded between 1951 and 1970 was 101; death among the unvaccinated for the same period was 37 or 2.73 times as among the immunized.

In 1870-71, Germany reported 124,948 smallpox deaths among a 96 percent vaccinated population. Bismarck, the Chancellor of Germany at the time, wrote, "The hope placed in the efficacy of the cowpox virus as prevention of smallpox has proved entirely deceptive." Dr. Parry wrote of this distressing reality, "How is it that in Germany, the best vaccinated country in the world, there are more deaths in proportion to the population than in England?" (which, at the time, had achieved less than a 50 percent vaccination rate?)

**Thus we see that there is no direct scientific correlation between immunization and a decreased incidence of smallpox.** What can be documented, however, is that smallpox died out as the city ghettos that spawned it were eliminated.

Such records show an apparent failure of smallpox immunization. Why, then, is it still not general knowledge over 150 years later? This is a critical question. One worthy of additional investigation because it motivates the scientific mind to wonder about the validity of other immunizations?

## WHY DISCUSS SMALLPOX

Since smallpox is now considered to be eradicated in the United States and inoculations are no longer required, why discuss it? Because it is accepted as the scientific benchmark for the theory of all other immunizations. However, there is one critical difference between smallpox and all of the other dis-eases against which our public health laws require immunizations. **Smallpox immunizations are derived from Veriola Vaccinae, a very similar but not identical and much milder dis-ease of cattle, and not the products of the identical human dis-ease as are all other immunizations. Therefore, since all other immunization rational and practice is based upon this assumption rather than well-controlled scientific facts, all current immunization practices come under suspicion as to their validity.**

## POSITION

What then must the modern scientific position be regarding immunization? In 1943, Dr. Dauer, an epidemiologist stated, "If mortality (from pertussis - whooping cough)) continues to decline at the same rate over the next fifteen years, it will be extremely difficult to show statistically that (pertussis immunization) had any affect in reducing mortality from whooping cough." Mortimer, writing in the journal *Science* in 1978, noted that "Morbidity and mortality from infectious diseases in the United States have declined more than 90 percent since 1900. Factors believed to be responsible for this decline include changes in the natural history of disease, sanitation (engineering), quarantine measures, control of non-human vectors, antibacterial drugs and immunization." To this list, we are obligated to add: increasing levels of patient education and personal hygiene; availability of a more varied diet and nutritional supplements; better protection from the elements; environmental and pollution controls; indoor plumbing; central heating and air conditioning; less taxing forms of transportation; shorter working hours; stricter immigration laws; better education of practitioners, a better understanding of and more respect for man's place in the ecosystem.

Obviously, from a scientific perspective, no one of these factors can claim exclusive credit for the reduction in the infectious dis-ease rates and yet, this is precisely what immunization proponents have repeatedly tried to have us believe for 150 plus years.

## ARE VACCINATIONS EFFECTIVE?

The side effects listed from a 1995 pharmaceutical company ad in a leading national woman's journal regarding measles vaccination include burning or stinging where the injection is given. Some individuals may develop moderate to high fevers (101 - 103 degrees F), rash or both, usually between the 5th and 12th day after vaccination. Very serious, severe allergic reactions have been reported following the administering of the vaccine. These may include convulsions, seizures, eye problems, complicated skin problems, blood abnormalities, inflammation of the blood vessels, temporary or permanent muscle paralysis, loss of feeling and encephalitis (inflammation of the brain), which may result in permanent brain damage and even death. The doctor can provide information about other possible side effects that have been reported following vaccination. **Vaccination may not result in protection against measles in every child.**

## POOR SCIENCE, POOR MEDICINE

When was the last time a proponent of immunization went over the side effects of immunizations prior to asking for your permission to immunize your child? Were you informed that one of these possible side effects of immunization was death? Were you told that the immunizations may not protect your child?

## RUBELLA

But what about the other components of the trivalent MMR immunizations? The rubella vaccine is under suspicion for a wide variety of serious complications as well. The 1996 (50th Edition) of the *Physician's Desk Reference (PDR)* states that the **first MMR is injected at 15 months, since prior to this, it is believed that circulating maternal antibodies will interfere with the immunization process.** It further reads, "Clinical studies of 279 triple seronegative children, 11 months to 7 years of age, demonstrated that MMR II is highly immunogenic and generally well tolerated. In these studies, a single injection of the vaccine induced measles hemaglutination-inhibition (HI) antibodies in 95 percent, mumps neutralizing antibody in 96 percent and rubella HI antibodies in 99 percent of the susceptible persons." If these figures are correct, then what is the scientific reason for administering a second or even a third immunization?

Even A. Guyton, M.D., considered to be a leading authority on the subject, writes, "Fortunately, the newborn inherits much immunity from its mother because many antibodies diffuse from the mother's blood through the placenta into the fetus. However, the newborn itself does not form antibodies to a significant extent. By the end of the first month, the baby's gamma globulins, which contain the antibodies, have decreased to less than one-half the original level, with a corresponding decrease in immunity. Thereafter, the baby's own immunization processes begin to form antibodies, and the gamma globulin concentrations return essentially to normal by the age of 6 to 20 months. Despite the decrease in gamma globulins soon after birth, the antibodies inherited from the mother still protect the infant for about six months against most major childhood infectious diseases, including diphtheria, measles, smallpox and polio. **Therefore, immunization against these diseases before six months is usually unnecessary**" (emphasis added). D. Tole, D.C., states, "It can take up to one year before the infant begins to develop a normal IgM titter and up to four years before some reach full IgA levels." Yet the PDR which was quoted as stated 15 months also reads, ". . . Vaccinations can be started at 6 weeks. . ." Pediatricians routinely push for such without individual considerations. Is this science?

Another question not being considered is why dis-eases like measles affect both the immunized and un-immunized. In 1993, during a measles outbreak in Cincinnati, Ohio, 82 percent of those who contracted the disease had three doses of the measles vaccine and 74 percent had four doses. A study done by the World Health Organization states that chances are about 14 times greater that measles will be contracted by those vaccinated against the dis-ease than by those not vaccinated. Although the overall incidence of measles in the U.S. has dropped from about 400,000 cases in the early 1960s to about 30,000 cases during the years 1974-76, the death rate remained between 2 and 3 percent.

## BY-PASS OF IMMUNE DEFENSE MECHANISMS

**Since an injected vaccine by-passes the majority of the immune defense responses based in tissues in the mucosal, tonsils, gut and lungs, these components are not stimulated to produce antibodies.** Compare this with natural immunity in which the barriers of the skin, gut, lungs, and lymphoid tissues that guard the portals of entry against microbes and trigger a full immune response before the infectious agent reaches the general circulation. Such by-passing of the natural defense mechanisms are certainly capable of producing profound and devastating effects upon the patient, but for all practical purposes they have been totally ignored by proponents of artificially injected immunizations.

## IMMUNOLOGICALLY (IATROGENICALLY) INDUCED DIS-EASE

Putting aside the questionable validity of immunization's effectiveness, vaccines have created whole new categories of dis-eases such as atypical measles, a highly virulent form of the dis-ease which **only effects the immunized with a considerably higher mortality rate than the naturally acquired dis-ease.**

But the problems do not stop there. A 1964 study, reported in the *American Journal Of Natural Medicine,* of 2,541 measles vaccinated individuals and 11,407 unvaccinated subjects documented a 3.01 times greater incidence of Crohn's Disease and a 2.54 times greater incidence of Ulcerative Colitis in the immunized group. **The issue is does the measles immunization prevent what is, in most cases, a rather mild, benign dis-ease, while at the same time laying the groundwork for more serious, chronic dis-eases such as Crohn's Disease and Ulcerative Colitis?**

## DEVELOPMENTAL DELAY CORRELATED TO IMMUNIZATION

*The Developmental Delay Registry* recently completed a multinational survey, reported in their publication, The Vaccine Registry, of 696 children, 449 of whom were delayed in their development and 247 who were normal in their development, and established that **children with developmental delays are 4 times more likely to have a negative reaction to vaccinations than children who were not developmentally delayed. This study also documented that delayed children are 27 percent more likely to suffer from repeated ear infections and 50 percent more likely to have been on repeated rounds of antibiotics (which are immune-suppressing in nature) for such infections.**

H. Coulter. M.P.H., extensively discusses the corollaries between immunizations and anorexia, autism, seizure disorders, asthma, Tourette's Syndrome, encephalitis, attention deficit disorders, dyslexia, stuttering and many more neurological and behavioral problems. He refers to an incident in **vaccinated children of 6 times more encephalitis which closely parallels the incidence of Attention Deficit Disorders (ADD) and hyperactivity (ADHD) and the use of the drug Ritalin.**

## TIP OF THE ICEBERG

V. Scheibner states in her book that she has **collected more than 55,000 pages of medical studies documenting adverse side effects from all forms of immunization.** She also documents that in 1975, the Japanese raised the minimal vaccination age to 2 years and this was followed by the virtual disappearance of Sudden Infant Death Syndrome (SIDS or Crib Death).

# PERTUSSIS

In 1950, published evidence that there was a definite correlation between administering the pertussis and/or pertussis-diphtheria-tetanus (DPT) immunization and the onset of poliomyelitis (within 90 days of immunization) with the majority of the paralysis occurring in the inoculated limb.

I. Gloden reports that, "A 1994 study of 446 children and adolescents demonstrated that **children who receive the pertussis vaccine are 5.43 times more likely to develop asthma in later years, over twice as likely to have recurring ear infections and significantly more likely to spend longer periods in hospitals than those not immunized.**

# POLIOMYELITIS

A Polio Vaccine Workshop, sponsored by the Institute of Medicine's Vaccine Safety Forum, featured a spirited two-day discussion among U. S. and international public health officials, physicians organization representatives, vaccine manufacturers, polio victims, parent groups and consumers about whether the U. S. should change polio vaccine policies to reduce the incidence of Vaccine Associated Polio (VAP - iatrogenically induced polio) caused by the mass, mandatory administration of the Sabin Oral Polio Vaccine (OPV). Unlike the Salk Inactive Polio Vaccine (IPV), which contains the killed polio virus, OPV contains a weakened but LIVE form of the polio virus.

# POLYIMMUNIZATIONS

If each of these "standard" childhood immunizations have so many negative side effects and so many unanswered questions remain, what happens when a child receives multiple vaccines at one time, the DPT-MMR-HIB-OPV for example? There are apparently no studies determining if this does or does not produce an overload on the immune system and yet this "immunological Russian roulette" is commonplace.

# GENETIC MUTATIONS

G. Buttram writes, "**Viral vaccines for many years have been suspected as agents which carry foreign genetic materials into the human system. Since the immune system must recognize and combat that which is foreign to 'self', this foreign genetic material may SET IN MOTION IMMUNE DERANGEMENTS IN THE FORM OF AUTO IMMUNE DIS-EASES**" (emphasis added).

He is not the only one to put forth such concerns. Laderberg, at the Department Of Genetics, Stanford University, said, "In point of fact we already practice biological engineering on a rather large scale by the use of live viruses and mass immunization campaigns. While these are thought to be of indubitable value for preventing serious diseases, their global impact on the development of human beings of a side range of genotypes is hard to assess at our present stage of wisdom. Crude virus preparations, such as some in common use at the present time, are also vulnerable to frightful mishaps of contamination and mis-identification. Live viruses are themselves genetic messages used for the purpose of programming human cells for the synthesis of immunogenetic virus antigens."

Viruses are suspect in bringing about genetic changes since they are made up of pure genetic materials, either DNA or RNA strands. Viruses are also uniquely susceptible to the process of "Jumping Genes". Mobile genetic elements (Jumping Genes) were first described by McClintock and there is now a large body of literature documenting the ability of viruses to bring about changes in host cells. However, the viruses themselves are also susceptible to genetic changes as they pass through different cell cultures during their production. Considering that viral vaccines must be incubated in some form of cell culture (chick embryo, monkey kidney, etc.) it would appear inevitable that the vaccines would carry these foreign imprints into the human recipient thereby causing a percentage of adverse genetic changes to take place.

In 1971, the Japanese described how bacteriologists discovered that bacteria of one species could transfer their resistance to specific antibodies to bacteria of a different species. Further research at the Department Of Plant Physiology at Geneva University has proved that the genetic transfer of information is not confined to bacteria but occurs also between bacteria and higher plants and animals. **This process involves the "shedding" of DNA material which may be taken up by other cells.** Turning from plants to animals, the research extracted frog tissue and immersed this in bacterial suspensions. They found that ribonucleic acid and deoxyribonucleic acid from the bacteria became "hybridized" with genetic material from the frog tissues. The results were explained thus: "Since we know that no bacteria got into the frog auricles, we can only conclude that the bacterial DNA must have been exuded from the bacteria and absorbed by the animal cells. This transfer phenomenon, or 'transcession' as it has been called, is very probably a general one, otherwise the synthesis of bacterial RNA would hardly have been successfully achieved with animal tissues at the first attempt."

A question has been posed in this text which has tremendous implications: **"What connection does transcession from bacteria to our own cells have with dis-ease?" Could heart damage that can follow after rheumatic fever and similar bacterial infections be the result of the body's immunological system reacting to its own production of alien RNA? From a scientific perspective, then, we are also forced to ask, could such damage also be the result of the viral immunizations?**

## CANCER

Research has continued along these lines and it has been confirmed that there does occur a spontaneous release of DNA by human blood lymphocytes in laboratory conditions. This process takes place, and has been consistently demonstrated, between a variety of different cells and species. DNA transfer occurs between bacteria and animals and man and also between cells of higher organisms. The possibility that all of this activity may have implications relating to the development of cancers cannot be dismissed. It is possible that DNA material could occur in free form, circulating in the blood stream and/or lymph, and that there may be a take-up of this genetic material by cells with implications relating to tumor development.

In 1975, the Nobel Prize was awarded to Baltimore and Temin for their work demonstrating that cancer-causing viruses used, as part of the process involved in the causation, an enzyme called "Reverse Transcriptase." This enabled the virus to attach itself to the DNA of the cells it infected. Thus incorporated into the genetic material of the cell of an animal, cancer development may begin. **Could immunizations be "seeding" humans with virus DNA?** At the present stage of research, we cannot definitely state yes or no. But wisdom should dictate, better safe than sorry.

## LEUKEMIA AND MULTIPLE SCLEROSIS

**Many hold the view that Salk and Sabin vaccines, being made of monkey kidney tissue, are responsible for the major increase of leukemia.**

In 1967, the *British Medical Journal* reported, "German authors have described the apparent provocation of multiple sclerosis by vaccination against smallpox, typhoid, tetanus, polio and tuberculosis, and after injections of antidiphtheria serum." Zintchenko (1965) reported 12 patients in whom multiple sclerosis first manifested after a course of anti-rabies vaccinations.

Weaver reported in 1967: **"Circulating antibodies are responsible for some destruction of the myelin sheath in MS. Moreover, cell culture tests reveal that an unidentified blood protein destroys the myelin, but when the protein factor is removed, the myelin is rapidly repaired. MS patients have probably had prior infections such as measles and mumps. A delayed autoimmune reaction in the central nervous system could be involved."**

It is interesting to note that the removal of the tonsils is yet another aspect of weakening the immune system which has been documented to increase the risk of MS in later years. Poskanzer of Harvard Medical School's Department Of Preventive Medicine and Neurology reports that **the risk of developing MS is doubled if the tonsils are absent.**

## PSYCHIATRIC DISORDERS

G. Buttram, et al., state, "Significant data implicates and relates viral infections in general to psychotic illness." Rabin, at Western Psychiatric Institute in Pittsburgh, has found evidence that approximately **one-third of all cases of schizophrenia are autoimmune in nature, with immune bodies attacking the brain cells.**

## MEDICAL DOGMA OR MEDICAL SCIENCE

The above is just a random sampling of the many volumes of data available questioning the validity of immunizations. In the past, immunity was reported if there were a certain number of antibodies to a specific disease present in the blood stream. However, the living being is designed to work as an integrated whole, not as a single system working in isolation. We now know that without the aid of the remainder of the defense system, antibodies cannot do their job properly. If antibodies were the exclusive key to immunity then it should be relatively easy to prove. However, this does not hold true under closer scrutiny. There are children who are born with agammaglobanemia and have not the capacity to produce antibodies. Yet these children show normal signs and symptoms of measles (for example) and recover with long-term immunity. They accomplish this without antibodies, indicating that there are a variety of factors involved in the immune defense system that are as yet little understood.

## DISCREPANCIES

AS previously noted **the PDR states a 95-99 percent finding of antibodies to MMR vaccine. Similar results are quoted for Haemophilis B vaccine. Such results might be questioned if it weren't for the fact that the reporting period following vaccination was a mere 48 hours! Everything, side effects, direct effects and antibody persistence after 48 hours was not examined (or the data was withheld). Yet an infant has about 26,000 days (70 years) ahead of him and all studies on HIB vaccinations look at only the first two days! Apparently no one knows what happens at 30 or 300 or 3,000 days; or perhaps the results are not good. If the values were good (high levels of persistent global immunity, with few iatrogenic side-effects) wouldn't the pharmaceutical companies want to trumpet it loud and long?** And if such research has not been done, doesn't that constitute extremely poor scientific procedure and even poorer government control of the pharmaceutical industry?

# THE POINT

There is a large volume of scientific data that contraindicates mass compulsory immunization. In fact, there is extensive scientific data that suggests that mass immunization, without regard to individual sensitivities, may be the single greatest health threat ever to be encountered by mankind. In a free society, the immunization choice must be the individual's, after having studied the pros and cons and giving informed consent. Under current mandatory public health immunization programs, the requirement of informed consent is totally ignored and, therefore ,there is a very strong legal position that such programs are in violation of the laws of free countries. In fact, they are characteristic of communistic countries in which individuals have no rights.

Proponents of mass, undiscriminating immunization obviously don't want to hear this and want to continue to force their viewpoint upon the rest of our society "for reasons of public safety". However, this is not scientifically rational; if immunizations are truly effective, they should protect immunized individuals in the event of epidemics. The second concept of proponents is the welfare of the non-immunized. But shouldn't a scientifically rational mind be just as concerned about the welfare of the immunized, considering all of the dramatic iatrogenic problems resulting from immunization? **In view of the conflicting and, in many instances, the absence of valid, scientific evidence relating to the effectiveness of immunizations, it is just as scientifically sound reasoning to reject immunization as it is to accept it.**

# Chapter 33
# THE ANTIBIOTIC QUANDARY

*"If I could live my life over again I would devote it
to proving that germs seek their natural
habitat - diseased tissue - rather than being
the cause of dis-eased tissue; i.e., mosquitoes
seek the stagnant water but do not cause the
pool to become stagnant."*
— Rudolph Virchow

## IN PERSPECTIVE

**The word "antibiotic" literally means "against life"**. Such a designation should alert every true healer to have great respect for and maintain an educated reservation about the indiscriminate use of these substances. In fact, Dr. H. A. Reimann of Hahnemann Medical College bluntly states, "90 percent of anti-biotics are given unnecessarily."

## PARASITES

Technically, a parasite is any organism that lives on or in another organism  upon  which it feeds. Bacteria, viruses (Latin for  "poisonous slime"), bacilli, prions (a minute particle of pure protein with a total absence of genetic materials and no known function other than to kill higher level organisms), fungi, yeasts, molds, protozoa and worms are, therefore, to some degree, parasitic in nature. Even cancers, in some respects, fit into this broad definition.

This concept is critical in order to understand the nature of such dis-eases and how to properly render care for them, but even more importantly how to prevent them. Traditionally, biologists have exhibited a peculiar quirk of using the term "parasite" in a much more severely restricted sense, mainly referring to protozoa and worms. It is this lack of broad scope understanding that in great part has led to the current antibiotic crisis.

## HISTORY

Secondly, and very unfortunately, the biologist's myopic perspective suggests to some that parasites are all bad. However, without them, life would not be possible since they constitute clean-up crews that break down and recycle materials so that another generation can be constructed from them. With no parasites (microbes, etc.), our environment would quickly become uninhabitable because  of undecomposed vegetable matter and corpses of every species of higher life littering our living space. Fortunately, over 97 percent of these clean-up crews are harmless or beneficial and less than 3 percent are problematic.

Even more intriguing, many of the beneficial ones, such as the bacteria in our guts, help to protect us from the other 3 percent. It is with these desirable organisms that antibiotics wreak havoc as they are in most cases indiscriminate killers of both the pathogenic and beneficial factors. For example, when the beneficial bacteria in the intestinal system  are destroyed, digestion and assimilation suffer. Additionally, antibiotics generally suppress the immune system (See Figure 13.2) and, therefore, the patient is more likely to have recurring episodes since the natural defense mechanisms have been rendered less effective. This is precisely the scenario being acted out with patients who have a long history of antibiotic treatment but continue to have recurring infections.

## OVER-PRESCRIPTION

Antibiotics are prescribed at an alarming rate. Obstetricians and gynecologists have been the biggest offenders, writing 2,645,000 prescriptions every week. Internists have been the next greatest abusers giving out 1,416,000 prescriptions in a week. But the new champions of iatrogenic prescribing are now pediatricians and family practitioners, prescribing over $500 million worth each year for the treatment of just one problem - ear infections in children. But that's not all. They write another $500 million a year to treat other pediatric illnesses. In fact, in the last 15 years, their prescription writing for antibiotics has increased a staggering 51 percent.

Congressional hearings have documented that 40 to 60 percent of all antibiotics are mis-prescribed and/or unnecessarily prescribed. In 1983, more than 51 percent of all patients seeing an allopathic doctor for the common cold were prescribed an antibiotic, even though it is common knowledge that almost all antibiotics are ineffective against the virus of the common cold.

## "CATCH 22"

**The catch is that these antibiotics can't tell the difference between something that should be killed and something that should not and does not want to be eliminated.**

In the 1960s the Surgeon General of the United States naively stated, "It is time to close the book on infectious diseases." Thirty years later, we are being overwhelmed by disastrous resurgence of virtually all classes of infectious and  parasitic dis-eases. This is because conventional medicine has failed to understand their so-called "enemy". Unfortunately, bacteria, viruses and other so-called "causative agents" are far more complicated, dynamic, tenacious, resourceful and adaptive than anticipated by the reductionistic mind.

## THE SHOCKING REALITY

**All parasitic agents, be they virus, bacteria, protozoa, fungus, yeasts, molds, bacilli, prions or worms can an do mutate. They freely mix genetic material from other species they come in contact with (as well as their hosts) and form new hybrid super species with totally different properties, resistance and virulence. However, the most distressing aspect is that the RNA based viruses (Ebola, HIV, influenzas, designer viruses) can mutate at the most rapid rates, about once every 1,000 replications, or once every two to three weeks.** This means literally that every two to three weeks, there is another antibiotic that is ineffective against them. Looking at this from a slightly different perspective, it means that they are becoming resistant to antibiotics faster than the pharmaceutical companies are creating new antibiotics. In other words, **pharmaceuticals are rapidly losing their "war" against dis-ease.** But it gets even worse. **Bacteria can mutate as much in 30 hours as it will take humans 2,000 years to achieve.** To put it bluntly, we cannot evolve fast enough to win the survival race by utilizing antibiotics. Antibiotics are, for the most part, a dead-end street.

By 1992, there were over 420 anti-infective products on the market in the U.S. Despite this impressive number, patients in hospitals die hourly in of incurable infectious dis-eases. Additionally, every year 2 million Americans develop iatrogenically-induced hospital infections and 80,000 of them die due to these antibiotic-resistance hospital super germs. R. Haley, M.D., head of the Epidemiology and Preventive Medicine Unit at the University of Texas Health Science Center states, "every piece of equipment, every invasive technique provides the opportunity for infection to develop." In fact, hospitals are now, statistically, one of the most dangerous and deadly places on earth due to such mutated super organisms. Think about this; 80,000 Americans die annually from iatrogenic super germs. We only lost 5,000 men a year from enemy bullets during the Viet Nam War. **That means our hospitals are sixteen times more deadly than modern combat.**

## DEMOGRAPHICS

Poor medical practices are not the only cause of this ticking biological time bomb. Closely-packed humanity also provides the ideal environment for the spread of dis-ease. Today, over 200 million people live in poverty in 15 mega-cities, mostly in poor third-world countries without adequate nutrition and sanitation, the victims of local and global politics that prevent solutions from being achieved. Scientific studies repeatedly document that when a population of any living entity reaches a "critical mass", dis-ease and death spread like wildfire.

Unfortunately, first-world cities are not immune to similar nightmares. The New York City Health Department announced that the life expectancy for a man living in the inner city had declined from 68.9 years in 1981 to 61.9 years in 1993. Interestingly, in non-metropolitan New York State, the life expectancy for the same year had increased to 73.4 years. In Harlem, the life expectancy was just 49.0 years. Compare this with the average life expectancy of 65.1 years for a man in Bangladesh, one of the world's poorest nations.

Numerous studies show that as many as 25 million Americans in 1993 were suffering from hunger and malnutrition. The same reports indicate that in 1993, one in ten Americans were forced to stand in a bread line, eat in a soup kitchen or received food from a charitable organization. Federal documents reveal that Americans living below the poverty line between 1982 and 1992 increased three times faster than the population. In 1992, 14.5 percent or 37,500,000 Americans lived in poverty. The Children's Defense Fund sadly documents that the United States ranks 19th in the world in infant mortality, 29th in low-birth weight, and 22nd for mortality under the age of five. **For tens of millions of Americans, America is a third-world country, with all of the third-world potential for disastrous epidemics.**

## TRANSPORTATION

It is estimated that by the turn of the century, one billion people worldwide will travel by air, allowing infected and infested individuals to spread their dis-eases globally within a matter of hours. Add to this those moving by less rapid and less regulated means such as automobiles, trucks, busses, shipping companies, railways, etc., and dis-eased individuals can literally travel, with very minimal restrictions, throughout the planet in hours to days.

# THE ENVIRONMENT

Within the past 50 years, mankind has changed the environment of the planet more than in all previous times combined. We annually dump hundreds of millions of tons of toxic waste into our air, water, land and foodstuffs. Items that in many cases can take thousands of years to degrade to non-toxic or non-lethal levels, some of which being biological in nature have the ability to multiply and mutate in and of themselves.

For example, in the United States between 1991 and 1992, federal agencies reported thirty-four outbreaks of drinking water-borne dis-ease in systems meeting federal drinking water standards. Of these, 27 percent were caused by identifiable agents but an astonishing 68 percent have never had their etiology identified in the most technologically advanced nation in the world. The Natural Resources Defense Council documents that over one million Americans fall ill every year from water contamination and 900 of them die. This same organization has documented over 250,000 violations of federal drinking water laws nationwide. Additionally, they estimate that 8 percent of the nation's drinking water, especially in smaller towns and rural areas, goes without monitoring by any state and/or federal agency.

# THE FOOD SUPPLY

With standardization of agricultural crops (hybrids), the vast majority of crops worldwide share the same genetic basis. Therefore, a crop dis-ease is capable of spreading without genetic restraints through the world's food supply and is capable, in very short order, of decimating entire crops and thereby producing world-wide famine and a corresponding decline in health.

Honey bees pollinate 80 to 95 percent of all food crops. A Reuters' news story states, "Utah's honey industry is feeling the effects of parasites that can kill an entire hive of bees in a few weeks. In fact, so many bees died last year that honey production for 1995 is less than half the previous year, and bee keepers are in danger of going out of business. When this hit, some bee keepers experienced total loss. One in Box Elder county had only six swarms out of 200 remaining." The world's population cannot survive on 3 percent of its current food supply and yet without bees there can be no pollination of crops and therefore no food.

# SUPPLEMENTATION

There are many who feel most of these woes can be circumvented by nutritional supplements; unfortunately, it is not as simple as they would have us believe. For example, Zulu men regularly drink beer made in iron pots and very frequently have serious liver infections caused by amoeba. In contrast, less than 10 percent of the Masai tribesmen have amoebic infections. They are herdsmen and drink large amounts of milk. When a group of Masai were supplemented with iron, 88 percent developed amoebic infections. In another study, well-meaning but poorly educated humanitarians gave iron supplements to increase the low levels of minerals found in Somali nomads. At the end of one month, 38 percent had infections as compared to 8 percent in the control group. It's an example of, "Medicine rushing in where angels fear to tread." A study by Kluger and associates reported only 11 percent of physicians and 6 percent of pharmacists knew that iron supplementation is contraindicated for patients with infections.

# NATURAL DISASTERS

Nor are first world countries immune from the effects of natural disasters such as hurricanes, typhoons, floods, drought, tornadoes, earthquakes, snowstorms, avalanches, volcanic eruptions and monsoons, all of which can disrupt utilities and sanitary services and thereby produce conditions that will allow those with lowered resistance to fall ill.

# ANTIBIOTICS IN ANIMAL FEEDS

For over 40 years, feed companies have known that antibiotics in their feeds cause animals to grow faster. Jude found that chicks, after only 25 days, were three times the size of the controls. With 30 times as many farm animals, fish and fowl as humans in the United States, this becomes a major problem of unnecessary and unwarranted antibiotic contamination for the consuming population. This agriculture source amounts to 20 million pounds of antibiotics a year or twice the human therapeutic usage.

It is estimated that the average cow excretes about 100 times the fecal and urinary matter of a human each day. This excretion is loaded with microorganisms that have become resistant to antibiotics. When spread on crop land as fertilizer, these super organisms are incorporated into the soil in which our foods are grown. A 1980 study on East Germany swine farms documented that within six months, streptothricin-laced feed produced resistant strains in the swine. Two years later, the same resistant strains were identified in the stools of the farm workers and even those villagers who lived near the farms but had no direct contact with the farming activities.

# THE PRICE

Lappe summarizes this entire problem thus, **"Unfortunately, we played a trick on the natural world by seizing control of these (natural) chemicals, making them more perfect in a way that has changed the whole microscopic constitution. . . . We have organisms now proliferating that never existed before in nature. We have selected them. We have organisms that probably caused a tenth of a percent of human disease in the past that now cause twenty to thirty percent of the diseases that we're seeing. We have changed the whole face of the earth by the use of antibiotics."**

# HOPELESS?

The above review as well as that found in Chapter 32, The Immunization Question, paints an extremely dismal picture for a healthy future or for that matter any future for mankind. **Without doubt, mankind's greatest threat to life and health is iatrogenically produced dis-eases. Nothing nature has ever devised compares with the deadly threat mankind has created for himself.**

All of this iatrogenic nightmare is the direct result of the arrogance of the myopic, reductionistic, non-vitalistic and unscientific logic that naively believes nature's laws can be ignored. **Universal laws have been broken and we now are paying the price. And, unfortunately, as a society, we have been enamored of the iatrogenic misconception of treating of symptoms the dis-ease rather than caring for the totality of the patient who has the dis-ease.** This is the very mistake alluded to by Virchow at the beginning of this chapter, that Hahnemann addressed in his discussion of miasmas, Stephenson in his discussion of diathesis and of phases in oriental medicine and doshas in ayurvedic medicine. In other words, for 5,000 years, astute and dedicated quantum physicians have been sounding the warning and have been totally ignored. **We are now out of time, we must now learn to abide by natural laws or perish as a race. We can never treat enough symptoms, regardless of whether the treatment be quantum or allopathic, to cure the cause of dis-ease. The miasma, diathesis, dosha, phase is the cause of dis-ease.**

## ANTIBIOTICS' PLACE

Antibiotics obviously have a very important place in modern health care. However, their indiscriminate and iatrogenic use by practitioners who lack self-control and/or are inadequately educated in iatrogenic pharmacology **must be immediately and aggressively controlled, in the interest of public health and safety.** Standards of practice and ethics committees can no longer look the other way with regard to the flippant attitude that has been customary in the past. If such renegade practitioners cannot be regulated within scientific parameters, their licenses must be revoked. Not to do so is to betray the public trust placed in the various licensing professional organizations when they were founded.

## THE ANSWERS

Mankind's only long-term answer is to return to a rational, expansionistic, vitalistic science and its **related way of life and health care practice. The short-term answer is to accurately comprehend and apply the laws of this text and especially the concept of miasmatic, diathesis, phase, doshic dis-ease which proves to be the basis of all dis-ease.** To do otherwise is to inhumanely abandon the human race to suicide.

# Chapter 34
# THE PETROCHEMICAL AND HEAVY METAL QUANDARY

*"There are three kinds of lies,*
*lies, damned lies and statistics."*
— Mark Twain

## THE GOOD, BAD AND UGLY

A major chemical company's motto is, "Better living through chemistry." That is without doubt true, as many of our modern conveniences would not exist without chemistry but it is only half of the story. The other side of the coin is, "Devastated lives because of chemistry."

**Since man-made chemical substances do not exist in nature, nature has never had to evolve effective means to deal with their toxicity.** Such toxic effects occur primarily because these  foreign substances cannot easily be broken down and eliminated by living tissues. Also, they are very frequently cumulative in nature; **they are able to enter the body tissues faster than they can be eliminated, thus building up to critical toxic levels.** Another issue, having to do with the quote by Mark Twain at the beginning of this chapter, is that data is manipulated  to represent only the desirable, money-producing aspect of these substances by the chemical-industrial-pharmaceutical-media- political cartels which hold the patents for their manufacturing.

Local Poison Control Centers have literally hundreds of thousands of references in medical and chemical industry literature to document widespread toxic incidents. Furthermore, there are tens of thousands of environmentally ill patients searching for answers on the Internet, in libraries, and in support groups on how to rid themselves and their loved ones of the toxic side effects that have devastated their lives. The latest addition to the ever-growing legions are the Gulf War Syndrome (GWS) veterans who were deliberately given extensive batteries of mandatory immunization and, according to some sources, even experimental immunizations by the military. Many also have been exposed to chemical warfare agents that were specifically engineered to be "super toxic" for the express purpose of killing and incapacitating and to biological warfare agents deliberately or accidentally released during combat. Last, but by no means least, are those who were issued chemically impregnated clothing to wear during the conflict. Truly, these brave souls were exposed to a chemical-biological cocktail the likes of which few human beings have ever been required to endure.

In 1995, *National Magazine* estimated that 67 percent of babies born to Gulf War veterans who are ill have serious birth problems. According to the Doctors Nicolson, Ph.D.s, over one-half of all babies in Iraq today have deformities or major birth defects. Riegle studies conclude that 78 percent of wives of veterans who are sick are also likely to become ill as are 25 percent of their children who were born before the war and 65 percent of their children born after the war.

# LEGAL LOOPHOLE

Today fewer than 20 mega-corporations control over 90 percent of all major newspapers, magazines, radio and TV stations in America. By the turn of the century, if the trend continues, only about six could be in control.

An equally ominous trend is that reporters are relying more and more on public relations officers of these mega-firms for their information. When polled, 2,432 journalists said they relied on such sources 81 to 90 percent of the time. **Clearly, our news is managed by the mega corporations.**

Such controlled release of data also allows these cartels to take advantage of a major legal **loophole in our federal laws which allows hazardous chemical wastes to be recycled in pesticides and labeled "inert ingredients." These "legal toxic wastes" include many known carcinogenic, mutagenic and teratogenic (deformity producing) agents. These "inert ingredients" in pesticides are anything not registered as an "active  ingredient" or active poison. The typical amounts of "inerts" vary from 1 to about 20 percent by weight and 80 to 90 percent by volume. "Inerts" perform such functions in the formulation as softening the skin and thereby making it easier for the active poison to penetrate. Or they may be an oily substance that prevents the active poison from being washed away.**

**The chemical companies that manufacture these substances are not legally required to disclose their composition.** The Environmental Protection Agency  currently maintains a list of over 2,000 such inert chemicals which include carbon tetrachloride, toluene, xylene, cadmium and lead compounds.

Because the companies that manufacture them are "recycling" these toxins, they are exempt from RCRA regulations. A year's worth of such recycled waste bought by Grantech from the Fort Howard Paper Company in Green Bay, Wisconsin, contained the following; 301 pounds of styrene; 287 pounds of 2,4,6-trichlorophenol; 1,921 pounds of naphthalene; 5,629 pounds of dis(2-ethylheyxl) phthalate; 5,814 pounds of chromium; 1,643 pounds of lead; 33 pounds of mercury; 122 pounds of thallium; 278,897 pounds of zinc and small amounts of 2,3,7,8-TCDD (the most potent of the dioxins); 2,3,7,8-TCDF (a dibenzo furan); and a range of chlorinated pheols, chlorinated catechols, chlorinated guaiacols and chlorinated bensaldehydes.

None of these poisons are beneficial to your garden, your pets, or you but Grantech and other chemical companies put them in their products they sell to you with the legal blessings of our state and federal governments.

# HEAVY METALS

In addition to synthetically engineered substances, we also have a significant number of heavy metals that produce adverse effects upon living organisms. The adverse effects of mercury and other metals in dental amalgams used in the filling of cavities pose a dramatic and extensively documented health threat in dentistry. But, strangely, while governmental agencies such as the Environmental Protection Agency and the American Dental Association consider these amalgam fillings perfectly safe as long as they are in your mouth, they do, however, maintain stringent hazardous materials standards for the storage of unused amalgams.

The most frustrating part of this problem is that metal amalgams are a 150-year-old, antiquated technology that progressive practitioners are rapidly abandoning for more modern, far less toxic and much more cosmetically pleasing resin fillings. Interestingly, a metal amalgam filling has only about 30 percent of the strength of the healthy tooth. With bonded resins, the filled tooth reaches strengths close to the inherent strength of a healthy tooth.

## ABUSE

Numerous authorities such as C. Pfeiffer, Ph.D., have extensively documented the adverse side effect of overdosing on nutrients elements. For example, excessive zinc levels cause deficiencies of copper and iron. Cardiomyopathies can cause excessive cobalt. There are also studies of excessive aluminum's role in producing seizures. And, of course, adverse effects from metals such as lead, mercury, cadmium and arsenic are extensively documented. Schizophrenia and autistic symptoms have been documented from excess copper levels. Bismuth poisoning from cosmetics and habitual use of over-the-counter medications such as Pepto-bismol causing mental confusion, slurring of speech, arthropathies (joint problems) and muscular twitching are only a few examples of a significant but largely unrecognized problem.

# OUTDOOR POLLUTION

**Repeated studies document that the most widespread outdoor toxic hazard is from agricultural chemicals in general and pesticides specifically. Not only do such chemicals foul the air but they are an even bigger problem once they enter the subterranean drinking water where their presence can be detected in toxic amounts for years and even decades after their use is discontinued.** Diesel exhaust comes in second in the most hazardous category with toxic chemical waste dumps close behind in both air pollution and ground water pollution. Immediately following is the smog problem, not just in major metropolitan areas but even in moderate-sized cities, especially districts close to industrial areas, freeways, congested downtown traffic, airports and harbors. Natural gas and hydrogen-fueled vehicles provide the best track  records for non-polluting transportation.

# INDOOR POLLUTION FROM SMOKING

The National Research Council has been able to document that cigarette smoking constitutes the largest inhaled oxidant challenge to humans. Smoke contains nitrogen oxide at concentrations of approximately 3,300 ppm and generates a multitude of free radicals that rapidly deplete the body of antioxidants (especially vitamin C). Additionally, the *Journal of the American Medical Association* reports that second-hand smoke is responsible for 150,000 to 300,000 serious respiratory ailments each year in children under 18 months of age and 26,000 cases of childhood asthma and it aggravates the symptoms of over a million each year. But the real heart of the problem, as identified by F. Martinez et al., is that second-hand smoke produces miasmatic, diathesis, phase, doshic patterns of chronic dis-ease. ". . . elevated IgE and eosinophil counts in these children **with accompanying sensitivity to a host of allergans and this effect appears to be directly related to the total; number of cigarettes smoked by the parents."**

# INDOOR POLLUTION FROM CHEMICALS

The Ashford and Miller report on Environmental Protection  Agency tests conducted for pesticides in homes revealed a profile of multiple contaminants including some that had been applied years earlier. A significant number of these were products that had been banned years before because of harmful side effects.

Spengler of the Harvard School Of Public Health, in 1989, described what he calls "Pathogenic Buildings" constructed of materials which "off-gas" toxic chemicals that cannot be dissipated due to tightly-sealed modern construction. Such conditions have proven to be the cause of "Space" or "NASA Flu." Because of this problem, NASA now maintains an extensive list of materials not permitted for use in their vehicles, buildings and space-craft.

Ashford and Miller further report that gas chromatographic analysis of air samples from such structures reveals multiple spikes, each representing a particular organic compound. In fact, gas chromatography of indoor air commonly shows toxic levels of chemical compounds many hundreds to thousands of times more concentrated than in equal volumes of outdoor air.

In Japan, Muranaka, et al., documented that allergies are strongly tied to diesel exhaust emissions. They noted that the Japanese cedar tree, indigenous to the islands for millions of years, was unknown for causing allergies prior to 1964; they targeted diesel emissions as the sensitizing agent for Japan's epidemic of allergies to the tree during the last thirty years. They also strongly suspect diesel exhaust sensitizes individuals to numerous other previously non-reactive substances.

Ashford and Miller reported on Scandinavian studies that documented total volatile compounds in homes of environmentally-ill patients at 1.3 mg/m3 as opposed to 0.36 mg/m3 for non-reactive individuals.

In recent years, smoking has also been repeatedly documented to be one of the major causes of indoor air pollution and most state and local governments have taken legal steps to protect the non-smoker from the smoker's pollution in public buildings and on public transportation.

# ORGANOPHOSPHATES

Dursban is a member of a family of organophosphate (OP) type of nerve poison (pesticide) implicated in Gulf War Syndrome. OPs are the category of neurotoxins that have been used in the Tokyo subway attack (Sarin) and in Afghanistan to kill the Kurdish people. OPs were originally invented for use in Nazi concentration camps during World War II to kill the Jews and were subsequently "re-invented" by the petrochemical cartel for peacetime use as pesticides. One of their major problems is that they leave highly toxic residues which frequently can produce adverse reactions in living organisms for years after their application.

# CASE HISTORY

A local technician with a major national fumigation company while applying the insecticide Dursban inside a home spilled the chemical into the living room rug. When levels were tested in September and October of 1996 the following was found: 94.8 micrograms (mg) per square inch, which calculated to 18,651 micrograms per square foot, probably the highest level of Dursban seen inside a house. The safe level is only about 5 micrograms per square foot or 17,000 times lower than the lab reported in this carpet sample. The wall void (within the walls) samples also were extremely high with the highest sample containing 5,407.57 micrograms, indicating that Dursban had soaked into the 2x4s on the bottom of the wall void. Dursban also was found in the mattress cover, the attic insulation, vacuum cleaner dust, the air purifier filter, the return air filter, clothing, and the couch fabric. A very high level was detected in the entrance way (9,474 micrograms per square foot) indicating a spill or accident of some sort. Dursban is a neurotoxic pesticide that can cause toxic encephalopathy with repeated and prolonged exposures. It also can cause headaches, disorientation, in-coordination, spacy-like sleepiness, twitching, cramps, problems with equilibrium, memory loss, anxiety, depression, and confusion. The solvent for Dursban is xylene which can cause respiratory difficulties primarily such as hyperactive airways. The patients who had inhabited this home currently suffer from every symptom on the foregoing list.

## NEURO-ENDOCRINE-BEHAVIORAL DISORDERS

In 1995, 17 of the world's leading medical authorities on nervous, endocrine and behavior disorders issued a statement in Erice, Italy, as follows: "**New evidence is especially worrisome because it underscores the exquisite sensitivity of the developing nervous system to chemical perturbations that result in functional abnormalities. Endocrine disrupting chemicals can undermine neurological and behavioral development. . . . Many endocrine disrupting contaminants, even if less potent than the natural products, are presented in living tissue at concentrations millions of times higher than the natural hormones. . . . Exposure to endocrine disrupters can produce permanent changes.**"

## HEALTH EFFECTS DATA

In 1984, the National Research Council accessed all available data relating only to industrial and consumer chemicals. **No data relating to toxicity was available for 66 percent of pesticides, for 88 percent of cosmetics, 64 percent of drugs, 81 percent of food additives and 89 percent of chemicals in use. These figures do not mean these substances were harmless; they mean there is no data being compiled on their toxic effects.**

Of those substances for which data was available, in the pesticide category including 3,350 substances, only 10 percent had complete assessments for health hazards, 24 percent had partial assessments, 2 percent minimal assessments, 26 percent had some sketchy references and 38 percent had no assessment. In the cosmetic category including 3,410 substances, 2 percent had complete assessments, 14 percent had partial, 10 percent minimal, 18 percent sketchy and 56 percent no assessment. In the drug category including 1,815 items, only 18 percent had complete assessments, 18 percent partial, 3 percent minimal, 36 sketchy and 25 percent none. In 8,627 food additive items, 5 percent had complete assessments, 14 percent partial, 1 percent minimal, 34 percent sketchy and 46 percent none. In commercial chemicals in excess of one million pounds production in a year, including 12,860 items, 0 percent complete assessments, 0 percent partial, 11 percent minimal, 11 percent sketchy, and 78 percent none. Chemicals under one million pounds per year production, 13,911 items, had 0 percent complete assessments, 0 percent partial, 12 percent minimal, 12 percent sketchy and 76 percent none. Commercial chemicals total amounts produced annually unknown, 21,752 items, had 0 percent complete assessments, 0 percent partial, 10 percent minimal, 8 percent sketchy, 82 percent none.

## CHLORINATED DRINKING WATER

Chlorine is a highly active chemical, which is one reason why it makes such a good disinfectant even in parts-per-million. However, in addition to killing germs, chlorine reacts with organic substances found naturally in drinking water (humic acids, for example) and causes the formation of a class of chemical compounds called trihalomethanes (THMs). Some THMs have long obscure names like bromodichloromethane (a carcinogen in rodents), dibromochloromethane, dichloroethylene and dichloroethane, but others are better known, such as chloroform, benzene, carbon tetrachloride and toluene, all of which are known or strongly suspected to be carcinogens. Chlorine also forms chlorofluorocarbons used in aerosol sprays which are destroying the protective ozone layer of the earth.

With study, it becomes clear that **the majority of chemicals in use today are chlorine based and/or chlorine derived.** In fact, so much so that the American Public Health Association, a professional association founded in 1872, passed resolutions 8912 and 9709 with the wording "Recognizing and addressing the environmental health problems posed by chlorinated organic chemicals." It has been noted that virtually all chlorinated organic compounds that have been studied exhibit at least one of a wide range of serious toxic effects such as endocrine dysfunction, developmental impairment, birth defects, reproductive dysfunctions and infertility, immunosuppression, and cancer, often at extremely low doses. Many chlorinated compounds, such as methylene chloride and trichloroethylene are recognized as significant workplace hazards as well as having major effects upon aquatic and terrestrial food chains.

Since 1974, no less than 18 studies based on 8,063 subjects in areas as diverse as Atlanta, Detroit, New Orleans, San Francisco, Seattle, New York, Chicago, Connecticut, Iowa, New Jersey, New Mexico and Utah have documented that those who drink 8 cups of chlorinated tap water a day for 40 to 59 years had a 40 percent greater risk of bladder cancer than those who drank un-chlorinated water. Those who drank chlorinated tap water for 60 years or longer had an 80 percent greater incidence of bladder cancer. Interestingly, Europeans have recognized and banned chlorine in water treatment; instead, they use more modern and far less harmful ozone.

# DIOXIN

In 1976, an explosion at the Hoffman-LaRoche chemical plant in Seveso, Italy, sent a cloud of herbicide 2,4,5-T over the surrounding countryside, contaminating 37,195 people. Dioxin is created as a byproduct of the manufacturing of 2,4,5-T so the population was exposed to this toxic compound. For years, dioxin (Agent Orange defoliant of Viet Nam fame) manufacturers had been claiming it did not cause cancer in humans.

The area around Seveso was divided into three zones, A, B and R. Zone A was the most heavily contaminated containing 13 to 494 micrograms of dioxin per square yard and all 724 residents were evacuated. Zone B with contamination of up to 43 micrograms per square yard had 4,824 residents who were not evacuated. Zone R with an average of 4.3 micrograms per yard contained 31,647 residents who were not evacuated. Another 181,579 people lived beyond the R zone and inadvertently served as the control group.

In zone A residents, the increase in cancer incidence was so small as to be of no significance. In zone B, there were significant increases in the cancer rate including biliary (gall bladder/liver), bladder, multiple melanoma and myeloid leukemia of the blood-forming system and lymphoreticulosarcoma, but not until years after exposure. In the 1970s, Swedish researchers also began reporting 3- to 6-fold increases in cancer rates after exposure to phenoxy herbacides (2,3-D and 2,4,5-T). (All phenoxy herbacides are contaminated with dioxin during manufacturing.)

The FDA recently published a draft report of all scientific knowledge relating to dioxin and cancer rates. It included four separate studies of workers exposed to dioxin with an overall increase in mortality from all forms of malignancy. The EPA indicated that dioxin can mimic hormones, giving it the ability to cause cancer in many different organs and body systems. Based upon these reports, the EPA stated for the first time, "Dioxin does cause cancer in humans."

O. Axelson, an epidemiologist says, "The biological effects of TCDD (Dioxin) are of the first order public health concern." He continues, "There seems to be an urgent and costly need to change or improve industrial and other processes so as not to produce dioxin (and the toxicologically similar chlorinated dibenzo-furans). For example, there is a need to restrict the use of chlorine in paper bleaching. Incineration of waste material at too low temperature should be avoided as well as the 'combustion' of organochlorines compounds in general."

Dioxin is produced by every municipal solid waste incinerator ever tested; it is produced by all hazardous waste incinerators, cement kilns and BIFs (boilers and industrial furnaces) that burn chlorinated wastes. It is also produced in the manufacturing of 85 percent of all pesticides. It is a byproduct of all smelters and paper mills and probably of other common industrial processes.

The American paper industry, for example, produces 150,000 tons of such toxic waste in a single year and a good-sized paper mill can contaminate up to 70 million gallons of water with this waste in a single day. Additionally, the paper industry uses nearly 5 billion kilowatts of energy a year in order to produce unneeded chlorine for bleaching. This unnecessary waste of energy is just one of the reasons why European TCF (totally chlorine free) paper production is able to underprice their American counterparts by 30 percent in the world market. Additionally, European firms sell their chlorine-free mill sludge as mulch which produces additional revenue instead of mountains, rivers and lakes full of toxic wastes which kill fish, animals and people.

In other parts of the world, such as Germany, the paper industry was TCF by 1990. But in the United States, no major efforts have been made to eliminate the 150,000 tons of cancer-causing toxic chlorine waste a year produced by the paper industry.

Dioxin and other chlorine-containing and chlorine-derived compounds are the most widespread and some of the most dangerous and ignored chemical pollutants in our environment. They range from chemical production, PBC oils in electrical transformers, to chlorine water treatment, to paper production, agriculture and plastics and, thus, it is virtually impossible to live a life free of their devastating long-term adverse effects in a society that has chosen to ignore their presence.

# Chapter 35
# THE ELECTROMAGNETIC QUANDARY

*"Long distance cell-to-cell or organism-to-organism
communications may be accomplished by transmission and reception of electromagnetic signals
through membrane receptors or enzymes."*
— Tian Y. Tsong, M.D.
Deciphering The Language Of Cells
In Trends in Biological Science

## PERSPECTIVE

We are currently wrestling with dis-eases that were unknown only a short time ago. Most of these conditions are unexplainable based upon the reductionistic chemical concept of dis-ease. They are likewise unexplainable based upon the reductionist structural concept of dis-ease. Only when we begin to look at the quantum aspects of magnetoelectric pollution can we begin to make scientific sense out of the dis-ease pictures.

## PROMOTIONAL HAZARD

For a number of years a company has been promoting the therapeutic use of magnets through a multi-level sales program. They sell adhesive magnets, magnetic insoles for shoes, magnetic mattresses, magnetic seat pads, magnets to fit in belts, etc. Unfortunately for their customers, none of their promotional literature, their in-house experts nor their lay sales force seem to comprehend the potential for the adverse side effects from over-exposure to magnetic fields.

Likewise, some practitioners are now utilizing devices that generate electromagnetic and/or magnetoelectric fields based upon the work of Abrams and others. Others embrace the work of Becker using electrical currents to promote healing. We also have electro-acupuncture units, TENS units, and others available. The list goes on and on.

## IATROGENIC COMPLICATIONS

There is available significant data relating to overdosing the living being with electromagnetic and/or magnetoelectric fields. Unfortunately, it seems to be ignored in the desire to sell magnetic products.

Boericke addresses such iatrogenic symptoms under the heading of X-ray (an energy produced by the stream of negatively charged electrons from the cathode hitting the positively charged anode or target) with comparison remedies listed as Electricas (under normal circumstances it is not possible to generate a magnetic field without an electrical field also being generated), Magnetis Poli Ambo (the north and south poles combined), Magnetis Polus Articus (the north pole) and Magnetis Polus Australis (the south pole).

Hahnemann writes of such overdosing, **"These self-inflicted disturbances go away on their own with improved living conditions if no chronic miasma (diathesis, dosha, phase) is present. . . ."** This of **course means that the patient must be removed from the adverse influence;** in this case, the adverse effects of the electromagnetic and/or magnetoelectric fields. This is in complete harmony with Soviet research conducted since the 1950s. **Former Soviet-block scientists now consider that any electromagnetic and/or magnetoelectric radiation or intensity not present in nature has some adverse effects upon living tissues.**

**Only when the above protocol fails to resolve the dis-ease pattern should the prescription of additional therapy be considered.** And then, of course, only the therapy that most closely matches the chronic miasmatic (diathesis, dosha, phase) totality of the case should be administered.

## THE INVERSE SQUARE LAW

The research of R. Becker, M.D., et al, with electromagnetic fields documented that the intensity and therefore the effect of a magnetic field on living tissue complies with the "Inverse Square Law" of physics. In other words, the therapeutic value at a distance of 1mm is 1/4th that of its effect on a tissue that is in direct contact with the magnet. At a distance of 2mm, its effect is 1/16th that of tissue in direct contact with the magnet. At 3mm or approximately 1/8th inch, a mere 1/64th; at 4mm, 1/256th; and at 5mm or 3/16th of an inch, 1/1,024th the therapeutic effect. Becker found this 5mm distance to be the outer limits for therapeutic success in his laboratory research.

Scientifically speaking, when properly indicated, it would make far more sense to prescribe therapies having a magnetic influence, but not magnets themselves, internally instead of by surface application, such as homeopaths have done for the last 200 years and as ayurvedic practitioners have done for the last 3,000 years. With this route of administration, every cell of the body comes into equal contact with the therapeutic agent equally.

## THE GAUSS LAW

H. Brown and S. Chattopadhyay, at Woods Hole Marine Biological Laboratory, documented that the gauss strength of the earth's magnetic field is _ gauss with a daily fluctuation of less than 0.1 gauss plus or minus or so slight that it will not affect the needle of a compass. Yet their work clearly shows that living organisms are capable of sensing such slight changes and timing their biological cycles to them. They have further shown that living organisms with such subtle mechanisms can be totally disoriented by as small as a 200 gauss magnet used to hold a cupboard or refrigerator door closed.

The question then must be asked is what iatrogenic problems are created when strong magnets are worn for therapeutic purposes for extended periods of time, or when they are slept on in the form of magnetic mattresses, or worn as insoles in shoes for extended periods? This issue seems to be entirely ignored by promoters of magnetic healing. Furthermore, different gauss strengths seem to exhibit different physiological responses. If such questions cannot be answered, then how scientific can the current approach to magnetic therapy be?

## A SECRET OF LIFE

Extensive research has led us to the inescapable conclusion that electromagnetic and magnetoelectric fields are one of the major secrets of life. After all, all chemistry functions because of electrical-magnetic valences. All neurology is based upon the principle of a reciprocal electromagnetic charge conducting the neurological message. Clearly, this quantum aspect of life should be receiving a much greater emphasis in modern research and healing.

Walcott, at the State University Of New York, found that our brains are far more sensitive to magnetic fields than the very best magnetic compass. And Baker, at the University Of Manchester, located our "magnetic organ" in the posterior wall of the ethmoid sinus, just anterior to the pituitary gland. Becker's work also implicates the pineal gland. He states, "The pineal gland produces a veritable pharmacopoeia of active chemical substances. Some regulate the operations of all other glands in the body (including the pituitary, the former 'master gland'); others are major neurohormones (such as melatonin, seratonin and dopamine), which regulate the level of operations of the brain itself. . . . The pineal is the 'clock' that the machinists postulated was the source of biological cycles. The cyclic pattern of sleep-wakefulness is dependent upon the level of melatonin secretion by the pineal. . . . More recently it has been shown that the pineal is also sensitive to the daily cyclic pattern in the Earth's magnetic field. Melatonin secretion in human subjects may be changed at will by exposure to steady magnetic fields of the same strength as the geomagnetic field (_ gauss)."

## RACEMOSES

Complex, synthetic, organic molecules exist in mirror-image structural forms (racemoses): a right-hand and a left-hand configuration. See Chapter 25. The amino acids and sugars that compose proteins and other important biochemical structures, such as DNA, are only of one type in all living organisms, the left-hand or levo configuration. Amino acids and sugars can be made synthetically in laboratories but we always obtain a fifty-fifty mixture of dextro (right-hand) and levo (left-hand) molecules. As stated, living organisms only produce levo molecules. **This is vitally important as only levo molecules can form DNA and proteins that work efficiently in living organisms.** In fact, German research termed "Spin or Rotation  Therapy" has documented that dis-eased tissues experience a reversal of the normal levo spin pattern and that the dis-ease process cannot be resolved until the abnormal dextro pattern is abolished. According to their research, this reversal is  accomplished by exposing a blood sample to a properly oriented magnetic field and then re-injecting it into the patient. Blood prepared in this manner appears to act as an energy template, much like a homeopathic remedy, reorganizing the magnetic fields and protein and DNA helix patterns to their proper levo rotation.

## ELECTRIC FIELDS

Most modern electrical utility systems are either 50 Hz or 60 Hz frequencies that have never been a component of the Earth's normal  electromagnetic spectrum. Nor is it any longer necessary to have wires to transmit electrical currents. Today, microwave transmitters bombard the atmosphere with literally hundreds of millions of impulses. Thus, the entire atmosphere and surface of the planet are bombarded from satellites; even the surface of and the physical mass of the Earth is used to transmit messages by the military. It is impossible, regardless of the remoteness of one's location, to escape this electromagnetic pollution and its effects upon our health. Becker boldly states, **"The exposure of living organisms to abnormal electromagnetic fields results in significant abnormalities in physiology and function."**

The worst sites for this problem are communications centers, radar sites, power-generating stations, substations, radio and television stations, MRI and X-ray labs, computer facilities, airports, military installations, warehouses and manufacturing facilities that produce, store and use magnets, buildings with extensive wiring, sites receiving and transmitting to satellites, navigational beacons, electrical advertising signs, electric power lines, cellular telephones, electric blankets, household appliances, fluorescent lights, electric clocks, electric heating, microwave ovens, radio and telephone head sets, and microwave towers.

## MICROWAVE HISTORY

As early as 1928, Hosmer, at Albany Medical College, was aware of the problems relating to exposure to electromagnetic fields at the General Electric plant in Schenectady, New York. Her research documented that workers exposed to 27 MHz for only fifteen minutes experienced a two degree elevation in body temperature and became ill with vague flu-like symptoms.

In the 40s, Richardson, at the State University Of Iowa, found that within three days of exposure to microwaves, test animals exhibited early signs of cataract formation. This was followed by impressive numbers of studies from the 1950s to the mid-1970s repeatedly confirming Richardson's results.

In 1953, McLaughlin, at Hughes Aircraft Corporation, documented large numbers of cases of unexplained bleeding in workers exposed to low-strength microwaves. The next year, Heller and Teixeira-Pinto of the New England Medical Research Institute documented chromosomal defects of plants exposed to 27 MHz radio frequencies.

The U. S. Air Force in the 1980s, through their School of Aerospace Medicine, funded research by Guy at the University of Washington in which rats were continuously exposed to high-frequency microwaves of 2.45 gigahertz and .5 mW/cm2 (which was twenty times lower than the set thermal safety levels). This research found that primary malignant tumors developed in eighteen of the exposed animals but in only five of the controls or 3.6 times the cancer rate of that of the controls.

The power line scandal of 1987 in the state of New York was the next major revelation regarding the inadequacy of the prevailing 3 milligauss safety standard. Values measured at the edge of the power company's 50 feet from the center line right-of-way measured 100 milligauss or 33.3 times the acceptable levels. J. Phillips, et al., of the Cancer Research and Treatment Center in San Antonio, Texas, found that a 60 Hz field caused human cancer cells to increase their growth rate by 1,600 percent.

Salzinger, at the Polytechnical University of Brooklyn, found that fetal rats exposed to a 60 Hz field experienced significant learning disabilities in later life as compared to control groups. Selzman of the State University of New York found that monkeys exposed to a 60 Hz field demonstrated disturbed biological cycles for months after the exposure. Wolpaw of the New York State Department of Health documented that this disturbance was in part due to abnormally low levels of the hormones seratonin and dopamine.

J. Delgado's work demonstrated that, "The electrical currents produced within the brain by exposure to such fields were hundreds of times lower in intensity than those required to electrically stimulate a nerve. . . ." Becker writes, "The mechanistic concept of the brain is essentially that of a 'hard wired' system, but one that could alter its wiring patterns through learning and experience. In this system, information is carried only by nerve impulse, which is basically the same whether it is transmitting vision, hearing or information between parts of the brain. **The different sensations are the result of signals that are routed from specific organs to specific regions of the brain, A system such as this, based solely on a single type of signal cannot be perturbed by exposure to ELF (extreme low frequency) fields of the extremely low strengths used by Delgado."** Becker continues, **"A dual system with a primitive DC analog system and a superimposed, sophisticated, digital nerve-impulse system is strengthened by the observation of these ELF effects. If the digital nervous system - by which we see, hear, smell, taste, feel and move - is the child of a more** primitive system by which we grow, heal and obey the physical rhythms of our world, then there must be an intersection, a meeting place between the two." He then speculates that this is the site of the mind, memory, logic and creativity.

## MILITARY IMPLICATIONS

Becker reports that electromagnetic pulse (EMP) weapons are currently being evaluated by the military in the range of 1,200 MHz to 35 GHz with a power of up to 1,000 megawatts. He further states that reports from the Microwave Research Department at Walter Reed Army Institute of Research state, "Microwave energy in the range of 1 to 5GHz, a militarily important range, penetrates all organ systems of the body and thus puts all organ systems at risk. Effects on the central nervous system are considered very important. The testing program began in 1986 and was  divided into four parts: 1) promote debilitation effects; 2) prompt stimulation through auditory effects; 3) work interference/stoppage effects; and 4) effects on the stimulus-controlled behavior." Thus, the grand question for health care providers is why would the military want to develop such weapons systems if they were not a highly effective means of adversely effecting target populations and, further, can the effects be any different from general electromagnetic pollution?

# Chapter 36
# THE PSYCHOLOGICAL QUANDARY

*"The potentials of consciousness remain well-nigh
the last reachable domain for man not yet
explored — the Undiscovered Country."*
— Charles Muses
Mathematician

## PSYCHOLOGICAL STRESS IN PERSPECTIVE

H. Selye, of McGill University, writes, **"Stress is not even necessarily bad for you; it is also the spice of life, for any emotion, any activity causes stress. But, of course, your system must be prepared to take it. The same stress which makes one person sick can be an invigorating experience for another. Stress is essentially reflected by the rate of all the wear and tear caused by life."**

## CAUSES OF STRESS

Distress is most easily understood in terms of the classic "fight or flight" response as envisioned by a person walking through the forest and coming upon a very large and very angry grizzly bear. The person either responds by fighting or running away from the danger. However, a much clearer understanding of stress is obtained if we begin to sort out the different types of distress.

## MENTAL

Mental distress is a very broad category and can range from shock experienced at the violent death of a loved one to having one's feelings hurt by an offhanded remark. The complicating factor is that in modern society we frequently do not have opportunities to dissipate the emotions generated and are required to suppress them to the subconscious level of our minds where they begin producing adverse effects that we do not easily associate with the true emotional cause. Nervous breakdowns and job burnout are modern examples of this type of stress.

# PHYSICAL

Physical distress can be as basic as working too many hours, not getting enough sleep, lack of exercise, performing repetitive motions as on an assembly line, twisting an ankle, breaking a bone, spinal problems. In other words, pushing ourselves beyond our limits which results in irritability, restlessness, poor mental performance or injury.

# CHEMICAL

This is a very common form of distress in our modern environment. It consists of numerous areas of contamination which can have very subtle to very obvious effects upon our mental, emotional and spiritual ability to function properly. They include environmental pollutants, food additives, coloring agents, preservatives, medications, lack of elimination of auto-toxins, agricultural, industrial and household chemicals.

# THERMAL

Distress results when the person is exposed to extremes of temperature, drafts or extremes of humidity, which place the body and/or mind in a state of shock.

# THE LAST FRONTIER

Human beings, in general, understand very little about themselves. We frequently do not clearly comprehend why we experience the emotional responses we do. If we did, psychiatrists, psychologists, counselors, social workers, clergy, hypnotherapists, etc., would have gone out of business long ago. We will probably come to understand everything else in the universe before we totally master ourselves. This is because **the human mind is the most complex thing in the universe.**

# LAW OF LAWS

What we do know, however, is that the human mind, emotions and spirit are governed by laws just as everything else in the universe is. When we understand the laws, we can then begin to understand ourselves.

# MUSIC

Retallack's research was among the first to document the effect of music on plants grown in control chambers. Baroque instrumental music, featuring compositions for strings by Bach, Mozart, Vivaldi, Telemann, Corelli and Handel and Indian sitar music in the Vilambita style (with a rhythm of sixty beats a minute) produced lushly foliated plants which leaned toward the source of music as much as 60 degrees and exhibited extensive root systems.     Interestingly, the same music produces alpha brain waves in humans. The plants in the chambers where rock music was played shriveled and died. Jazz, such as Joplin, caused the plants to lean toward the speakers 15 degrees and show somewhat increased growth over controls in the silent chambers. Country and Western music resulted in no different effects on the plants from those grown in silent chambers. Unexplainably, the music of Debussy caused plants to lean away from the speaker at a 10 degree angle.

Research has documented that two-thirds of the inner ear's cilia (the tens of thousands of tiny hairs that lie flat like piano keys) resonate only at the higher "musical" frequencies (3,000 to 20,000 hertz). This indicates that humans are designed to do a significant portion of their communicating through song and tone. But, humans are not the only creatures that respond to music. Dairy farmers know that milk production goes up when relaxing music is played in their milking barns.

Washington State, Department of Immigration and Naturalization play Mozart and baroque classics during English classes for new arrivals and report that it speeds up their learning. The city of Edmonton, Alberta, Canada plays Mozart string quartets in public squares to calm pedestrians and have documented that crimes such as drug dealing have diminished in these locations. Ohara Brewery in Japan plays Mozart to its yeast to increase, by a factor of ten times, the density of the colony in brewing traditional rice wine. R. Bahr, M.D., Director of the Coronary Care Unit at Saint Agnas Hospital in Baltimore, Maryland, finds, "Half an hour of music produces the same effect as ten milligrams of Valium."

In 1993 at Michigan State University it was documented that listening to relaxing music for fifteen minutes increased subjects Interleukin-1 (a proteins that provide cells protection against AIDS and cancer) increased by 10 percent. Scientist at Washington University demonstrated that the accuracy of ninety copy editors increased 21.3 percent when they listened to light classical music. In 1996 research on expectant women printed in the *Journal of the American medical Association* reported, "Music stimulation increases endorphin release and decreases the need for medication."

G. Shaw, a theoretical physicist, states Mozart music seems "'warm up' the brain" and in *Cymantics* H. Jenny, a Swiss engineer and doctor, describes the science of how sound and vibration interact with matter. Jenny has established that intricate geometric figures can be formed by sound.

The challenge is to accurately understand what effects sound has upon cells, tissues, organs and organisms. It appears that sound vibrations form patterns and create subtle energetic fields of resonance and movement in space. Living things, and very likely inanimate objects, absorb these energies, and they cause the organism to alter their physiological processes.

## WHY MOZART?

This phenomenon of music healing has been termed the "Mozart Effect" because, Mozart compositions, of all of the types and styles of music most consistently produces the desired results, even in anesthetized subjects. It appears that Mozart compositions bring the organism back into an energy and physiological balance. This phenomenon appears, in part, to take place through the autonomic nervous system.

## THE SOUND OF THE UNIVERSE

Andrews, a chemist, commenting on his research stated, "We are finding that the universe is composed not of matter but of music." When subjects heard sounds made at specific ratios, the rhythms of their bodies and minds would synchronize to the very same rhythm as the planets and plants, earth and sea. Ostrander, et al., found, **"The mathematical Baroque music affects people by aligning, harmonizing and synchronizing their minds and bodies to more harmonious patterns."**

Ancient mathematicians likewise recognized such relationships in music and architecture and referred to this as the "Golden Mean" or mathematical formula in Greek architecture that produces its pleasing balance and proportions. This "mean" was also utilized in relation to the body. In other words, the Greeks, 2,500 years ago, were designing buildings and furniture ergonomically.

## THE PSYCHOSOMATIC LINK

Burr of Yale University states of his research, **"Changes inside the body, changes in one's brain waves or heartbeat, were the  result of changes in these energetic fields, not the other way around."** Lozanov demonstrated that, "The rhythms of the body - heartbeat, brain waves, and so forth - tend to synchronize themselves to the beat of music." In his work, people were monitored during concerts by means of physiological instruments. The pattern was very revealing. It was the identical pattern Wallace and Benson found on individuals during meditation. Heartbeats slowed by an average of five beats per minute. Blood pressure was down slightly. Brain waves showed beta waves decreased (over 13 per sec.) and brain waves slowed to the alpha rhythm (7 - 13 per sec.). Slow theta (4 - 7 per sec.) and delta waves tended to decrease, showing that this relaxation state is not a sleep pattern but similar to that found in hypnosis.

## BREATHING

Soviet block research has demonstrated, **"When between inhaling and  exhaling, you go on holding for a few seconds, mental activity stabilizes and the mind can focus in on a single point or idea."** These studies showed a primary, but diabolical, interest in using such procedures to accelerate brain-washing techniques and a more noble secondary desire to accelerate learning rates.

All of this, of course, has been known and practiced by Yoga, Tai ch'i and Sufi Masters for hundreds and even thousands of years but was ridiculed as "unscientific" by the closed reductionistic western mind, another prime example of the "arrogance of ignorance". Ramacharaka distills all of this in *The Science Of Breath*. He says, "Rhythm brings the whole system, including the brain, under perfect control and in perfect harmony and by this means the most perfect condition is obtained for unfoldment of . . . latent faculties." **Such procedures produce more effective and less stressful ways of arriving at the true potential of the individual.**

## RESULTS

S. Ostrander, et al., found that synchronizing the breathing to the material spoken during a learning session significantly helped enhance memory of the data presented. Addition of the proper low volume music at the same cadence still further enhanced the learning process. However, an even a more interesting fact was obtained when subjects were retested at extended intervals of six months; such a protocol documented a dramatically increased retention of the materials.

## THE DIFFERENCE

Bruner, of Harvard, says of these practices, "We are only now on the threshold of knowing the range of educatibility of man - the perfectibility of man. We have never addressed ourselves to this problem before." Schwartz, a psycophysicist, continues the thought, "We are hoarding potentials so great that they are just about unimaginable." (That is, to reductionist solid state science, but expansionistic quantum science has known of, researched and applied them for centuries.)

Caycedo, at the University of Madrid, conducted research utilizing the human voice, rather than instrumental music, with the material to be  memorized  presented in what Plato the ancient Greek described as, "A smooth, soft, soothing, monotonous, melodious tone, something like an incantation" which he termed "Terpons Logos". Caycedo further states that his research has determined that this method is what is instinctively used by mothers to soothe their children by singing lullabies.

## LIGHT

J. Ott writes of his early research. "I found that I could create radical changes within the cells by changing color in the microscope. I could increase their metabolic activity, I could kill them. Working with live animals - laboratory mice - I discovered that various kinds of lighting conditions could affect them physically. Not only did the changing lights cause external physical changes, the lights had a definite effect on their sex lives and life spans." In later years, Ott's research documented that pink lights on fish eggs would produce predominately, more than 80 percent, females.

Additional research led Ott to conclude, "In what I have learned about viruses, **no consideration been has given to the possibility of a virus originating within the living cells. . . .** The metabolism, or life itself, that goes on within a living cell is the utilization of the nutritional factors present by the energy of light. The nutritional factors are like the coal or oil used for fuel to fire a boiler, and the light could be compared to the fire that burns it. Another comparison would be the gasoline used in an automobile engine and the spark that ignites it. If the draft in the boiler is not adjusted correctly, or the carburetor is giving too rich a mixture, there will be incomplete combustion. This can result in both the boiler and the engine giving off not only obnoxious smoke and fumes but also partially consumed fuel. In a similar way, it seems quite possible that a chemical substance of a poisonous nature could result as a by-product from an incomplete or unbalanced metabolism within the cells of a leaf.

"This could result from either a nutritional factor as in the case of wheat virus or light deficiency as with the tomato virus. If so, **then this chemical by-product would fit all of the various descriptions of a virus. It would not be capable of reproducing itself but, if injected into the cells of other leaves, it might throw the metabolism of these cells off balance so that they would in turn produce more of the same chemical substances of a poisonous nature. It could be easily transmitted from one plant to another either by direct contact or some intermediary carrier. It could also be isolated and crystallized. It could fit all the various descriptions of a virus and still originate within the affected plant itself. This might also explain why too much plant  food could kill a plant faster than not enough - simply too much of a good thing."** (Emphasis added.) Exactly as D. D. Palmer said, "Too much or too little is dis-ease."

Ott's research continues, "**. . .some of the abnormal biological effects produced by placing a blue filter in the microscope light source closely resembled the effects of cells being attacked by viruses."**

## INCANDESCENT VS. FLUORESCENT

The electromagnetic spectrum varies from less than one trillionth of an inch in length for cosmic rays to 454 meters (1,500 feet) for the longest radio waves to 3,100 miles for electrical currents at 60 cycles per second. **Natural sunlight is a continuous spectrum but peaks in the blue-green range and cuts off abruptly in the ultra-violet range** at about 2,900 angstroms (an angstrom is 1/10 billionth of a meter) because of the filtering effect of the earth's atmosphere.

The ordinary incandescent light bulb contains virtually no ultraviolet and produces its maximum energy in the infrared range (approximately 10,150 angstroms) which is well beyond the visible range of the human eye (approximately 5,250 to 6,400 angstroms) but does produce large amounts of heat. In fact, the tungsten filament operates at roughly twice the temperature of molten steel or about 5,800 degrees F.

The fluorescent light operates on quite a different concept. It is filled with argon gas and mercury vapors. At each end of the tube is a cathode. When the electrical current is applied, the cathodes discharge electrons and a flow of current moves through the mercury vapor producing an electrical arc. This arc produces shortwave ultraviolet light concentrated at the particular wavelength of 2,537 angstroms. This wave length causes the phosphorous coating inside the tube to fluoresce and converts the ultraviolet to a longer visible light. Different phosphorous coatings cause different wave lengths, or colors, of light to be emitted.

Each wavelength of visible and ultraviolet light, and/or its absence, produces different physiological and psychological effects on biological organisms. Interestingly, the human eye sees far less than 1 percent of the electromagnetic spectrum but there is an overwhelming amount of evidence documenting that these unseen ranges exert profound influences upon many aspects of human health.

## BIOLOGICAL CLOCKS

Ott next quotes the research of Van Allen to explain why plants react to certain areas of so-called general nighttime background radiation in a positive way, rather than merely to the absence of the visible light during the dark nighttime period. He states that it is "derived from Van Allen's suggestion that the solar winds, consisting of charged particles emitted continuously from the sun at velocities varying from 670,000 to 1,600,000 m.p.h., compress into a rounded thin layer on the daylight side of the earth and sweep into a long tail on the night side. Van Allen further suggests that the earth's magnetic field causes a positive electrical charge on the morning side of the boundary and a negative charge on the opposite or evening side." Such emissions are significantly affected by the mass of structures and the topographical location of such structures.

For example, an individual living in a basement apartment of a reinforced concrete building near the foot of an easterly mountain range who sleeps at night would receive far less exposure than an individual residing in a wood-framed structure at the base of a westerly-situated mountain who sleeps during the day. Ott demonstrated that such "background" light radiation had significant effects on nocturnal animals. Thus the individual in the first example living in the basement of the concrete building at the base of an easterly mountain would receive less exposure and tend to be more lethargic and to sleep longer.

Geller, then chairman of the Department of Experimental Pharmacology at Southwestern Foundation For Research And Education, found that abnormal lighting and darkness affect the pineal gland, one of the master glands of the entire endocrine system. He found that rats placed under stress preferred alcohol over water. When left in continuous darkness for weeks, they went on alcoholic binges similar to many people with Seasonal Adaptive Disorder (SAD). Axelrod, a Nobel Prize winner, found that a pineal gland produces more of the hormone melatonin during periods of darkness. When Blum, at the University Of Texas, returned rats to equal periods of light and darkness, he found that the alcoholic rats retained their alcohol dependency indicating that a percentage of alcoholics may have a pineal-related light deficiency dis-ease as the root of their problem.

# HYPERACTIVITY/HYPERSENSITIVITY

Feingold of Kiser-Permanente Medical Center found that diets devoid of artificial coloring and flavoring agents brought about dramatic improvements in 60 percent of hyperactive children he studied. This suggests the strong possibility of an interaction between light wavelength absorption bands of synthetic pigments and the energy peaks and mercury vapors in fluorescent lights. For example, two children in the same family subjected to the identical source of low-level radiation can react differently if one prefers to consume cherry or strawberry soda pop while the other likes lemon-lime greenish-yellow drinks.

At the molecular level, all substances have a maximum wavelength absorption band or resonance. Some are within the visible portion of the electromagnetic spectrum, but others are of longer or shorter wavelengths than the visible range. For example, iron has a specific wavelength in which it functions. If a child won't eat spinach or raisins, good sources of iron, altering the wavelengths of the light spectrum to which they are being exposed may in some cases cause them to begin to eat the previously disliked food with a degree of relish.

# ADDITIONAL RESEARCH

Clearly, there is a great deal of research correlating numerous aspects with a patient's mental, emotional and spiritual health which has been ignored by reductionist medicine but which nonetheless has profound effects upon mankind's health. The sheer volume of the data to date would indicate that these areas are worthy of additional intense investigation. Unfortunately, such is not happening to any great degree within the reductionistic scientific community. Therefore, it falls to the quantum expansionistic community to safeguard the continuation of such vital research.

# Chapter 37
# THE PHARMACEUTICAL QUANDARY

*"I find the medicine worse than the malady."*
— Shakespeare

## THE MONUMENTAL QUESTION

Eli Lilly, founder of the giant drug cartel that still bears his name, stated, **"A drug without toxicity is no drug at all."** R. Williams, et al., reported in 1977, "This means over 1,500,000 people are sent to the hospital each year as a result of drug therapy. And after a patient is admitted to the hospital, his chances of falling victim of drug-induced sickness more than doubles. Drug sickness in hospitals causes suffering to well over 3,500,000 patients each year." Data published in the *Journal of the American Medical Association* in 1998 by J. Lazarou, et. al., indicates that **FDA approved, double-blind-tested prescription drugs are the forth leading cause of death in the United States. For the year 1994 alone, the number of adverse drug-related fatalities was estimated at 106,000.**

All of this is merely a restatement of the Law Of Hormesis discussed in Chapter 19 and the Arndt-Schultz, Koestschau and Wilder's Laws discussed in Chapters 7 and 12. Thus, the grand question every conscientious practitioner must repeatedly ask is, **"Is the potential harm that can be done by this drug outweighed by the potential benefit of prescribing it?" This is quite simply another way of stating the First Law of Healing, "***Primum, Non Nocere*** - First Do No Harm."**

Dr. D. G. Friend of Harvard Medical School said, "From among the 8,000 drugs available, it is utterly impossible for the medical physician to have enough information (about each of them) to select the drugs he uses in the treatment of his patients wisely." Dr. D. Console, the then Medical Director of Squibb Laboratories, added, "Doctors and the public are subject to a constant 'barrage' of new drugs, some worthless and others with greater potential for harm than good."

## THE CRITERIA

In 1938, the United States Congress passed the "Food, Drug and Cosmetics Act" requiring that before marketing a drug, the developer must provide the FDA with adequate evidence of its safety. The 1962 Kefauver-Harris Amendment added significantly to the original act by requiring "substantial evidence" - i.e., adequate, well-controlled clinical studies - that the new drug was effective with regard to all claims made for it in labeling and advertising.

All drugs first marketed after 1962 must be approved by the FDA under this added authority. Drugs in continuous use since before 1938 are not subject to such requirements; however, drugs developed between 1938 and 1962 are subject to evaluation. Studies have been done on over 16,000 claims for more than 4,000 drugs and mixtures of drugs and have been categorized as follows:

1. Effective: **The drug has been found effective for at least one of its claims and no questions regarding its continued marketing have been raised.** (The problem is the manufacturer may make numerous claims for its effectiveness.)

2. Probably effective: **The presumption is that the drug is probably effective for the claim(s) made but adequate scientific data is lacking.** The manufacturer is given one year to establish an acceptable research protocol during which time the drug remains on the market. If the research protocol is approved by the FDA, the drug in question can remain on the market for many years while the research is being conducted.

3. Possibly effective: **There is little evidence of its effectiveness and little expectation that scientifically supportable data will be forthcoming.** The manufacturer is given six months to establish an acceptable research protocol during which time the drug remains on the market. If the research protocol is approved by the FDA, the drug in question can remain on the market for many years while the research is being conducted.

4. Ineffective: The data is available and documents that the drug is ineffective or harmful. **The pharmaceutical will be removed from the market.**

5. Ineffective in mixed combinations: **The data is available and documents that the drugs are ineffective or harmful in combination.** They will not be permitted to be sold in combination but may continue to be used independently of each other.

## SCIENTIFIC CONTROLS?

Unfortunately, such noble goals are not infrequently trodden underfoot in the race for drug patents and the huge profits to be made. Meyers, et al., tell us that, Reserpine 0.25 mg tablets, offered as a generic preparation, cost $0.99 per 1,000 tablets to produce, but the most familiar brand name preparation costs $39.50 per 1,000 or a profit margin of 4,000 percent over and above the profit margin made when selling the generic product.

In the 3 November 1975 issue of the *Journal of the American Medical Association* there appeared a report on the scandal of falsifying drug research reports. A commission of distinguished scientists, including four Nobel Laureates, studying the problem concluded that such lack of scientifically controlled research was the norm. **In fact, FDA spot checks revealed 20 percent of the cases investigated guilty of a wide range of unethical practices including giving incorrect dosages and altering records to reflect accepted dosages. In 33 percent of the cases, there was no substantiating documentation showing that the tests had ever been conducted. In another 33 percent, the required protocol was not followed, invalidating the results. In only 33 percent of the cases investigated could the FDA document that the research met the minimal research standards.**

## SCIENTIFIC SHORTCOMINGS

Believe it or not, it is possible under current American drug laws to have a pharmaceutical substance approved for human use without having administered it to a single human being if the animal studies are favorable.

Herein lies a major problem. No animal study can compare with human studies for numerous reasons. For example, how does an animal relay to the researcher that it has been depressed since having the drug administered to it? Yet, one of the unanticipated side effects of that drug for humans will be depression. Or let us say the animals chosen for the study are dogs. Assume, for the sake of discussion, that this test drug destroys vitamin C. All members of the canine family internally produce vitamin C. Because the test animals simply replace the destroyed vitamin C, no side effects are revealed until the drug is given to humans who cannot produce endogenous vitamin C. We now have a iatrogenically-induced drug scurvy as one of its major complications.

## CHAIRMAN MAO'S SOLUTION

Chairman Mao of the People's Republic Of China addressed this very issue of drug testing in 1973 when he said, "**It is my thought that doctors should not prescribe new drugs until they have exhaustively tested them on themselves. I think doctors are best qualified to detect and describe side effects experienced first hand, and to be more responsible for the drug when given.**" Interestingly, this is precisely one of the standards of homeopathy provings (testing) implemented by Hahnemann over 175 years ago.

## HOW SAFE ARE DRUGS?

In 1976, in Bogota, Colombia, there was an allopathic doctors' strike that lasted for 52 days. The *National Catholic Reporter* documented that the death rate decreased 35 percent during that time period. In Los Angeles County in 1976, allopathic doctors also went on strike; Dr. Roemer, Professor of Health Care Administration at the University Of California, Los Angeles, studied seventeen hospitals during this period and found a significant decrease in deaths accompanied by a 60 percent reduction in surgeries. At the end of the strike, the death rate returned to its "norm". In 1973, in Israel, allopathic doctors went out on strike and there was a 50 percent drop in the death rate, the lowest it had been in over twenty years. But again, the death rate returned to "normal" once the strike was over.

This is disturbing; if drugs are properly administered, the death rates should sky-rocket when allopathic practitioners go on strike instead of falling by such dramatic percentages. There can be only a few explanations for this phenomenon:

1. Mistakes in compiling the data. Since the data has been compiled by different researchers at different locations working under the auspices of different organizations, the likelihood of each making the same mistakes is statistically extremely remote.

2. Allopathic pharmacology has an inherent flaw in its philosophy and/or application. Were this an all-pervasive flaw, allopathic therapy would have no consistent success rate. Obviously, this is not true as many patients respond predictably to pharmaceuticals and have few side effects but there is also a significant percent who are not so fortunate. Therefore, the problem must lie in the philosophy of administration. A lack of adherence to the universal laws described throughout this text is, in fact, the answer to this quandary. **A practitioner cannot ignore the universal laws of health and healing, as taught in this text, and not do harm.**

# AN EXAMPLE

The following illustrates this abandonment of these universal laws and philosophy not only within medicine but throughout our society at large. We put drug pushers in prison for selling "speed" to our children on the streets but, in many cases, our public schools and allopathic practitioners aggressively encourage parents to give it to their attention-deficit and hyperactive children in which case it is called Ritalin. Scientific logic must ask, "If it's bad on the streets how can it be good in the schools?"

# THE PHYSICIAN'S DESK REFERENCE (PDR)

The *PDR*, published annually, is a text consisting of between 2,000 and 3,000 pages of information. There is also a companion volume of approximately 1,000 pages titled *Drug Interactions and Side Effects Index*. And the same company publishes a third text, *Physician's Desk Reference For Non-prescription Drugs* of between 800 and 900 pages. Approximately 3,800 to 4,000 pages of these texts deal with "contraindications, warnings, precautions, adverse reactions, drug interactions, over dosage, drug abuse and dependence, and hypersensitivity." **That means 70 to 80 percent of all known data relating to drugs deals with the adverse side effects referred to by Lilly in the opening paragraph of this chapter and only 20 to 30 percent of all knowledge regarding drugs is therapeutic in value.**

# ANOTHER GRAND QUESTION

This brings us to the next vital question. **Is it scientifically and philosophically logical to require a patient whose system is already malfunctioning to handle an additional 70 to 80 percent toxic assault upon his system in order to obtain a 20 to 30 percent beneficial result? Reason would suggest that in situations short of life threatening, the risks of prescribing drugs very frequently far outweighs their benefits.**

# EXCESSIVE USE PROBLEM

There are numerous over-the-counter preparations for eliminating head lice which used to work extremely well. Currently, however, the public schools are experiencing an epidemic of head lice and these products are no longer effective for dealing with the problem. After being repeatedly exposed to these commercial preparations over an extended period of time, the lice have mutated and have become resistant to them. Unfortunately, the symptom (the presence of lice) and not the cause was repeatedly addressed. The cause is lack of personal hygiene in some of the students which allows them to serve as hosts to the lice which then infest the remainder of their classmates. If an effort had also been made to correct the personal hygiene problem, the dis-ease would not have continued to re-present itself and the lice would not have had the opportunity to mutate to a more virulent form. **Such is, and always will continue to be, the result when the universal laws are not known and/or are ignored.**

# ANTIBIOTICS AND VITAMIN INTER-RELATIONSHIPS

Antibiotics represent a major category within allopathic pharmacology not only in the total amounts prescribed but in the number of dollars spent by patients and insurance carriers. See Chapter 33. Unfortunately, most practitioners do not clearly understand the inter-relationship of antibiotics with other substances such as vitamins.

In microorganisms, an enzyme usually catalyzes a single reaction. The substrate attaches to the enzyme's center to be activated, metabolized and released. The biochemical rationale for an anti-microbial, then, is a compound similar to but not identical with the substrate that is able to combine with the enzyme's active center but is not metabolized and released. This compound remains attached to the enzyme's center and blocks its combination with the true substrate.

For many microbes, paraminobenzoic acid (PABA) is an essential metabolite. It is used by the microorganism as a precursor in its synthesis of folic acid (pteroylglutamic acid or PGA), a vital step in the synthesis of puren. Purens are obtained from the hydrolysis of nucleic acids found in the nuclear proteins of living cells.

The specific mode of action of PABA involves adenosinetriphosphate (ATP), dependent condensation of a pteridine with PABA to yield dihydroptroic acid, which is subsequently converted to folic acid. The sulfonamide and sulfone classes of drugs are structural analogues of PABA. See figure 37.1.

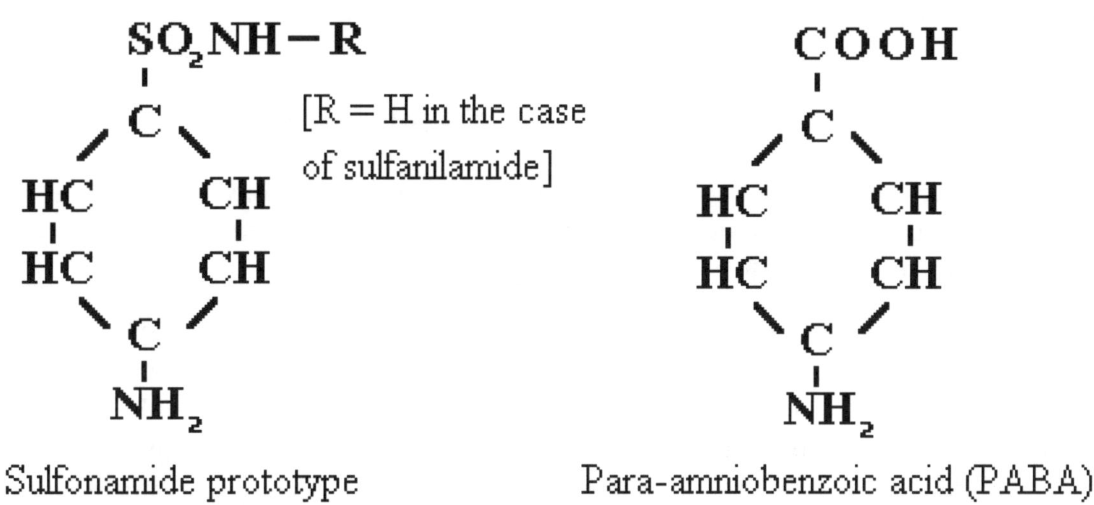


*Figure 37.1 — The sulfonamide prototype and its structural relationship to PABA*

## THE PROBLEM

Any practitioner not aggressively restricting dietary and/or supplementary sources of folic acid and PABA is encouraging the growth of the pathogenic microorganism. Meyers, et al., report, "Animal cells (and some bacteria) are unable to synthesize folic acid but depend upon exogenous sources and for this reason are not susceptible to sulfonamide action. Other cells which produce a large excess of PABA are resistant to sulfonamides, and still others may actually destroy sulfonamides. Sulfonamides-resistant mutants occur in most susceptible bacteria populations and tend to emerge under suitable selection pressure. Thus, the widespread therapeutic use of sulfonamides against gonorrhea has resulted in the establishment of sulfonamides-resistant strains throughout the world. The widespread use of sulfonamides against beta-hemolytic streptococci similarly aided the emergence of resistant strains. Most recently, sulfonamide-resistant meningococci have appeared in military - and have spread  to civilian - populations. Other types of microorganisms - e.g., many coliform organisms - are also commonly resistant. It should be specifically mentioned that ricketsiae not only are not inhibited by sulfonamides but are actually stimulated in their growth."

Unfortunately, there as many such idiosyncrasies throughout pharmacology that are not well known among practitioners and, therefore, are overlooked and thus become the source and/or enhancing agent of numerous iatrogenic problems.

## ACUTE TOXICITY

The LD50 represents the lethal dose in 50 percent of the test subjects to whom it is administered. The inherent problem is that not all organisms are of equal sensitivity. **Therefore, what may kill only 50 percent of the test animals in a normally sensitive group may kill 100 percent of the individuals in a hypersensitive group. The same holds true for human sensitivity. This concept contains no adjustments for the principles discussed under the headings of the Arndt-Schultz, Koestchau and Wilder's Laws discussed in Chapters 7 and 12.** Therefore, the LD50 is strictly a theoretical estimation and of very limited use in clinical practice.

## SUBACUTE AND CHRONIC TOXICITY

A **"subacute" toxicity test period is only 14-21 days duration.** The inconsistency here is that patients may be on the drug for months or even years before subacute toxicity manifests itself. Therefore, such short test periods are totally inadequate and of only very limited scientific value.

**Chronic toxicity test requires the experimental drug to be given to only two species for 90 days in only three dosage levels with no regard for individual idiosyncracies.** One of these levels is the proposed therapeutic dose and another is the lowest toxic level. At the conclusion of the study, only gross and histiopathological examinations are performed and there is no attempt at psychological evaluation even though adverse side effects are frequently registered in this area. Nor is there any attempt to evaluate for disturbances in the quantum energy fields. In the USA, chronic toxicity tests on dogs must continue for one year but early clinical trials on humans can be instituted after an initial 90-day period. The problem is there frequently is no long-term toxicity data available within 90 days. What happens when a living organism has been affected by the drug for 120 or 360 or 720 or 1,480 or 2,960 days? This information can be completely absent when human clinical trials are legally undertaken. These human subjects are thus provided inadequate, or at best very minimal, scientific data upon which to base their decision to become part of such an experiment.

## SPECIAL TOXICITY TESTS

If the drug is to be used in pregnant women or women of childbearing age, a teratogenicity test  must also performed. The drug is administered to both male and female rats throughout the production of two litters. However, these studies are of limited scientific value as rat genetics are not the same as human genetics. A second type of test can also be conducted on newborn animals if the drug is an anesthetic. The experimental drug is administered every three hours for five consecutive days.

# THERAPEUTIC INDEX

An ED50 (effective dose) is the amount that is therapeutically effective in 50 percent of the population. The LD50/ED50 is then determined as the "therapeutic index" or range. Unfortunately, few drugs have a direct relationship to the therapeutic index in both test animals and humans.

# EVALUATION OF TOXICITY IN HUMANS

As stated earlier, testing on volunteer humans may legally begin before chronic animal toxicity tests are even completed. This phase is designed to "determine any toxic effects on humans which did not become apparent during the animal tests." One must question the scientific advisability of being allowed to begin such tests on humans before the animal tests are completed.

# RISK OF DRUGS IN GENERAL USE

Meyers, et al., write, **"When a new drug is released for general use, information about its toxicity may be incomplete."** In fact, it is almost without exception **incomplete.** Meyer,, et al., further add, "There are 2 questions about many drugs that remain unanswered even after years of widespread use:

1. The absolute incidence of adverse reactions.

2. Whether all reactions are recognized or only those that cause obvious rather than familiar signs of disease."

They continue, "The reporting of drug reactions is grossly inadequate. Monitoring of hospital populations has shown that adverse reactions occur many times oftener than are recognized and reported. What is needed is a report of all untoward effects of a drug given to a representative sample of patients of diverse types. Such a system is not now available nor in prospect in spite of the efforts of the FDA to establish one.

Still further along in the text, the researchers comment, "Case reports and registry of drug reactions - e.g., the now abandoned registry of adverse reactions of the AMA - are not adequate for qualifying the risk with any degree of accuracy. Such registries depend upon volunteered information and there is no way of knowing what fraction of the total experience is represented. Certainly it is a very small fraction."

# RARE TOXIC EFFECTS

Next, Meyer, et al., comment, "Association of a rare toxic effect of a drug with that drug cannot be accomplished by the study of single cases but only by refined epidemiologic techniques." (Consider the similarity with the problem of establishing a causal relationship between cigarette smoking and cancer of the lung.) While their statement is correct from a strictly scientific standpoint, **does that mean that we have a moral obligation to completely disregard the obvious because science has not yet been able to document it?**

# ALLERGIC REACTIONS

To again quote Meyers, et al, "Signs and symptoms of allergic reactions are unrelated to the pharmacological effect of the drug but resemble instead those of other allergic reactions. . . . Drug molecules (except for those fewthat are proteins) cannot function as complete antigens but only as haptens - .i.e., they must chemically react with some homologous protein after administration or contact. The altered body protein is antigenic and the haptenic drug confers specificity."

# IMMEDIATE ALLERGIC REACTIONS

Meyers, et al, write, "The IgE or reaginic or tissue-fixed antibody specific for the drug hapten is bound to the surface of tissue mast cells or blood basophils. When the drug is subsequently reintroduced, the sensitized cells are degranulated by the reaction of the antigen and antibody on their surface, releasing histamine and other substances and causing an anaphylactic or urticarial reaction. At the same time, antibodies of the IgG and IgM (circulating) class are also formed. These may combine with antigen administered later to keep antigen from reaching tissue-fixed (IgE) antibody and thus block anaphylaxis, or the antigen-antibody complex may be deposited in blood vessels to cause serum sickness or vasculitis."

# ANAPHYLAXIS

Such an extreme reaction is due almost exclusively to mast cell degeneration. Human histamine release leads to bronchiolar constriction; localized edema, often in the laryngeal and glottal region; and vasodilatation with consequential hypertension and shock. **Antihistamine administration blocks further histamine reactions but does nothing to reverse the damage that has already taken place.**

Almost all drugs that are injected subcutaneously, intermuscularly and intravenously have the potential for causing anaphylactic shock, with the biological drugs that contain serums and other proteins (chymotrypsin, penicillinase, etc.) being the most dangerous.

# OTHER IMMEDIATE REACTIONS

1. UTICARIA AND ANGIONEUROTIC EDEMA - Hives and localized swelling are also frequently caused by food allergies and therefore can be confused with drug allergies.

2. ASTHMA AND RHINITIS - Usually occur in individuals with other allergies but drugs such as aspirin, quinine, sulfonamides and penicillin are frequent offenders.

3. SERUM SICKNESS - The incubation period for the antibodies is approximately 5 to 14 days; therefore, when the symptoms do begin to appear they may not initially be connected to the true source. This is especially true when the symptoms are primarily clotting and inflammation which closely mimic conditions such as phlebitis.

4. DRUG FEVER - Again, there is an incubation period of from 7 to 21 days before a fever of 104 degrees or higher manifests and continues for 2 to 3 days after the drug has been discontinued. Thus, the reaction can be misdiagnosed as a severe influenza or fever-producing dis-ease.

# AUTOIMMUNE REACTIONS

1. THEOMBOCYTOPENIA - This problem is caused by quinidine. In reality, it is not a true autoimmune reaction in that neither the platelets nor other homologous proteins function as the antigen. The antigen-antibody reaction is the result of quinidine being absorbed into the platelets of the sensitive patient and causing sudden agglutination with bleeding occurring under the skin.

2. DISSEMINATED LUPUS ERYTHEMATOUS - Long-term administration of drugs such as hydrazine, procainamide, phenytoin, trimethadione, isonizid and others can be followed by the appearance of classic lupus symptoms. Fortunately, the symptoms usually subside with discontinuation of these drugs.

3. HEMOLYTIC ANEMIA - Drugs such as phenylhydrazine may cause hemolytic anemia by acting directly upon the blood cells and producing hemolysis. In patients with an inherited deficiency of glucose 6 phosphate dehydrogenase in the red blood cells, administration of primaquine, nitrofurantoin, etc., will cause oxidative hemolysis. Methyldopa also causes hemolytic anemia which will give a positive Coombs test (the presence of antibody globulins on the surface of the erythrocyte).

4. AGRANULOCYTOSIS - is produced by an allergic reaction due to an abrupt peripheral destruction of granulocytes and is associated with a cellular marrow. The onset is abrupt and immediately severe.

# DELAYED ALLERGIC REACTIONS

The drug-protein combination is identified by small lymphocytes (antigen recognition cells) as foreign. Immune cells differentiate these allergic reaction cells and return to the antigen-containing cells to initiate an inflammatory reaction which generally takes 24-48 hours to become apparent.

# THE PHARMACIST VS. THE PHYSICIAN

Who then should logically be prescribing such complex and potentially dangerous substances? Obviously, the individual with the greatest amount of pharmaceutical training. Doctors spend the vast majority of time studying other subjects such as anatomy, physiology, pathology, physical examinations, laboratory diagnosis, endocrinology, neurology, histology, myology, osteology, lymphology, cardiology, proctology, psychiatry, records keeping, orthopedics, pediatrics, gynecology, obstetrics, surgery, anesthesiology, rheumatology, oncology, dermatology, internal diseases, gastroenterology, eye, ear, nose and throat conditions, emergency procedures, geriatrics, pulmonary diseases, occupational diseases, radiology, rehabilitation, obesity, manipulation, acupuncture, counseling, protocols, office management, nuclear medicine, forensic and public health requirements, and on and on. And somewhere among all of this, some classes on pharmacology are sandwiched in. The problem is with all of the other required subjects, allopathic practitioners routinely receive only a small percentage of the pharmaceutical training that the typical pharmacist receives. **This makes the pharmacists far more competent to prescribe drugs than the physicians even though the laws of every state and province prevent them from doing so.** Indeed a strange set of circumstances with which the legislatures, special interest groups and the legal system have saddled the sick and suffering.

# PRESCRIPTION WRITING FOR ALL PRACTITIONERS

As horrified as many of my quantum colleagues may be, I aggressively encourage prescription writing privileges for all health care practitioners. **The point being that one does not have the legal right to take patients off of prescription drugs unless he also has the legal right to prescribe them in the first place. If, as stated above, 70 to 80 percent of all responses to pharmaceuticals are adverse in nature, then the legal ability to take  patients off and/or reduce the dosage of prescription medications must certainly be one of the major factors in returning health to the patient in 70 to 80 percent of cases.** Why then would any conscientious healer object to having such a legal right to provide a greater degree of health to a patient?

# PALLIATIVE CARE VS. HEALING

Insulin does not cure diabetes, Synthroid does not permanently solve the problem of a malfunctioning thyroid gland, estrogen never repairs a malfunctioning ovary, phenobarbital never has permanently resolved an epileptic's seizures, Ritalin never permanently resolves hyperactivity or attention deficit disorders, anti-depressant drugs, such as Prozac, never resolve depression. **These drugs only mask symptoms, they do not heal.**

# THE LAW OF REBOUND EFFECT

True, an anti-depressant may help a person from sinking too deeply into depression but it cannot solve the cause of the problem. **The individual and his care giver must continue to work at making sense out of his life by sorting out and resolving the causative issues, regardless of whether they are  physiological, mental, psychological or spiritual in nature, that are not in harmony with the universal laws before the patient can be truly happy again. Drugs only mask and/or suppress the problem.** These statements are verified by the fact that when a patient is taken off of a drug, without resolution of the causative issue(s), the problem(s) re-manifest and very frequently are far more dramatic in their adverse impact than they were during the initial incidence. This is called the "Law Of Rebound Effect".

# LAW OF SHUT-DOWN

A patient may be placed on a 1-grain-a-day dose of thyroxin replacement therapy and feel fine for a year or two. Then, he doesn't feel as well as he did and is re-evaluated. The laboratory tests indicate that he is again experiencing hypothyroidism and the dose needs to be increased to 2 grains per day. In other words, the patient is getting worse in spite of the therapy. The therapy has been only palliative in nature. If the thyroid were healing, the patient should need less and less exogenous (external source) thyroid supplementation or insulin or Ritalin or whatever the tissue, function and/or drug in question might be.

**In reality, what is happening is that such therapy has placed that particular function of the body on a welfare system. The body is thus saying, "Why work? I get what I need whether I work or not." The result is like any welfare system, the recipient gets lazier and lazier and needs more and more of the prescribed therapy.** We are in reality making the patient sicker not healthier by utilization of replacement therapies.

## LAW OF CHEMICAL CONFIGURATION

If a pharmaceutical firm manufactures a naturally occurring substance, it cannot obtain a patent, cannot lock out competition, and cannot charge the highest possible price for the drug. Therefore, once the chemical structure of the naturally occurring substance is identified, the firm requires its chemists to find a way to alter the molecular configuration to one that has never existed before in order to obtain a patent.

If 20 percent of the chemical configuration of the molecule has been changed, then there is the potential that 20 percent of what the new synthetic drug does differs from that of the naturally occurring substance. This is another reason why synthetic drugs cause side-effects that natural occurring substances do not.

Allopathic practitioners have gotten careless and frequently call these synthetic substances by the same name as the naturally occurring ones. This is un-scientific. **In chemistry, if two molecules do not have *exactly* the same configuration, they are not the same substance.**

Never having had prior exposure to these synthetic drugs, the living system is placed under increased stress trying to deal with their alien chemistry. In other words, the therapy is part of the challenge to the patient's health.

## TEACH THE CHILDREN

The adverse effects of our Madison Avenue advertising, pharmaceutically-based society are increasingly being visited upon our children. They have accepted the false idea that there is a drug for everything. If you are sad, take an upper; if you're hyper, take a downer; if you can't sleep, take a pill; if you have indigestion, take a pill; if you want to escape the pressure, take a drug. Consider the most recent findings of adolescent drug use from the 22nd annual Public Health Service survey: Marijuana use by 8th graders in 1991 was 3 percent; in 1996, 11 percent or an increase of 370 percent. Marijuana use by 10th graders in 1991 was 9 percent; in 1996, 20 percent or a 220 percent increase. Cigarette smoking by 8th graders in 1991 was 14 percent; in 1996, 21 percent for a 150 percent increase. Cigarette smoking by 10th graders in 1991 was 21 percent; in 1996, 30 percent or a 140 percent increase. Alcohol consumption by 8th graders in 1991 was .5 percent; in 1996, it was 1.0 percent or a 200 percent increase. And worst of all, children who smoke cigarettes are 500 percent more likely to become addicted to (prescription and/or street) drugs.

## DRUGGING OF STUDENTS

Ritalin is the drug of choice for psychiatrists and school administrators for control of students. The key word being *control.* In 1997 schools dispensed it to over 3 million children a day. Some schools report as many as 90 percent of their students on this mind altering drug.

What you may not know is Ritalin is the number one "Speed" drug sold on the streets. A recent study of adult drug addicts found that 90 percent were forced to take Ritalin or a like mind altering drug as a child. The Food and Drug Administration classifies Ritalin as a Category II drug requiring a special narcotic prescription pad to be dispensed. This is the same classification as cocaine, morphine, opium, methadone, amphetamines, Dexedrine, Desoxyn, Preludin, Percodan, Dilaudid and Demerol. Ritalin is a synthetic analog of codeine. The *Physician's Desk Reference* (PDR) states that Ritalin should not be given to any child under the age of six. In 1995 the United States dispensed five times as much Ritalin as the rest of the world combined. Studies show that students on Ritalin make better daily grades but on standardized tests their scores, over the years go down or making smaller than average improvements and they show little or no long term retention of subject matter.

If administration of such volumes of dangerous mind altering drugs to similar numbers of people were undertaken in Nazi Germany, Soviet Russia or Red China it would be considered "mind control" but in American public schools it is encouraged "good administrative, educational and medical procedures". What is wrong with this picture in Figure 37.2?

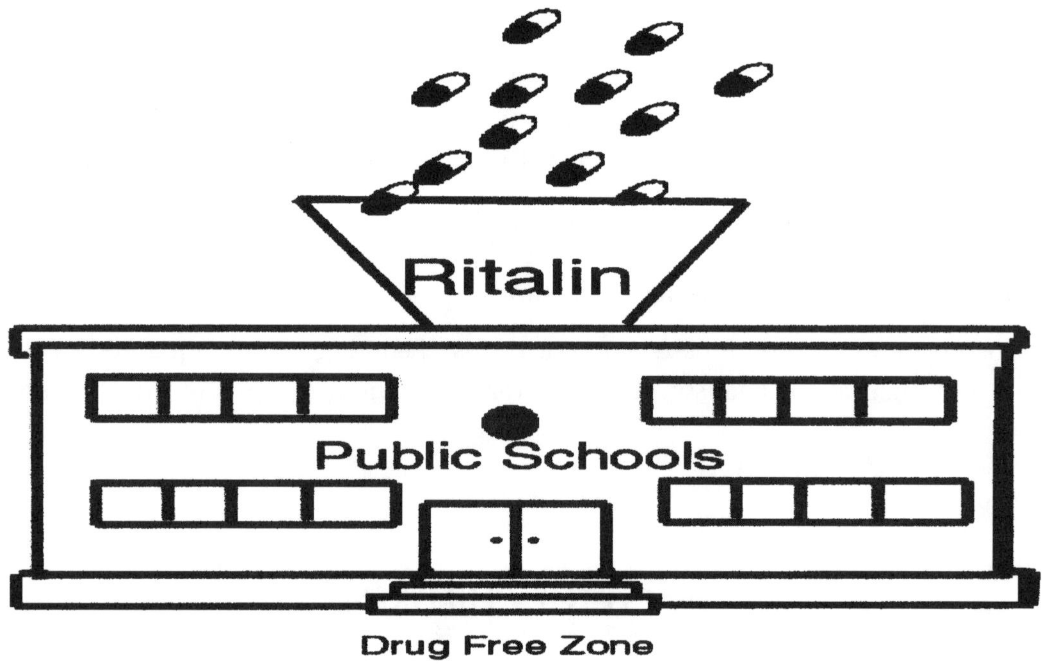


*Figure 37.2 — The Paradox of Ritalin*

## A MORE RATIONAL APPROACH

Therefore, as healers we should be looking for not just a palliative or band-aid pharmaceutical but rather an agent(s) that assists the patient to enter the self-healing mode; an agent(s) that will allow the innate intelligence of the being to strengthen and repair the injured and/or malfunctioning part(s); a therapy that ideally will allow the patient to arrive at the point at which the practitioner can say, "You don't need this anymore. Go and enjoy life without being tied to a practitioner and/or pharmaceutical company."

In many cases, this is what knowledge of the philosophy and application of complementary health care can provide that can never be provided by pharmaceuticals and this is why every conscientious healer should be devoting his/her life diligently to studying these more natural reparative forms of healing.

## DRUGS IN YOUR DRINKING WATER

In 1998, the publication *Chemosphere* reported that more than 100 research papers have been published worldwide confirming the fact that we are getting toxic and/or physiologically-altering amounts of drugs in our drinking water.

It is estimated the approximately 90 percent of all prescription drugs pass through the body and are eliminated in the urine and/or feces. Unfortunately, sewage treatment plants are equipped to deal with only bacteria, viruses and a few toxic chemicals but not prescription drugs. Many scientists are now convinced that this is one of the main reasons why so many pathogenic microorganisms are mutating and becoming antibiotic resistant. S. Levy, director of the Center for Adaptation Genetics and Drug Resistance at Tufts University confirms this position by saying, "Our (American) concentration of antibiotics is 1,000 times higher than in German water . . . causing the bacteria to become medication resistant."

T. Ternes found lipid (triglyceride and cholesterol) lowering drugs, analgesics (pain killers) including OTC (over the counter) ibuprofen, chemotherapy (cancer) drugs, 30 different antibiotics, beta blockers (heart drugs), anti-seizure medications, contrast agents for X-ray, and numerous hormones in tap water.

According to A. Hartman, "a class of broad spectrum antibiotics in drinking water is causing toxicity to human DNA." The *Nugent Report* documents, "Estrogen-like chemicals are rampant in the environment." L. Guillete, a reproductive biologist from the University of Florida, indicates these include the PCBs (polychlorinated biphenyls and dioxins) and DDEs which are metabolites of DDT. Guillete states, "DDT, dioxins and dozens of other chemicals . . . trick the body into thinking they are hormones." He further states, The amount of estrogen needed to feminize a human embryo - essentially turning a baby boy into a baby girl - is the same ratio as one drop of gin in 700 railway cars full of tonic water." In other words a homeopathic dilution.

S. Snyder of Michigan State University, in his study of the water in Lake Mead, Nevada, found that the level of estrogen was so high in the lake water that male fish were producing female egg protein! He repeated his test 30 times to be certain of the results. In this study, Snyder was not talking about estrogen-like toxic chemicals, he was measuring the amounts of pharmaceutical estrogen which had passed through the bodies of women who were on estrogen replacement therapy, through the sewage treatment plant without being altered, and back into the lake. Lake Mead is a major reservoir for the southwest United States with tens of millions of Americans drinking its drug contaminated water.

The challenges, then, are to find ways to aid our immune systems to become strong enough to successfully resist drug-mutated microorganisms and to find more pro-biotic (life-friendly) and scientifically rational ways of dealing with infections, hormone imbalances, pain, etc.

# Chapter 38
# THE RADIATION QUANDARY

*"All matter is composed of elements, all elements are composed of atoms. All atoms are composed of the basic particles of physics. Living forms use atoms to build biologic structure for chemical molecules. Radiation disrupts and destroys these molecules and hence destroys life."*

— Sears

## RADIOACTIVITY

Elements that are heavier than iron have a characteristic of emitting radiation (radioactivity) which is nature's way of converting those elements into lighter elements. This conversion takes place at constant rates that is the same for a free element as for compounds and is also independent of influences such as temperature and pressure which can dramatically affect the elements found at the lighter end of the atomic scale.

## RADIOACTIVE PROPERTIES

The radioactive elements emit three distinct types of energy known as alpha (positively charged), beta (neutrons - negatively charged) and gamma rays (no electromagnetic charge) but have very high vibrational frequencies. This quality imparts to gamma rays an impressive ability to penetrate solid objects to far greater depths than X-rays. In fact, gamma rays can penetrate several inches of solid lead.

## THE ACTINIDE SERIES

This group consists of all elements above thorium on the periodic table. Only thorium, uranium and very small amounts of plutonium occur in ores; the rest are made by means of cyclotrons or similar man-made means and all are highly radioactive meaning they want to give off alpha, beta and gamma rays.

# NUCLEAR FUSION

When this energy is rapidly released, we experience a nuclear explosion; with controlled release, we have a nuclear power plant; and when even smaller controlled amounts are being released, we have nuclear medicine. **These processes also produces hundreds of radioactive isotopes. (An isotope is an element of identical chemical character as another element occupying the same place on the periodic table but differing from it in other characteristics such as radioactivity levels or in the mass of its atoms.)**

In order to appreciate this conversion from matter to energy it is helpful to use the following example. Assume that only 1/1,000 of the mass of a pound of uranium (or 0.016 of an ounce) is converted into energy. The release would be equivalent to 1,140 tons of coal or 11,400,000 kilowatt-hours of electricity.

# THE CHAIN REACTION

A chain reaction takes place when this process becomes self-sustaining. A neutron from the above exploding mass strikes another atom of un-exploded material causing it to also explode. This sustained process of releasing energy will continue at a steady rate as long as there is additional material to be struck by neutrons. Thus, huge amounts of kilowatt-hours of energy can be released from a radioactive substance or the energy can be released within a very small period of time resulting in a bomb with the destructive power of hundreds of millions of tons of TNT. (A 100-megaton bomb would equal the force of 100 million tons of TNT.) But this is only the immediate effect; there are  also residual effects of the isotopes of the matter exposed to the blast.

# INDUSTRIAL AND MEDICAL USES

Vast stores of energy have been tapped through the use of nuclear energy but with this we have inherited almost incomprehensible problems and dangers of nuclear waste which we bequeath to future generations. For example, **radium takes 1,590 years to decrease its radioactive emissions by 50 percent. Thus, if an exposure of 4 hours will produce a lethal dose in 1,590 years, it will still prove lethal with an exposure of 8 hours. In 3,180 years, only 16 hours exposure would be necessary to receive a lethal dose of radiation. In 4,770 years, 32 hours of exposure would prove lethal. In 6,360 years, 64 hours; in 7,950 years, 128 hours; in 9,540 years, 256 hours which is only a little over ten days. Giving each generation 25 years to reproduce 9,540 years equates to 381 generations. By continuing to work this mathematical progression we can see the huge time frames required before such materials become harmless.**

**And yet, each year, worldwide, we produce tens of thousands of tons of such radioactive toxic waste that will have to be stored and monitored for from tens of thousands to hundreds of billions of years. It is not at all inconceivable that a cost equal to or even greater than the gross national product of the entire planet may be needed at some point in the future just to safely contain this ever-growing volume of radioactive waste. At that point, it will cease being maintained in safe containment and future generations in its vicinity will be exposed to lethal doses of radiation. Consider uranium which has a half-life of 4 billion years! The human race could well be extinct before the natural process of hormesis can render it harmless.** Figure 38.1 shows how these radioactive contaminates gain entry and become more and more concentrated as they move up the food chain.

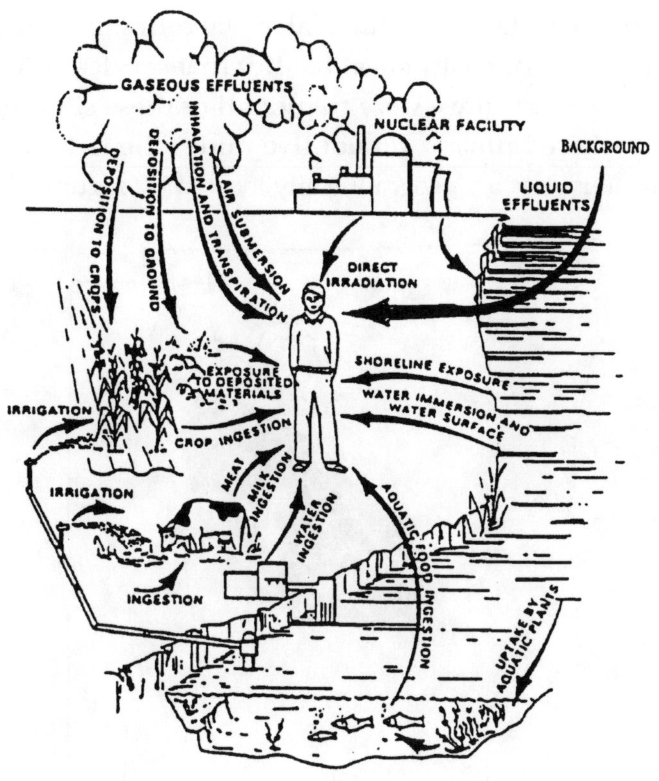


*Figure 38.1 — Potential dose pathways*

# RADIATION SICKNESS

Radiation sickness is a variety of symptoms produced by damaging exposure to radiation. The source of this radiation exposure may be nuclear fallout, medical and industrial use of radioisotopes, particle accelerators or X-ray machines. The various types of radiation produce increasing degrees of biological damage. This damage is graded as Relative Biological Effectiveness (RBE) and indicates the extent to which it damages cells compared with equal doses of other ionizing radiations. To illustrate, the dense tracks of ions formed by alpha particles can cause about 20 times (an RBE of 20) as much  damage as the thin ion trails generated by electrons (an RBE of 1).

The amount of radiation absorbed by the tissue is measured in rads. A rad is 1/100 joule of radiation energy per kilogram of mass. Another unit called the rem measures the biological damage to the living cells by different types of radiation. The number of rems equals the number of rads multiplied by the RBE of radiation. Another frequently used unit of  measurement is the millirem or 1/1,000 of a rem.

It has been estimated that the average American now annually receives about 180 to 200 millirems of radiation from a combination of natural exposure from the sun and other celestial objects (which is steadily increasing as the protective ozone layer around the Earth continues to be destroyed), fallout from nuclear explosions, fallout from nuclear accidents, meteors impacting on the Earth, nuclear research, color TVs, nuclear military propulsion systems, storage and maintenance of nuclear weapons, computer screens, smoke detectors, airport X-ray machines, industrial X-ray machines, units irradiating foods, black market sales with improper shielding, transportation of nuclear materials, nuclear power plants, microwaves, nuclear waste dumps, contaminated drinking water and from nuclear medicine and medical X-rays.

Nor are these the only sources; every railway, highway, seaport and airport that handles and/or transports nuclear materials is a potential disaster area with a radius of several hundreds of miles depending on directions of prevailing winds and water flow. Hospitals and universities, usually situated in congested areas of cities, that have a nuclear medicine department or are doing nuclear research must receive, store, use nuclear material and dispose of their nuclear waste. **Any population within 200 to 500 miles of a nuclear arsenal, power plant, nuclear manufacturing facility, waste deposit, naval facility that services nuclear ships or food processing plants that irradiate foods. In short, if we were to plot all of these sites on a map there would be very few places in the United States where humans do not live under the risk of a potential accident.** To illustrate, three of the more notorious sites are geographically located by Figure 38.2, 38.3 and 38.4.

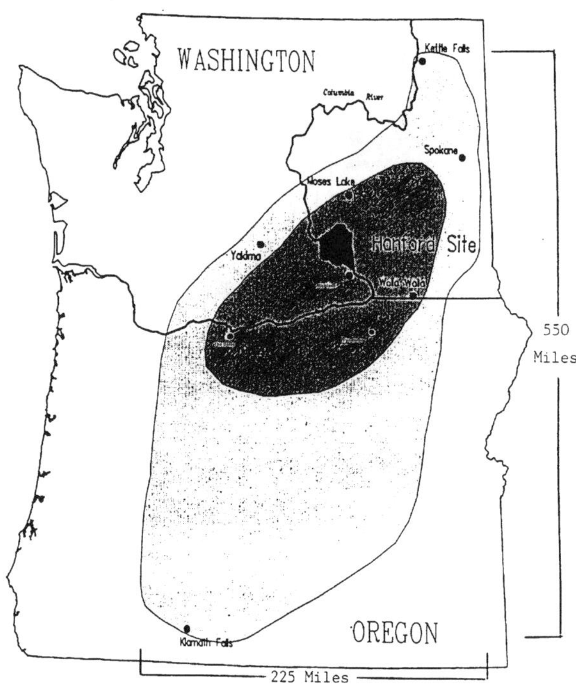


*Figure 38.2 — Hanford Site radioactive contamination map*

Extent of iodine-131 contamination from the Hanford Site. Little or no data was collected outside of the 75,000-square-mile shaded area. From Klamath Falls, Oregon, to Kettle Falls, Washington, is approximately 550 miles and from the area's eastern to its western boundary is approximately 225 miles.

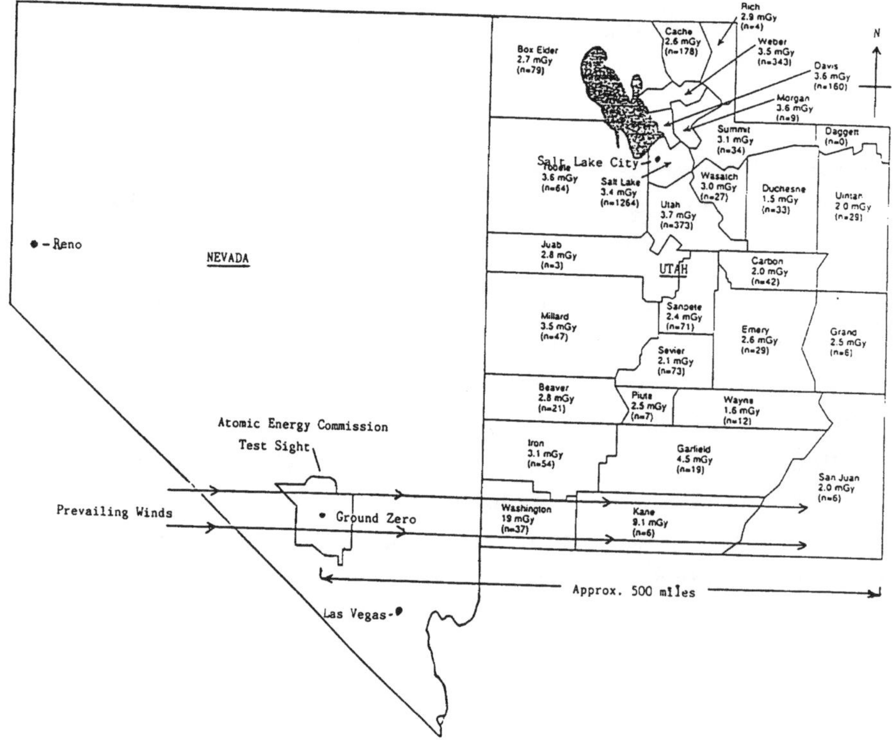


*Figure 38.3 — Utah bone marrow dose map*

The map of Utah showing the average bone marrow dose to subjects who remained in a single county during the 1952-1958 activity at the Nevada nuclear weapons test site. Washington, Kane and San Juan counties lie 200 to 500 miles directly east of ground zero and in the prevailing wind paths.

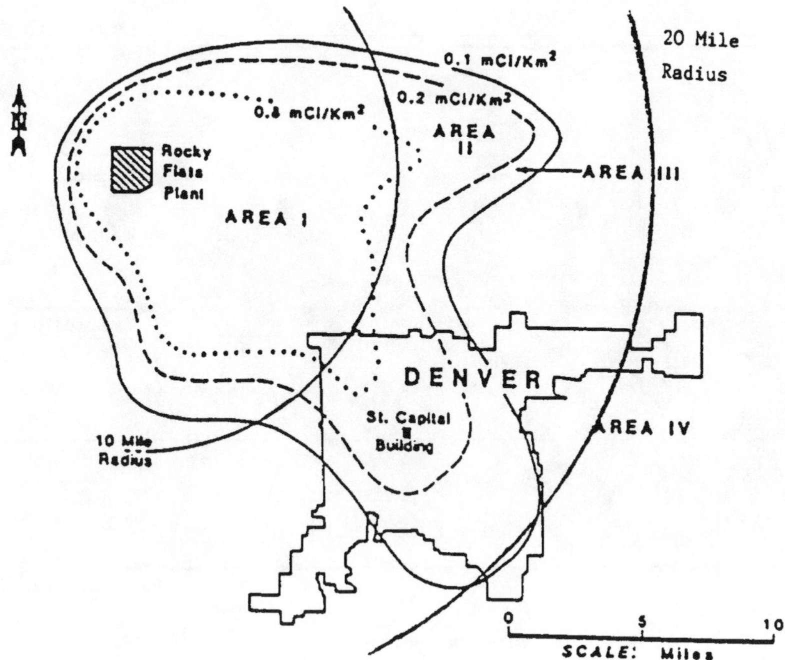


*Figure 38.4 — Rocky Flats Contamination Map*

The map of Denver for 1981 showing plutonium in soil in concentration contours over a 440-square-mile area of metropolitan Denver from Rocky Flats nuclear weapons plant. Note that Denver has a metropolitan population of over one million people being routinely exposed to the cumulative radiation levels.

Figure 38.5 illustrates the cumulative effects of living near nuclear power plants. While technology and stricter safety standards are slowly reducing annual emissions, the cumulative amount continues to steadily increase and will do so for many years (hundreds to tens of millions) into the future due to the half-life of these radioactive emissions. The ultimate question Figure 38.5 does not address is how many tens of thousands to tens of millions of years will need to pass before the striped bar graph at the far right will finally level off?

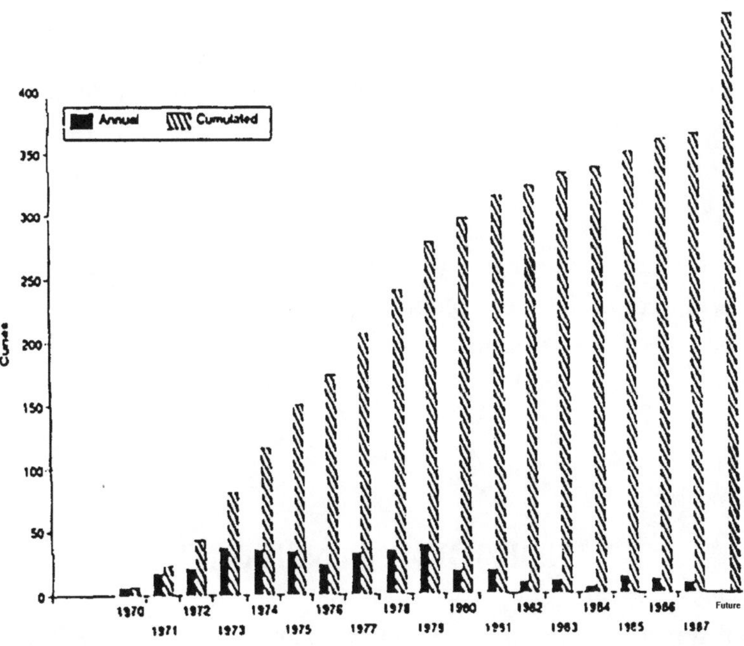


*Figure 38.5 — Annual and accumulative airborne I-131 and other fusion products released from United States nuclear power plants 1970-1987.*

Nor is the United States the only country with such problems. Figure 38.6 shows the legacy inherited from the former Soviet Union.

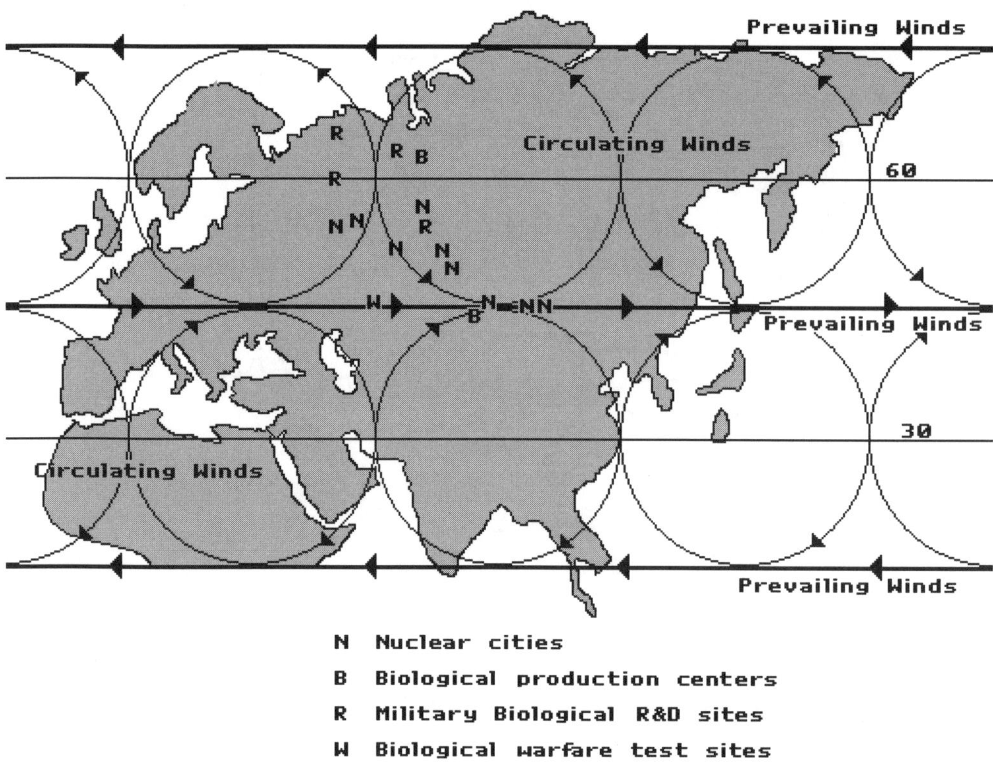



*Figure 38.6 — Map of former Soviet sites*

Location of former secret Soviet nuclear, biological and chemical research, production and testing facilities. Note that below the 30th parallel, the prevailing winds are east to west; between the 30th and 60th parallels, the prevailing winds are west to east; and above the 60th parallel, they blow east to west. With such prevailing wind patterns, these sites in the western half of the former Soviet Union are capable of literally blanketing the majority of Europe and China with deadly radioactive, biological and/or chemical fallout. Then add nuclear power plants such as Chernobyl, notorious for antiquated technology, nuclear weapons storage sites, and nuclear waste dumps. The problem then takes on menacing parameters for 750 million Europeans, one billion Indians and over one billion Chinese, totaling one-half of the human race. Nor does this map plot similar activities in the People's Republic of China, Canada, Japan, India, France, England, Iraq, Sweden, Belgium, Taiwan, Israel, Korea, the South Pacific test sites, and numerous other countries with nuclear weapons capability, research, nuclear power plants, and nuclear waste sites.

By the mid 1980s, there were 235 nuclear power plants operating in 22 countries producing over one billion watts per year of power; 15 other countries were planning or building at least one or more nuclear power plants. In short, the planet is literally dotted with potentials for nuclear disasters from these facilities and their nuclear wastes. Thus a map similar to figure 38.1 could be constructed for the western hemisphere also.

## INDIVIDUAL SENSITIVITY

An individual of normal sensitivity can receive approximately 25 rems of radiation without demonstrating immediate adverse effects but in a hypersensitive individual, about 12 rems can produce immediate effects. About 100 rems will usually produce symptoms of radiation sickness in the normal individual, 100 to 400 rems produces severe radiation sickness, more than 400 rems proves fatal in 50 percent (LD50) of humans and 800 or more rems is fatal in all cases.

## BERONIE-TRIBONDEAU LAW

Immune cells and cells in the active state of division are more sensitive than those that have acquired adult morphological and physiological characteristics. This law, of course, is the basis of therapeutic irradiation of cancer cells. Since they are a more immature cell in the process of a higher rate of cellular division than non-cancerous cells, they should be more susceptible to destruction by radiation therapy. Unfortunately, a second fact is ignored, that being that cancer cells will also be more likely to further mutate and become even more malignant from irradiation than the non-cancerous cells. Thus, radiation therapy's greatest strength is also its greatest weakness and this makes it a scientifically questionable mode of treatment.

## ACCUMULATIVE EFFECT

The cumulative effects of radiation frequently take years to manifest and although they result in shortened life spans and increased possibilities of developing leukemia, osteogenic sarcoma, fibrosarcoma, epidermoid carcinoma and other forms of cancer, necrosis, thyroid abnormalities, hemorrhage, cataracts, adverse lymphoid and hematopoietic, dermal, pulmonary and gastrointestinal changes, lowered immunity with increased infection rates, sterility, birth defects and/or genetic chromosomal damage as well as further  mutations that transfer harmful and weakening traits to the individual's progeny.

## MUTATIONS

Here we encounter possibilities of deformed, retarded, and potentially non-functional beings who to varying degrees will have to be cared for throughout their entire lifetimes and the attending drain that will place upon the available resources. Statistically, 25 percent of all mutations are lethal; another 15 to 20 percent are sterile. That still leaves a dramatic percentage of beings who will need to be wards of the productive members of society.

Boyd states, "If the mutation is recessive, requiring a double dose to become  evident, hundreds of generations may intervene before the damage occurs."

## HANFORD

For over 40 years, Hanford Nuclear Reservation released almost 23 million curies of radiation into the air water and soil of eastern Washington and Oregon and western Idaho. Radioactive Zinc 65 was detected in oysters 300 miles away at the mouth of the Columbia River in Willapa Bay, Washington. Some 350,000 people live within 80 miles of Hanford and are exposed to this residual radioactivity on a daily basis.

## CHELYABINSK

In 1957, the nuclear waste dump at Chelyabinsk (Mayak), U.S.S.R., exploded following a cooling failure, releasing 20 million curies into the atmosphere. All the pine tress within a 12.5-square-mile area died within 18 months. Only 11,000 of the 272,000 humans exposed were evacuated. In 1990 alone, 391,000 tons of such nuclear waste and other pollutants were released into the atmosphere. Lake Karachay within the Mayak facilities, called "The most polluted spot on earth", contains another 120 million curies of which 93 percent has entered into the soil and 60 percent now has entered the water table. Another 76 million cubic meters of radioactive waste was dumped into wells and the Techa river resulting in radioactive pollution being detected hundreds of miles downstream in the Arctic Ocean.

All of this was done secretly in order for the Soviets to catch up with the west in nuclear weapons technology and armaments. By comparison, Chernobyl, 30 years later, ejected about twice as much radiation affecting 750,000 victims who received about as much exposure as that from the 1957 waste dump explosion alone. Of the 272,000 Chelaybinsk victims, health records have been kept on only 66,000 in which there is at least twice the cancer rate of control populations.

## OAK RIDGE

Oak Ridge, Tennessee, is one of the oldest nuclear facilities in the United States. Unfortunately, precise records have not been maintained of exactly how much radiation the plant has released into the atmosphere, soil and water during its 54 years of operation. (One wonders, from a scientific perspective, how some of the most intelligent and most highly trained scientists in our world could have overlooked such record keeping or could have lost such records. It also makes the truly scientific mind wonder about the in-house safety standards and about the credibility of their managers for maintaining such a dangerous facility.) We do know from the fragmentary records that at least 2,400,000 pounds of mercury was "lost" into the environment between 1953 and 1977. From 1949 to 1987, Oak Ridge "lost" 1,197.8 curies of strontium-90, 693 curies of cesium-137 and 175.3 curies of iodine-131 into the local water supply.

However, changes in age-adjusted cancer mortality rates between 1950-1952 and 1987-1989 are available for 600,000 people in the area and these have been analyzed to determine if radioactive emissions have had any adverse effects on the population living within a 100-mile radius of the Oak Ridge facility. The results indicate that downwind cancer mortality rate definitely exceeds the regional and national averages. See Figure 38.7.

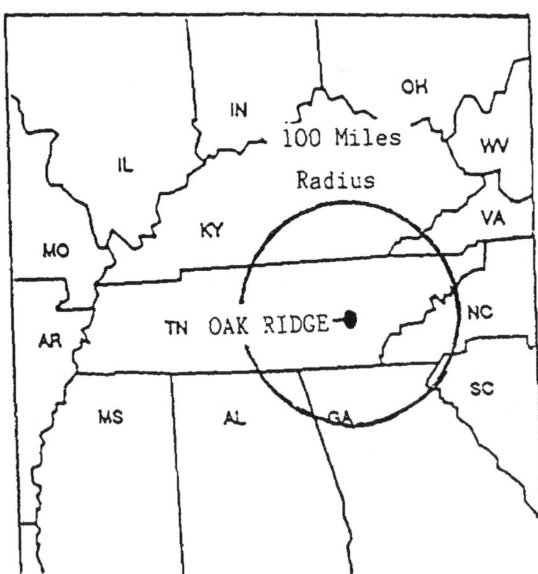


*Figure 38.7 — Location of Oak Ridge 100-mile radius*

## THREE MILE ISLAND

For comparison purposes of the discharges from the above sites, the 1979 Three Mile Island nuclear disaster in Pennsylvania released between 15-24 curies into the atmosphere and was considered a major incident. The difference was that Three Mile Island was a known accident relating to a public utility and could not be kept from public knowledge under the guise of national security and military secrets.

## UNIVERSITY OF CHICAGO

On 2 December 1942, the world's first man-made nuclear chain reaction took place at the University of Chicago as part of the Manhattan Project. If late 20th Century technology still is producing Three Mile Islands, Chernobyls, Chelynbinsks, Hanfords, Oak Ridges and Nevada Test Sites, what was the extent of the nuclear emissions from the University of Chicago in the 1940s? It is not scientifically logical to believe that with their primitive technology they were able to achieve 100 percent containment of the radiation produced. At that time, the nuclear danger radius around the Chicago area probably contained 3 million people.

## FULL EXTENT

It makes true scientists wonder what the total worldwide nuclear contamination and potential contamination actually is in terms of human suffering if all data were readily available. Obviously, nuclear power is not going to go away as mankind's thirst for electricity continues to increase every year and nuclear energy is very efficient. For example, as cited earlier in this chapter, one pound of uranium produces the energy equivalent of 1,140 tons of coal, without the smoke and other non-nuclear pollutants.

The world is unlikely to ever again be nuclear weapons-free. There are simply too many individuals who have the miasmatic, diathic, phase, doshic tendency to take advantage of and destroy their neighbors regardless of the cost to the rest of the world and themselves. Nor is the waste from nuclear medicine and industrial nuclear waste likely to be stopped. In 1997, it was  estimated that there was 64 million pounds of contaminated materials in the United States alone.

In reality, it is likely that the danger of nuclear waste will continue to grow. Mankind must, therefore, find more efficient means of dealing with it. Failure to do so is to live with a death sentence hanging over the heads of the entire human race.

# Chapter 39
# THE SURGICAL QUANDARY

*"When we have to resort to our skills as a surgeon
we have failed in our skills as a physician."*
— Anonymous

## THE LAW OF SURGICAL REMOVAL

The above aphorism must be permanently emblazoned upon the heart and mind of every healer. To do otherwise would be to offer the patient a severely distorted concept of what healing is and to allow healers to mislead themselves.

If you remove one wheel from an automobile, even though you may counterbalance it to run on the remaining three wheels, it will never be able to run as effectively as it was designed to do on all four wheels. Such is the reality of surgery. For example, a cholecystectomy (surgical removal of the gall bladder) alters the body's ability to assimilate fats, greases and oils in the diet. Surgery forces the patient to go from a concentration reservoir mechanism to an un-concentrated drip system. Never again will the patient digest fats, grease and oils quite as efficiently as he did when the gall bladder was properly concentrating the bile. Thus, a greater stress is placed upon the intestinal tract.

So it is with any surgery that removes a tissue or an organ. The universal and/or innate wisdom that formed the living being placed all parts within the system for specific purposes. It is not scientifically logical to believe that the organism can function just as efficiently and effectively without all of its designed parts. In some manner, any surgical removal of body parts or portions of body parts must place a greater burden upon other aspects of a living being's constitution. Therefore, it is a far wiser, when possible, to assist the patient's being in the repair of the unhealthy tissue than to surgically excise it.

The exception to this law, of course, is the surgical repair of injured tissues. In this case, we are allowing the tissue or organ to more effectively heal and resume its normal physiological functions. In such situations it is also vital to provide a complete complement of the basic minerals, vitamins, amino acids, essential fatty acids and indicated phytotherapeutic agents to ensure the most rapid recovery and minimize post-surgical shock and trauma.

# THE SHIFT

It must constantly be kept in mind by the surgeon and all subsequent practitioners that this shifting of demands on the various levels of the total being, as a consequence of eliminative surgery, results in an irrevocable change in the innate manner in which that patient is capable of responding under any set of given conditions or stresses. See Chapter 17, and Figures 12.1 and 17.5.

Because of such shifts, the patient may no longer respond to various forms of therapy in the same manner that he did prior to surgery. In fact, it may be necessary to completely re-evaluate the patient on all levels of his being and prescribe a therapy more compatible with the new symptom picture.

# Chapter 40
# THE SPIRITUAL QUANDARY

*"No one breaks the Ten Commandments;*
*they only break themselves against them."*
— Cecil B. De Mille

## THE GREAT CHALLENGE

Without doubt this chapter has been the most demanding to write of the entire text for numerous reasons. First, because western, reductionistic, non-vitalistic science refuses to even consider the possibility of the existence of the spiritual aspect of the total being and its influence. Secondly, it is because this chapter must be written without embracing the doctrines of any particular religious sect. Thirdly, because many individuals, even ones highly educated in other disciplines, have failed to achieve a spiritual education or discipline and are therefore completely unaware, or only vaguely aware, of its impact upon their lives. Fourth, because the "spiritual aspect" discussed in this chapter encompasses a more specific definition than the term "spiritual" used elsewhere in this text.

Many people, even many highly educated ones, feel ill at ease at the mention of the subject because religion is an "unknown" to their experiences. It is common knowledge that the unknown is one of mankind's greatest fears. Therefore, one must have the courage to acknowledge this void and address it intelligently and without preconceived prejudices in order to fully understand what is being discussed in this chapter.

Fifth, because it was much more difficult to reference this chapter in the same manner as with all of the others. Frequently, the references deal with the topic in an abstract manner that takes far greater reflection to understand. And finally, because I want to avoid any judgmental and/or sermon-like connotation.

## THE FOUNDING FATHERS

Perhaps the best way of broaching this topic is to refer to the founding fathers of the United States of America. One of the things that was uppermost in their minds was that the new government they were forming be in harmony with the universal laws. They constantly wrestled with these "spiritual issues" as they framed the Constitution and Bill of Rights and they came to some very interesting conclusions.

# THE PURPOSE OF LIFE

Unfortunately, in our western society, it is a question that many people don't want to slow down long enough to think about. For many, this is because they must confront the reality of their own mortality. Others are fearful of dealing with an issue to which is attached so much uncertainty in their minds. Are we here simply to experience the joy of good food, sex, comfortable clothing and attractive shelters? While these things do contribute to our overall well-being, there are many individuals who have them all and more but who are not happy. Hence, in and of themselves, they cannot be the answer to our inquiry.

Is good physical health the elusive answer that we seek? As healers we might initially think so, but there are many persons who experience good physical health but are not truly happy with their lot in life. Again, it proves to be only a small piece of what we are seeking.

Are friends the answer? Many individuals have numerous friends and spend  much time and money with and on them but find that they still have the craving for something more. Therefore, friends prove not to be the answer either.

How about achieving our goals and realizing our potentials? There are people with several Ph.Ds and/or millions of dollars in assets who are not happy. There are individuals with great power and influence and they are not necessarily happy. There are great artists with well developed talents, especially in Hollywood, who are not happy. Thus, achieving goals cannot provide the answer we seek.

True happiness and contentment is something more than any of the above is capable of providing either independently or in combination. What then is the answer we are looking for? It is that **we have to be living in harmony with all, or as many as we are currently aware of, of the universal (divine) laws. In other words, we must begin to address the universal science of true religion.** I say "true religion" because there are many dogmas, bigotries, prejudices, and traditions that are cloaked in the guise of spirituality but have little or nothing to do with universal laws.

# THE UNIVERSAL RELIGION

In their writings and discussions, the Founding Fathers referred to John Locke (1632-1704) who proposed something called "The Universal Religion" in his publications, *Concerning Civil Government* and *Essay Concerning Human Understanding*. As startling as it may seem to those who have not studied this subject, the Founding Fathers went so far as to say that only members of this "universal religion" could be citizens of the new nation they were founding! **They also made it abundantly clear they were founding a government based upon universal laws such as "the inalienable rights of men" and "freedom of religion" not freedom from religion, as many have erroneously interpreted it.**

They outlined the following seven requirements of this "universal religion" that each individual would be required to embrace before he or she could become a citizen of the new nation. Failure to abide by these doctrines was grounds for revocation of citizenship in their minds. This unusual step was taken because the Founding Fathers understood that this higher form of government they were instituting required a moral or spiritual awareness and self-control on the part of its citizens in order to make it work. Individuals lacking in this spiritual maturity would not be able to adequately govern (control) themselves and ultimately would prove to be the downfall of the nation (and, in a larger sense, the world).

1. That a Universal Intelligence (God) exists and that all things were created by this supreme entity.

2. This supreme intelligence holds humans responsible for their treatment of one another under universally revealed moral codes.

3. That mankind continues to exist after this life.

4. That mankind will be judged and held responsible in the next life for conduct in this life.

5. That the Universal Intelligence has given to mankind certain inalienable rights that are required for proper government of self and nations. These are:

    a. The protection of human life.

    b. The protection of human liberty.

    c. The protection of private property.

    d. The protection of the right to pursue happiness in a private, individualized manner, so long as the rights of others are not violated and/or infringed upon.

The second great influence upon the Founding Fathers was Baron Charles Louis de Montesquieu (1589-1755) from whom they gleaned the following:

6. That there can be no permanent reliance upon the benevolence and integrity of human beings placed in positions of power. As Lord Acton said, "Power tends to corrupt; and absolute power corrupts absolutely." Therefore, all men must take care of themselves (including their health care) in order to be truly free.

7. That human nature is a combination of good and evil, virtue and vice. Good standards of personal conduct and good institutions will provide for the first and prevent the latter.

## WHO QUALIFIES?

Can an individual professing the Islamic faith qualify under this "universal religion" for citizenship? Yes, indeed. Can a Jew qualify? Absolutely. Can a Christian? Yes. How about a professor of a Native American religion? No problem. Can a Buddhist? Again, yes. How about a Hindu? Yes. How about a member of a Native African religion. Again, no problem.

How about an Agnostic? No, because they assert that "all knowledge is relative (therefore, there can be no fixed universal laws by which to govern themselves) and uncertain." Therefore, they have a fluxing value system which does not insure that they will act in a consistent and predictable manner. Under one set of circumstances, they may act with sincere human compassion and yet, on another similar occasion, they may ruthlessly strike out against their fellow man.

How about an Atheist? No, for the reason that they believe there is no such thing as universal laws and, therefore, they have no moral and/or ethical restraints with which to govern themselves. They are highly predictable in the manner in which they will act. It will always be beneficial to themselves even when it may be injurious to others. Theirs is the Law of the Jungle. They have numbed their human compassion to the point that they experience no guilt for their acts.

## SPIRITUAL POLLUTION

**Anything that leads us away from the universal principles is "spiritual pollution" and causes us to become unbalanced and dis-eased on this highest level of our being.** This includes false and/or distorted principles, deceptions, and even honest misunderstanding of the true nature of Universal Intelligence (God), pornography, profanity, immorality, dependence upon addictive substances, any form of abuse of another human being, animal life and even the planet itself, disrespect, irreverence, uncontrolled lusts, desires and appetites, lack of self-control on any and/or every level and much more.

True, many different peoples, cultures and religions have vastly different ideas about Universal Intelligence. However, one thing is clear. There can be only one Universal Intelligence. More than one would produce confusion, conflict and chaos. (Even polytheists [many gods] have a hierarchy of deity with one supreme being governing over the others.) Therefore, we must all eventually come to the same understanding of universal intelligence in order to achieve spiritual wellness. To do less **is to fall short of a total understanding of universal intelligence and to remain spiritually polluted.**

## THE TEXTBOOKS OF UNIVERSAL LAWS

Obviously, all scientific textbooks that contain correct principles and understandings can be utilized on the material level. Additionally, the writings of all religions, if in harmony with Universal Intelligence (God), are textbooks of universal spiritual laws. Thus, the Bible, the Koran, the Torah, the Bhagavad Gita, the Tripitika, the Book of Mormon, the Mahabharata, the Vedas and the other sacred writings can be utilized as textbooks of universal law.

Now, lest some gain an incorrect understanding of what is being said here, let us clarify. **All truth is universal law and as such we are obligated to abide by it, regardless of its secular origins and our own bigotries, prejudices and discriminations; but what is not truth places no obligation upon the truth seeker. The real challenge, then, is to have the inspiration and wisdom to successfully separate truth from tradition and fallacy and then to have the courage to abide by it.**

## THE UNIVERSAL LAW OF LAWS

Some may say, "I don't believe that" or "That's not part of my faith" or "I don't believe in religion". However, the scientific reality is that it does not matter if an individual, a group of individuals or even all individuals fail to accept a universal law; it has no universal significance. **The law remains operative in spite of ourselves, our opinions and our organizations. If we do not comply, we must and will pay the price of failing to abide by it. True, this price may not be paid immediately, but it will be required to be paid sooner or later. That is simply another of the Universal Laws.**

## THE MEASURING STICK

The problem is essentially one of a measuring device. If we have no fixed values for measuring something, everything becomes relative and hence constantly varying and meaningless. If people and/or organizations do not have a fixed value system (which more consistently than anything else is what true religion provides) they tend to be erratic in their actions and thoughts and, therefore, unreliable and unpredictable, able to justify any conduct regardless of its inappropriateness. There can be no consistent justice and fairness emanating from these individuals  nor their organizations and/or governments.

**Laws, even Universal Laws, must be fixed in order to dispense equity and justice at all times and in all things.** This is the inherent problem with *"Lex Regina"* or *"Ruler's Law"*. The ruler could change the laws any time he/she  pleased. People were never sure what the current law was, and whether they were performing a legal or illegal act. This produces a state of chaos and often results in a revolution undertaken to achieve a more just and equitable environment.

## LAW OF UNIVERSAL JUSTICE

**Universal (Divine) Laws are unchangeable, unless suspended by a higher law, and are therefore predictable and just in all times, places and under all  circumstances.** One always knows what to expect exactly in the future because it is exactly what happened on each occasion in the past. This is the very reason that these laws can be used with such precision in healing; we can rely on them time and time again. When we do not achieve the desired response, it is because we are unaware of or have ignored a collateral and/or higher law. **Nor is one universal law ever in conflict with another. All form a harmonious whole.**

## THE PURPOSE

Here is the grandest of truths. **The purpose of all Universal Laws is to teach us to live in harmony with the Universal Intelligence (God).** When this is achieved, there can be no dis-ease, no injustice, no prejudice, no discrimination, no bigotry, no inequity, no dissatisfaction. **When we are out of harmony with the universal spiritual laws, they begin to have a detrimental effect upon us and our total health, just as the quote by De Mille at the beginning of this chapter implies. Conversely, when we are in harmony with Universal Laws they begin to have a constructive effect upon our entire being and all around us.**

These are irrevocable decrees. **Even the Universal Intelligence must abide by them or it would cease to be the Universal Intelligence. Therefore, we can always be 100 percent certain of these laws and their effects. They have been, are and always will be constants. The catch is, we have to learn them and abide by them before we can use them to the advantage of the entire human race.** This has always been mankind's greatest challenge: To bring ourselves and our society into harmony with the universal laws. When this is accomplished, nothing will be impossible to us. This is the science of the spirit or the science of religion. **Without it we cannot succeed; with it we cannot fail.** We each simply have to decide if we are willing to pay the price required.

# Chapter 41
# THE BIG IDEA

*"Get the Big Idea and all else follows."*
— B. J. Palmer, D. C.

## THE FIRST STEP

As we come to understand the vast number of factors that can have an adverse affect upon a patient's health, it would be very easy to become disheartened. This need not be the case if we have mastered the "Big Idea". First of all, there is data indicating that very small amounts of pollutants actually stimulate our defense mechanisms. This should come as no surprise considering our discussion of the Arndt-Schultz Law in Chapter 7. But Wilder's Law, discussed in Chapter 12, must also be considered.

## WHY DO WE MISS IT?

If the "Big Idea" is as important as Palmer implies why are there so few who master it? Collier answers thus, **"A science with all the answers and no more  questions atrophies into mere technology."** Unfortunately, such is the state of most of our professions; we have become technicians doing the same thing over and over without using our reasoning powers to advance our science. For example, an allopath who repeatedly writes the same prescription, a chiropractor who repeatedly adjusts the same vertebra, an acupuncturist who repeatedly needles the same point, a homeopath who repeatedly utilizes the same remedy, and so on.

It's so easy to just follow accepted protocol which is exactly what the "Big Idea" is not. The "Big Idea" requires constant effort, constant humility, constant learning, constant re-evaluation and constant self-correction. We must overcome **"The arrogance of our own ignorance."**

## THE OVERVIEW

The previous chapters have discussed the serious scientific quandaries relating to immunization, antibiotics, petrochemical, electromagnetic, psychological stresses, nuclear radiation, structural, nutritional, auto-toxins, genetics, surgery, pharmaceuticals, over-treatment, spiritual and numerous other adverse impacts of our modern world and it is quite likely that there are more factors we have not yet identified that have a detrimental impact upon our own and our patient's total health.

See Figure 41.1 — Note this is the same mathematical progression appearing in figure 8.1 but in this situation representing a different principle) assists us in seeing **the multi-pronged, accumulative, interacting and synergistic threats to human life and health. Add to that the knowledge accumulated from our previous discussions of miasmas, (diathesis, dosha and phase) and we are beginning to comprehend and appreciate the true prophetic genius of the individuals who originated these concepts.**

## LACK OF SCIENCE

Yet, even today in our so-called "scientific Age" there is very little hard data on multiple drug interactions, multiple heavy metal interactions, multiple petrochemical interactions, multiple electromagnetic interactions, multiple auto-toxic interactions, multiple carcinogen interactions, multiple sources of radiation interactions, multiple surgical interactions, multiple allergens and so on. And the hard scientific documentation is even more minute to non-existent when we consider the interactions of each category with another or multiple categories.

In view of this glaring lack of scientific data, much of so-called "modern medical science" is nothing more than pure guesswork. Upon critical analysis, we find that **there is nothing scientific about it** (see Chapter 47, Research, for further details.) Such a total lack of scientific controls should alarm a scientifically-oriented culture such as ours but our western, solid state, reductionistic, pseudo-scientific culture conveniently chooses to ignore our greatest scientific weakness, western medicine.

## THE ORIGINATORS OF THE MIASMA, DIATHESIS, PHASE, DOSHA

Truly, the individuals who conceived the miasmatic, diathesis, doshic, phase were correct in their prophetic vision of the "Big Idea". They foretold with complete and uncanny accuracy the disastrous outcomes of ignoring natural (universal) laws and polluting the planet while in pursuit of science for science's sake.

$1 \times 1 = 1$

$1 \times 2 = 2$

$1 \times 2 \times 3 = 6$

$1 \times 2 \times 3 \times 4 = 24$

$1 \times 2 \times 3 \times 4 \times 5 = 120$

$1 \times 2 \times 3 \times 4 \times 5 \times 6 = 720$

$1 \times 2 \times 3 \times 4 \times 5 \times 6 \times 7 = 5{,}040$

$1 \times 2 \times 3 \times 4 \times 5 \times 6 \times 7 \times 8 = 40{,}320$

$1 \times 2 \times 3 \times 4 \times 5 \times 6 \times 7 \times 8 \times 9 = 362{,}880$

$1 \times 2 \times 3 \times 4 \times 5 \times 6 \times 7 \times 8 \times 9 \times 10 = 3{,}628{,}800$ possible adverse interactions on the total health of an individual impacted by just 10 different antagonistic factors.

*Figure 41.1 — Multiple interacting factors adversely affecting health*

Yet another way of comprehending this is that our present health problems are an accumulation of all of the various positive and negative influences upon our total being on any and all levels. **Hence, no one thing can be THE CAUSE of dis-ease.** We learn with ever greater clarity that **the miasma, (diathesis, dosha, phase) is in fact the origin of all dis-ease but for multiple reasons.** It may manifest in various forms, a skin rash, a vertebral subluxation, a fever, paralysis, asthma, depression or any combination of symptoms, but **it is the cumulative positive and negative circumstances encountered on all levels of our total being, even before birth, and in our ancestors, and upon our individual genetic make up that determines what dis-ease symptoms (miasma, diathesis, dosha, phase) will express themselves as the total dis-ease (strengths and weaknesses) patterns in any given individual.**

**The "Big Idea" is to precisely understand this individual expression of dis-ease and how to deal with it in the most efficient individualized manner.** This literally means that there are 6,250,000,000 different protocols for the 6,250,000,000 individuals currently living on the earth. And when there are 50 billion or even 100 billion individuals on this planet, there will of necessity be 50 billion or 100 billion individual protocols necessary to achieve the potential for healing each of them.

This means that **canned health care with routine protocols is as antiquated as the dinosaur and so are practitioners and health care organizations (such as insurance companies, medicare, health maintenance organizations, preferred provider organizations, etc,) who persist in practicing in such an unscientific manner. To be a cookbook practitioner and do exactly the same thing to every patient is to be a major part of the problem, allowing miasmatic (diathic, doshic, phase) dis-ease to advance unchecked while only caring for isolated symptoms. Such ignorance of the universal laws of healing, if not corrected, will eventually destroy the individual and the human race - in fact, all life on this planet.**

## THE MIASMATIC, DIATHESIS, DOSHIC, PHASE INFLUENCE

Truly, mankind is on a suicidal course, as Hahnemann taught, unless the effects of the taints of life can be reversed and eliminated. Unfortunately, health care, regardless of the type, is nothing more than symptom chasing if this is not clearly comprehended and applied routinely in clinical practice.

Centuries of man's trials and errors, education and technology have not only failed to halt the progress of the miasmatic, (diathesis, doshic, phase) problem but have actually accelerated the problem. To prove this point, the world at the start of the 21st Century is far more polluted and hostile to life than at any time in human history.

**Obviously, man is incapable of saving himself. We have made a science of every aspect of health care except the one that will ultimately prove to be the answer. The spiritual aspect. The handwriting is on the wall. Mankind is not intelligent enough to solve his major problem. In order to survive, we must return to the God who made us and learn to keep his Universal Laws. Failure to do so is for the human race to have a death wish. Theo-science must become the ultimate science if the race is to survive and prosper. Otherwise, we will slowly continue to commit genocide. The entire human experience conclusively proves that scientists, and the race in general, must become men and women of deep religious faith.**

I realize that many will scream, "Such things are not science" for so has our materialistic, reductionistic, non-vitalistic oriented educational system taught us. **But the reality is that system has missed the grandest of all universal truths, the one that allows all other truths to come into clear and proper focus, order and execution. There is a being who rules the universe and that being's universal laws must be obeyed if we are to survive long-term. If we do not do so, we will be forever learning but never able to come to a knowledge of the truth.**

# COMBINATIONS

As we continue to study the issues that determine the survival of the human race, we see that many of these problems are the result of groups and individuals entering into agreements for the purposes of gaining wealth, power and/or monopolistic or cartel control. In the past, when such undesirable situations have been exposed to the public, the response tactics of these entities have included gaining legal exemptions from or simply ignoring the laws, bribing, belittling, confusing the issues and discrediting the sources  of the information in the public media (which, incidently, they also own and/or control).

Since these approaches have worked repeatedly in the past they will no  doubt continue to be the tactics of choice but that does not change the reality of cartels and monopolies which see us and our loved ones as mere pawns. As they seek to totally control our health, minds, bodies, assets, institutions, education, food supply and governments, they are actively striving to become our dictators.

# THE INTERNET

With the advent of the Internet and Freedom Of Information Act, it is becoming more and more difficult for the controlling interests to maintain and hide their activities. The Internet and computers now allow the average citizen access to hundreds of millions of pages of information that can be reviewed, organized and consolidated to establish a clearer picture of how and why all of these interwoven cartels and monopolies are manipulating our world.

This is precisely how many of the facts included in this text were found, documented, organized, and inter-related. This book is only the tip of the iceberg. Hopefully, there will be many thousands of similar revealing works in the future. As the old saying states, **"Truth shall make you free."**

# THE FUTURE

Henry Ford also once said, **"If you give no thought to the future, you have none."** This is exactly what will happen to the human race if the diabolical combinations are not successfully combated; the human race will have no future. We will be the mental, emotional, financial, political, educational, social, spiritual and healing slaves of Madison Avenue and the cartels and monopolies that are trying to attractively package their control over us. Therefore, it becomes a moral as well as a self-preservation act for every healer and every citizen to aggressively combat these pernicious influences. In the words of Thomas Jefferson, "Rebellion to tyrants is obedience to God." and "Enlighten the people generally, and tyranny and oppression of body and mind will vanish like evil spirits at the dawn of day." **Thus, the true healer is forced to move far beyond the traditional doctor-patient role if he or she is to be successful in establishing health in the fullest sense of its definition. This requires a courage not needed in the past to be merely a solid state, reductionist, non-vitalistic practitioner.** Are we equal to the task at hand? Each of us must find the answer to that question in our own hearts and minds. If, yes, then lets get on with it; if, no, then please get out of the way because you are part of the problem.

# BOOK V

# THE POST-DOCTORAL TEXT

# INTRODUCTION TO THE POST-DOCTORAL TEXT

*"It is easy in the world to live after the world's
opinion, it is easy to live in solitude after your own;
but the great man is he who in the midst of the
crowd keeps with perfect sweetness the
independence of solitude."*
— Ralph Waldo Emerson

## WHERE LEARNING BEGINS

Post-doctoral education is, unfortunately, most frequently construed and constructed for the purpose of getting those annoying continuing education requirements out of the way so that the practitioner can fulfill the legal requirements for license renewal.

Few seem to realize that it is instead the genesis of true professional education. As undergraduates, students are so busy memorizing materials for examinations that they do not have the luxury of time for reflective examination of the data being presented. If a so-called "Post-graduate Course" is more of the same pattern of lectures, exams and cramming for specialty certification, then it has sadly missed the mark.

True post-doctoral education should cause the student to reflect upon and separate the "ash and trash" accumulated in the student's undergraduate and graduate educations from the "pure gold" of true healing knowledge and clinical experience. It should open the mind to new vistas of knowledge that  undergraduate and graduate programs had neither the time for nor the understanding of. It should re-vitalize our understanding of, love for and dedication to healing. To do anything else is to simply re-hash our undergraduate and graduate programs and is a counterfeit of the true post-doctoral educational experience. With this in mind, let us then begin the post-doctoral experience.

# Chapter 42

# WHEN DOES EACH SYSTEM EXCEL?

*"To everything there is a season, and*
*a time to every purpose under the heaven."*
— Ecclesiastes

## PERSPECTIVE

To this point we have reviewed the universal laws of healing and the strengths and weaknesses of each system of complementary healing. Now we must learn how and when to combine them and how to determine when one is preferable to another. **When this ability is mastered we move beyond the scope and limitations of any one system and in fact become the eclectic quantum healer.**

This is not easy to achieve, however. We all have prejudices created by our particular professional training. A chiropractor tends to think of all illness in terms of neuro-mechanical subluxations. An acupuncturist, in terms of where to insert a needle for energy balance. A naturopath, in terms of what herb, vitamin or mineral to administer to the patient. A physical therapist, in terms of what exercise to prescribe. A surgeon, in terms of what to cut out. An allopath, in terms of what drug to prescribe. A psychologist or counselor, in terms of how to talk out the problem, and so on.

**L. Timberlake in his book** *Born To Win* **continues to develop this concept. He writes, "our minds absorb thousands of bites of information every second, much of it we do not need or even want, so the subconscious mind filters out the unnecessary data received by using 'Scotomas' or 'blind spots'". The problem is the subconscious mind can also use these scotomas to filter out truths perceived as false-hoods, based upon previously accepted prejudices. Thus, we begin to accept what we want to believe as truth and then base our reasoning and research upon distorted and, therefore, scientifically invalid data. This, in turn, produces scientifically invalid research data.**

The goal is to be able to accurately determine when each is the therapy of choice or how and when to successfully combine the various disciplines. In the past, some have claimed, for example, that homeopathy and acupuncture do not mix. Or that Ayurveda and allopathy are not compatible. There is great truth in these statements, but not for the reason(s) generally believed by those making such remarks.

The challenge is finding that rare individual who has taken the time and effort to become **competent in multiple disciplines. The point being, if we are not highly competent in each of the disciplines we seek to combine we cannot hope to be successful in the effort.**

# THE KEY

Marsh once said, **"In these pages it is no part of my objective to save my readers the labor of observation or thought."** We will do well to remember these words for the eclectic, vitalistic, quantum practitioner must constantly sift and evaluate data relating to **each individual patient.** What may work for one will not for another and what worked yesterday on a particular patient may not be correct for that individual today. Many practitioners tend to get in a rut about the care they render and succumb to a "canned care" style of practice establishing programs in which all patients are forced into a routine office procedure. While this approach is efficient for office management, it produces individual healing results that are far from ideal. In fact, allopathy's endorsement of the concept that all patients with the same diagnosis should receive the same treatment is the primary reason why quantum health care is flourishing today. Patients have tried the allopathic method, have not gotten well, and have instinctively gravitated to the individualization of care that quantum health care provides.

Thus, the quantum physician (QP) must never allow his/her mind to rest. We must be constantly re-evaluating patients with respect to their histories and their response to the care rendered. **If the primary mode of care is not documenting definite improvements within two or three visits then the patient should be re-evaluated for a change of therapy or inclusion of additional forms of therapy.** If we are using the proper therapy(ies)we should see improvements or at the very least aggravation patterns indicating that improvement is eminent. See figure 42.1 for an illustrated representation of this inter-relationship. Please be aware that this diagram is only meant to be a representation and the placement of each discipline may not reflect the ideal relationship under all circumstances.

To illustrate the inter-relationships of figure 42.1, we will use the example of allopathy. On the graph, allopathy with its reductionistic, materialistic philosophy is situated opposite spiritual healing which is an expansionistic, vitalistic concept. Notice that the arrow moving from allopathy narrows as it approaches spiritual healing until it reaches a point. At that point, allopathy has no relationship with spiritual healing.

Additionally, chiropractic is positioned next to allopathy and, in fact, has an overlap with it, forming yet another arrowhead that reaches a point in Native American and Oceanic healing and vice versa. This illustrates that current-day, reductionistic solid state chiropractic science and philosophy and reductionistic solid state allopathic science and philosophy have much in common in their scope of practice. (Such was not the case with chiropractic as envisioned by its founder. In fact, this is diametrically opposed to what D. D. Palmer taught. (See Chapter 17.) At the same time, current reductionistic solid state chiropractic has reached a point where it has little or nothing in common with the expansionistic, vitalistic concepts of native American and Oceanic healing. And so it goes around the figure 42.1.

The next point of consideration involves the more central areas of the graph where all healing arts begin to overlap. **Here is the great balance of cooperative healing in which each contributes its unique expertise and is respected by all others for what it has to offer. At this point, the "turf battles" have been abandoned in favor of what is best for the patient. Equally importantly here is the great balance in which each system has abandoned its dirty politics, smear campaigns, unscientific dogmas, prejudices, discriminations and pseudo-religious fanaticism and has progressed to a true science which has as its only goal the greatest degree of benefit to suffering humanity. A truly healthy positive healing environment finally has been achieved.**

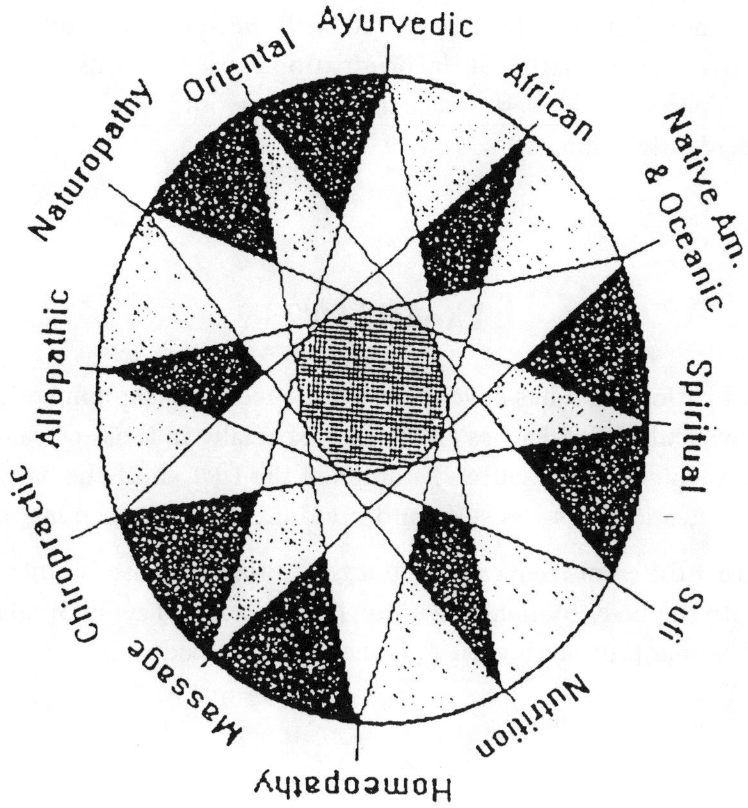


*Figure 42.1 — Overlapping and interacting scopes of practice*

## LAW OF SIMILARS

A condition resulting from physical trauma will most likely respond best to a similar (but not identical) controlled force of a chiropractic adjustment. A condition caused by a failing organ may respond to similar (but not identical) organo or phyto therapy; one of energy deficiency, to the similar (but not identical) energy of acupuncture. One of an emotional disturbance, to a similar (but not identical) controlled emotional response of counseling.

## EXAMPLE #1

Let us consider a much more involved case. A patient with physical trauma from an automobile accident who has not had a normal energy level since the accident. There has also been major emotional disturbance causing loss of sleep, vivid dreams reliving the crash and a nervous uticaria. The patient has numerous large and severe hematomas resulting from being thrown around in the vehicle because he was not wearing a seat belt. The patient has experienced epileptic seizures since the accident and complains of cervical pain even though the hospital emergency room found no problem. Yet, an X-ray examination reveals a retrolordotic cervical curvature and the trapezius and sternoclydomastoid muscles are functioning at only 20 percent of their normal functional capacity. The patient is also experiencing, for the first time, asthmatic attacks that are ameliorated when the uticaria is aggravated. He is also very restless, nervous, irritable and depressed since the accident.

How do you determine the priority for care? Homeopathy certainly could deal with many of these symptoms. Numerous acupuncture meridians could be associated with the symptoms. But using the Law of Similars, the true healer must ask, "What was the nature of the originating cause?" In this case, it was physical forces encountered in the accident. Therefore, the best choice in this case would be a chiropractic adjustment which constitutes a similar (but not identical) force.

## EXAMPLE #2

A second case involves a patient who has never been well since receiving immunizations. She complains of lethargy, asthma, numerous musculoskeletal aches and pains, especially in the cervical area. She has had severe epileptic seizures and uticaria which started within 24 hours of the DPT shot. She has been nervous, irritable and depressed since the immunization. Restless sleep and vivid dreams are becoming more frequent.

The symptoms are not that different from case #1 but the initiating cause is quite different. In case #2, the cause is toxins introduced into the body by immunization. Therefore, the Law of Similars indicates that case #2 will likely respond best to a similar (but not identical) homeopathic remedy.

## EXAMPLE #3

This patient is dragging, has no energy, is restless, anxious, depressed and irritable. He is having headaches in the morning that last until about 11 A.M. The headaches are aggravated in damp weather. The patient has asthma in late summer and fall. He exhibits marked muscular discomfort and has herpetic -like eruptions in and around the mouth and there is a yellow coating on the tongue.

Again, there are many similarities to case #1 and #2. Many of the symptoms are also identifiable rubrics in homeopathic repertories but the case centers around a lack of energy rather than a mechanical injury or a toxic condition. This case is a classic picture for the earth phase disturbance in acupuncture. Acupuncture will produce a similar (but not identical) response and should be the first choice of therapy in this case.

## THE ART FORM

If a hundred art students were trained in the identical laws of perspective, composition, primary and secondary colors, harmony, lighting, shading, etc., and then all painted the same still life, none of their pictures would be exactly the same. This our culture accepts as art. The same is true of the healing professions. **The art of healing is to be able to determine when one protocol will produce superior results to another that is very similar but not identical. In the vast majority of cases, this can be achieved by applying the laws that we have been studying in this text but, on occasion, a more intuitive factor comes into play.**

For example, a chiropractor may evaluate a case; palpation indicates the segment is structurally deviated to the left, X-ray examination collaborates the finding, the subjective symptoms are all left-sided and the neurological and orthopedic tests further confirm the impression. Upon setting up for the corrective thrust, the practitioner receives the distinct impression to contact the segment on the right side. Having learned to rely on such "inspiration", the practitioner makes contact on the apparently contra-indicated side and the vertebra literally falls into juxtaposition without a thrust being necessary.

**This is the art form.** Every other discipline will from time to time experience similar promptings, the acupuncturist, the naturopath, the ayurvedic practitioner, etc. Each must learn to "go with the flow" so to speak. These are the miracle cases. There is a power higher than the practitioner, the Universal Intelligence, working through the healer. This intelligence understands how all of these indications can be apparently ignored and yet the patient can be completely healed. **Learn to accept this gift and strive to cultivate it so that it will happen more and more often.**

## MULTIPLE MODES OF CARE

Let us return to case #2 now and assume that dramatic progress was made with a properly selected homeopathic remedy but the case has now come to a standstill and it is primarily the musculoskeletal problem that persists. At this point, we may want to shift our focus toward a more neuromechanical chiropractic approach.

Let us now reconsider case #1. All the symptoms have improved with the exception of the hives. At this juncture, we might want to consider homeopathy or acupuncture as the primary therapy since this symptom is not responding well to chiropractic care.

## THE TOOL BOX

The quantum practitioner has a tool box that allows him/her to pick and choose the tool (therapy) that best suits the situation. A carpenter would be quite handicapped if he/she only had a saw. Just imagine trying to pound nails with a saw or trying to use it as a screwdriver. Yet that is precisely the mistake that mono-therapy practitioners are making as it concerns the health of their patients' bodies, minds and spirits.

A chiropractor who can only adjust has just one tool in his/her toolbox. The same is true for the acupuncturist who is only trained in needling or a naturopath who only knows how to prescribe herbs. For the practitioner trained only in surgery, the knife is his only tool. There is an old adage, **"When your only tool is a hammer everything must be treated as if it is a nail."** What we should be thinking about is the damage that is done as a result of trying to pound a screw into a board. What iatrogenic damage is done to the patient when a saw (surgery) is used when a level (acupuncture needle) is the tool of choice? Or a weld (orthopedic fusion) when a plum-bob (chiropractic adjustment) is what is needed.

**The quantum, expansionistic practitioner must be trained in all of these tools, or know when to refer, in order to obtain maximum results from each of them.** Not to do so is to reduce ourselves to the unscientific chaos of present day reductionistic, non-vitalistic, solid state pseudo-healing.

## LAW OF NON-SUBSTITUTION

**There is never something just as good as the needed specific therapy. To practice as if there is, is to deceive ourselves, our patients, and their third-party payers and to abandon our integrity and self-respect.** In summary, we are either healers or we are not. And if not, that makes us a major part of the problem and is contrary to all of the universal laws and principles being taught in this textbook and by the universe itself.

# LAW OF SUPPRESSIVE THERAPIES

**Suppressive, inappropriate and/or excessive therapies adversely alter the normal expression of the vital or life force, innate, ch'i causing iatrogenic dis-ease. Iatrogenic causes of dis-ease tend to be far more disruptive to the patient because they tend to be more forceful than naturally occurring causes.**

# THERAPEUTIC LAW OF TIME

An average of **one month's healing time should be allowed for each year that a dis-ease has existed.** For example, if properly cared for, a patient with an asthmatic condition of ten years duration should be given ten months to reach a cured state.

# LAW OF CORRELATION OF SYSTEMS

Ayurvedic, Chiropractic, Homeopathy and Oriental Medicine each have a well-established method for the categorization of dis-ease. If properly understood, these various systems can be correlated into one whole.

The Ayurvedic doshic system uses the Vattic representation of motion or increasing function; the Pittic, a heat-producing state; and the Kaphaic, a lubricating or decreasing function.

The Chiropractic diathesis classify dis-ease a Motor/motion in-coordination, Sensory/interpretation in-coordination, Spasm/improper function or relational control, Fever/improper thermogenesis or thermolysis, Poison/improper elimination or secretion, Anemia/abnormal nutrition, reparation or repletion, Tumor/cells not physiologically useful and Degenerative/decomposition of tissues. Additionally there are Prolapse and Contracture.

Homeopathy divides dis-ease into three grand miasmas; the Psoric or hypo-functional, the Sycotic or hyper-functional, and the Syphilitic or erratic or dysfunctional dis-eases. Additionally, Tubercular and Cancerous states are discussed but are not as extensively indexed.

Oriental medicine utilizes a Five Phase heading; Wood relates to hyper-functional or growth, Fire to maximal hyper-function or heating, Earth to a balance or neutral state, Metal to a hypo-functional or decreasing state, and Water to a minimal hypo-functional or cooling state.

Let us graphically superimpose these disciplines. See figure 42.1 and 42.2.

Such a correlation should come as no surprise to the informed healer and should actually have been anticipated. Remember, "universal" applied in all times, places and conditions **unless superseded by a higher law. Therefore, locales as diverse as India circa 2,000 B. C., China circa 400 B. C. and Germany circa 1790s should have developed somewhat similar systems if they were functioning under the same Universal Laws.** It is simply a matter of each group applying the Universal Laws within a slightly different context which prevents a 100 percent correlation.

With adequate data, there should be a similar correlation possible with the other forms of quantum healing because they too are working within the framework of the Universal Laws.

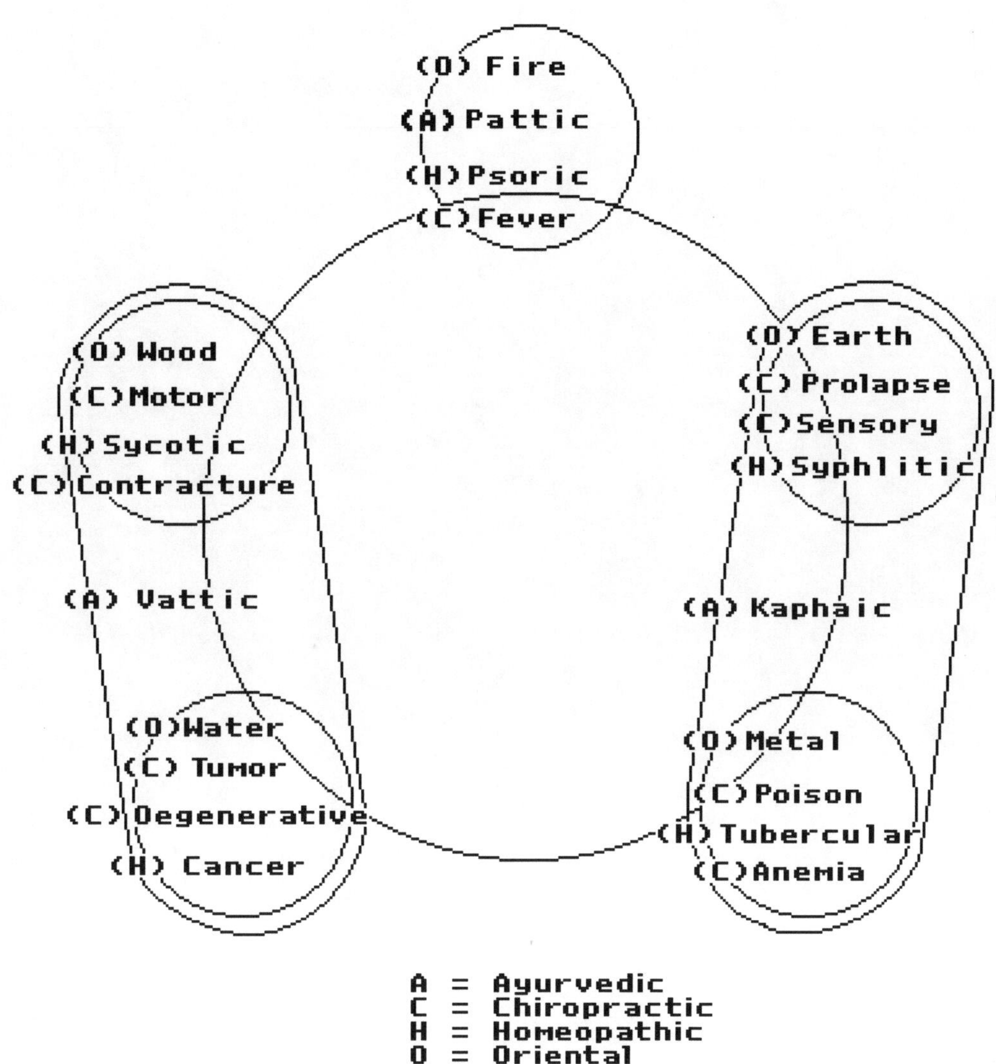


*Figure 42.2 — Correlation Of Systems*

# Chapter 43
# A NEW PERSPECTIVE ON INHERITED DIS-EASE

*"To preserve health is a moral and religious duty for
health is the basis of all social virtues. We can no
longer be useful when we are not well."*

— Anonymous

## THE CONCEPT

One of the most difficult concepts for the reductionistic-trained mind of the allopath, the limited neuromusculoskeletal chiropractor, and the cause- and-effect naturopath is the expansionistic, vitalistic miasmatic (diathesis, dosha, phase) principle of dis-ease. Yet, individuals such as Hahnemann and Stevenson indicated that the inherited principle of dis-ease, when properly understood, provides the basis not only for the proper care of the patient's present problems but much more importantly, for the totality of the patient and his posterity by removing dis-ease taints from the family genetic pool. (Farmers are constantly doing just this, producing hybrid crops and animals to overcome present weaknesses, breeding cattle to eliminate weaknesses and strengthen desirable characteristics.)

In a deeper sense, however, an accurate understanding of the miasmas, diathesis, dosha, phase proves to be an answer for the longevity of the race and in a very literal sense probably all living things. Thus, genetic engineering cannot reach its full potential without an understanding of miasmas, diathesis, dosha, phases. In the long run, it can only produce genetic disasters.

If the inherited concept of dis-ease is correct, then there is no hope for those members of the human race who do not have this taint resolved. They are doomed. In fact, if the taints are not resolved all life on the planet, is doomed. **The ultimate end result of all miasmatic, diathesis, dosha, phase dis-ease tends to be death by suicide.** One could say that contamination by the hereditary taint and the continual reinforcement by sexually-contracted dis-ease, suppressive application of both allopathic and natural remedies and the increasing stresses of modern society (remember stresses are the most frequent triggering mechanism of latent miasmatic, diathesis, doshic, phase tendencies) are subconscious affirmations of the basic taint's suicidal tendency. According to Hahnemannian concept, if not properly countered, these inherited  taints will continue to multiply in the human race until each individual will reach the point where life is no longer possible because of them.

## EXAMPLES

In many respects, this is probably why we are seeing such an astronomical increase in chronic dis-eases such as allergies. One hundred years ago the word "allergy" did not even appear in standard dictionaries. Today, however, it is rare to find individuals who are totally allergy-free. Sheraskin and Ringsdorf at the University of

Alabama Medical School have mathematically projected, based upon database studies, that in a few years it will be statistically impossible to find a human being who does not exhibit some form of chronic degenerative dis-ease process, including allergies.

From this perspective, AIDS appears to be nothing more than a more virulent form of a destructive miasma, diathesis, dosha, phase. Cancer likewise appears to be nothing more than a combination of several of these inherited weaknesses.

## A POSSIBLE ANSWER

At first it may be difficult or even impossible for some to accept all of the implications of the above statements. If these are indeed accurate comments, they may well prove to be the **most important healing arts principles ever conceived by the mind of man,** even more important than the subluxation for chiropractors, or the meridian for the acupuncturist or detoxification for the naturopath. This is not necessarily because the **inheritance of dis-ease type provides answers to why some patients are so prone to certain types of subluxations, or weaknesses in certain meridians, or why the certain types of toxins seem to accumulate so much more readily in certain individuals. The most important principle, however, is that the miasma (diathesis, dosha, phase) dis-eases can be eliminated, or at the very least dramatically limited in the production of genetic and familial weaknesses which produce fertile soil for degenerative dis-ease, cancer and familiar dis-eases such as diabetes and heart problems, to name only a few.**

Why is it, then, that so few practitioners of the healing arts have been able to master the vitalistic, expansionistic concept of inherited weakness?

## THE BASIS

**The basic miasmatic, diathesis, doshic, phase premise is that all dis-ease affecting not only man but all living things can be traced to and categorized under one or more primordial dis-ease causes or categories.** Of all the authorities on the inheritance of dis-ease tendencies, Hahnemann, without doubt, wrote the most extensive, concise and best-preserved treatises. We go to his writings in order to further expand our understanding of this critical issue.

To Hahnemann, psora is the mother of all other dis-eases. But to Hahnemann, the word psora, in addition to the classic dictionary definition of "itch", meant its effect on the psychic, physiological, biochemical, neurological, pathological and autoimmune systems, and its effect on sleep, sexual, spiritual and energetic changes which tend to be of a hypo-functioning nature and much, much more.

## ADDITIONAL FACTORS

In an attempt to explain miasmas, most authorities continue to utilize terminology similar to Hahnemann's; i.e., terms such as infestation, morbific agent, minute, invisible, animated being, dis-ease factor, etiology, etc. These tend to leave the distinct impression that we are exclusively discussing the effects of micro-organisms. **While in some cases the microbial influences are accurate, additional factors such as subluxations, imbalances of acupuncture meridians, poor nutrition, stress and lack of rest also must be considered in order to understand the totality of miasmatic, diathesis, doshic, phase dis-ease.** (See Chapters 23 through 41.)

In fact, **when such micro-organisms and others of the above-mentioned factors are properly understood, they are frequently demonstrated to be the result of miasmatic, diathesis, doshic, phase changes within the living being rather than the initiating cause of miasmas.** This is yet another reason why the reductionistic-trained, cause-and-effect practitioners struggle so with the miasmatic concept. They cannot successfully extract their thought process from the severely limited reductionistically-oriented immediate cause-and-effect response.

## A MOST CHALLENGING QUESTION

What is antecedent to the miasma? It is the pre-miasmatic, pre-diathesis, pre-doshic, pre-phase influence. **What changed in order to allow the initial miasma to become operative in the first living beings and, subsequently, in every person descending from them.** For the ultimate answer, it is necessary to go back to the parents of the race, Adam and Eve (to place the example within the Judean-Christian context that most Americans and Europeans are familiar with).

First: The original parents of the race lived in a state free from dis-ease, degeneration and all other adverse influences so far as the health of their bodies, minds and spirits was concerned. In other words, they were immortal or could have lived indefinitely.

Second: All that changed when they partook of the fruit, apple, pear, whatever it actually was. But the simple act of eating a fruit was unlikely to have been  the true deciding factor. Rather, the fruit appears to be a literary symbol.

What then actually took place? **The parents of the race were given a spiritual or higher order, non-corporal law which knowingly or unknowingly, depending upon your particular theological viewpoint, they violated. The penalty for the violation of this spiritual law was mortality and susceptibility to dis-ease, dis-function, degeneration and death. In order to reverse these degenerative processes, there must be an equally powerful spiritual law. It is extremely unlikely that lower order substances and/or forces, such as drugs, herbs, adjustments, homeopathics, acupuncture therapy, etc., could approach this spiritual or energy level. Remember, one cannot truly heal from below up but rather by Herring's (Palmer's) Law which requires true healing from "above down".**

## THE GRAND QUESTION

The grand question is, then, can any corporal process or therapy counteract these original universal spiritual laws? This is extremely unlikely from any of the healing philosophies covered in this text or from a quantum or even theological viewpoint. **True, various therapies may significantly decrease aggravations and the dis-ease taint on the patient's total health but they apparently do not have the power to totally overcome death and degeneration.** In other words, no corporal therapy is capable of making human beings immortal again. Kent concurs, "The Soul, which is the most interior (and non-material aspect) of man, cannot be affected by drugs (or any other corporal therapy). This can only be affected by Man's own will." For example, a person who delights in immorality cannot be made moral by a therapy. **The individual must have the desire to change and be willing to pay the price.**

Interestingly, this was one of the major purposes of the physicians to the emperor in ancient China and most other ancient royal and/or imperial courts. Because the ruler was worshiped as a divine being, it was necessary for the attending physicians to render him immortal. Much of ancient phytotherapy was involved with such "youth or rejuvenation formulas". Unfortunately, for the rulers, in spite of their wealth, power and the skill of their court physicians, none of them was ever able to overcome aging, degeneration and death.

The question is then, **"What is capable of making such a change?"** Every major world religion, be it Judaism, Christianity, Buddhism, Hinduism, Islam and even tribal religions, believe that a "major or mighty change" must take place before mankind is capable of again becoming immortal. Christians believe that this change can only come through the atonement of Jesus Christ. The Jewish people are still waiting for their Messiah. Other religions believe that the individual is responsible for working out his own change or salvation. Still others believe if you aren't successful in this life, you will be reincarnated and come back for additional tries until you finally master spirituality

The important point is not the individual's or group's theological belief system but rather the apparent universal religious and philosophical understanding that **when a spiritual law is broken it is only capable of being compensated for, or counteracted, by another equally significant and/or higher spiritual law.** Therefore, as true healers, we must learn additional ways of guiding, without offending the patient's particular religious tenets, the healing at these higher spiritual levels.

As stated earlier, the culmination of all miasmatic dis-ease is death by suicide or the destruction of one's self, the antithesis of life and immortality. What could be sicker?

# APPREHENSION

I am sure that many of you are apprehensive and feel that this mingling of healing and spiritual tenets can be dangerous. In our western reductionistic society, such blending of theology and science is considered taboo. But in almost all early cultures, and even in some societies today, the healers were and are also the priests. It was, and is, not considered possible, in those expansionistic cultures, to segregate the two into distinct and entirely unrelated entities. A better understanding of quantum physics healing forces requires us to return to the eclectic approach of science and healing.

# THE PRICE

The lesson to be learned here is that **Universal Laws cannot be broken. This is the basis of natural healing. These laws may be ignored but they are still operating and we must and will pay the consequences sooner or later for our failure to heed them. This is what miasmas, diatheses, dosha, phases are all about and how they began to function in the first place. They are the price to be paid for a broken universal law.**

Thus, we see that in spite of race, culture, geography or religion there appears to be an inherent understanding in the entire human family of the miasmatic, diathesis, doshic, phase or inherited concept of degeneration, dis-ease and death. True, it may not be recognized in those particular terms but the basic concept appears with amazing consistency; it has survived the trial of time and when explained in terms that a particular culture is familiar with, it is readily understandable and easily acceptable to them.

# Chapter 44
# THE ANTI-MATTER COMPONENT OF HEALING

*"We are never justified in assuming a force to be
insignificant because its measure is unknown or
even because no physical effect can be traced to it."*
— George Perkins Marsh

## THE FACTS

Very little actually has been documented regarding the anti-matter role in health and dis-ease. Since anti-matter (or the parallel universe concept) is a relatively new concept in quantum, astro and theoretical physics (since the 1920s), all discussions about it were theoretical in nature until DeWitt documented the existence of the anti-electron. At that point, anti-matter became a reality of our existence, a reality that presents far more questions than answers but nevertheless a reality. Therefore, our philosophical thinking must be expanded to include this reality in order to maintain the leading edge position in health care. To ignore such would be to slip to a second-class status.

## LAW OF MATTER - ANTI-MATTER

The ancient oriental principle of yin-yang (or opposition in all things) may be one of the earliest references to what we now refer to as matter and anti-matter. If there is matter, there must be anti-matter to compensate and balance it. Yet, matter and anti-matter do not appear to be directly interchangeable. Each must pass through the intermediate step of conversion to energy (the quantum leap) illustrated in figure 18.2.

## LAW OF SIMPLICITY VS. COMPLEXITY

This concept of simplicity vs. complexity is the pattern that all knowledge takes. For example, we learned that the basic building block of all tissues is the cell. Then, it became more complicated when we learned that there were sub-cellular components such as the mitochondria and nuclei. Next, we began to study the molecular structure of these sub-cellular components. This, in turn, led us to yet more factors at the atomic and sub-atomic levels. Then, we simplified it all by stating that all solid state matter is simply closely compacted energy. Now, we have progressed to the anti-matter aspect. If the law continues to hold true (which it should do if it is a universal law), there will always be another new level to investigate.

Interestingly, since our minds are not capable of dealing with conceptsof ever-increasing complexity, we constantly re-evaluate and reorganize our knowledge into simpler or more consistent formats. The most striking thing about this pattern of simplicity-yielding-complexity and complexity-yielding- simplicity is that it is not limited to the human race. It is a Universal Law which has been repeatedly observed at all levels of organization from the most minute to the grandest.

## A NEW PERSPECTIVE

A very interesting statement provides us with a new paradigm for thinking about anti-matter. **There is no such thing as immaterial matter - all non- corporal (anti-matter) is matter, but it is more highly refined in form and therefore not discernible to our corporal five senses.** To place this concept in the theological format, it would mean that **spirit is anti-matter.** To place it in the philosophical arena, this would mean that the **vital force, life force, ch'i, innate intelligence, kung, kundalini is not energy, as stated in the undergraduate portion of this text, but is instead anti-matter.**

Such a prospect places an entirely new emphasis on the spiritual aspect of healing; it would be one of the few things, or quite possibly the only thing, we currently have available to us that would heal at the anti-matter level of our being. If so, **this quite literally makes anti-matter the substance of things not seen and very likely the most important aspect of healing yet discovered.**

## PHILOSOPHY OF ANTI-MATTER

Obviously, there will be some who do not agree with this concept and that is as it should be. By looking for the weaknesses of this theory, it will either be proven incorrect and in need of modification to make it more correct scientifically or it is a correct statement as it stands. If the latter is the case, then **we must begin to re-think what it means to be a healer in its purest sense.** After all, this is the purpose of philosophy to lead us to bold new worlds. What could be bolder and newer at this time than the world of anti-matter healing?

# Chapter 45
# THE POLITICS OF HEALING

*"The Constitution of this Republic should make
provision for healing freedom as well as religious
freedom. To restrict the art of healing to one class of
men and deny equal privileges to others will
constitute the bastille of medical science. Such
restrictions are fragments of monarchy and
have no place in a republic."*
— Benjamin Rush, M.D.
Signer of the Declaration of Independence

## THE REALITY

**Tragically, the politics of medicine have little or nothing to do with healing and the patient's best interests.** In general, medical politics (regardless of the school or system) are based upon the monopolistic concept of "turf wars". In other words, who will control the legislatures, procedures and protocols, suppliers, educational institutions, insurers, practitioners, facilities, government programs, public relations, finances and ultimately the minds and bodies of the patients?

As R. Mendelsohn, M.D., states, "The ultimate goal is that we would all become the wards of Modern Medicine." This is especially dangerous in expansionistic, quantum, vitalistic medicine because **such cartels and monopolies destroy independent thinking and innovation.** For example, while peer review does result in raising substandard practitioners up to a minimal level of competence, it must by its very nature also drag the above-standard practitioners down to the common level. "Politically safe health care" causes practitioners to degenerate to doing everything exactly as every other practitioner does it, regardless of there being a better way and/or of patient idiosyncrasies.

This is obviously in contradiction to the expansionistic, vitalistic concept of quantum medicine. One of the basic principles of quantum medicine is that allopathic assembly-line medicine (everyone with the same diagnosis gets the same treatment) has failed to meet the needs of a dramatic percentage of the population; in fact, the *New England Journal Of Medicine* in 1995 stated that one-third of all Americans were consulting some type of quantum practitioner for this very reason. It is the reason that quantum health care has been able to survive and grow. We are able to take many of these allopathic assembly-line failures and by applying individualized, quantum, vitalistic care achieve a return to health for that patient.

# LAW OF POLITICAL CORRECTNESS

Poorly conducted scientific research and/or bias of interpretation, which nevertheless is politically correct for the times, can frequently, but not permanently, suppress quality scientific research and interpretation that is not politically correct for the times.

# LAW OF DISPOSITION

**The true healer must not live by what is politically correct but by what is universally correct.** The grand trial of the character of a quantum healer in politics is therefore to be able to walk this political maze and emerge uncorrupted. This may mean MANY failures when dealing with legislators, insurance companies, the AMA, educational institutions, state medical associations. Even some quantum organizations are extremely resistant to change. One must not be willing to compromise for small political gains. It is said that, "The art of politics is compromise." In reality that means that no one gets what they truly need. We cannot afford to corrupt quantum healing by watering it down with distorted reductionistic, non-vitalistic concepts. To do so would be to betray the sick and suffering of the world. They don't need more political intrigue, they need health.

This is the great tragedy of socialized medicine, more and more politico-allopathic-pharmaceutical-academic-insurance-media bureaucracy and more and more paperwork at greater and greater cost with fewer and fewer citizens enjoying truly quality health. Quantum health care has made its reputation by remaining unpolluted by this politico-allopathic- pharmaceutical-academic-insurance-media intrigue. To retain the public trust, we must constantly distance ourselves from its taint. Failure to do so at some point in the future, exposes us to the wrath of an outraged citizenry and we will fall along with the corrupt politico-allopathic-pharmaceutical-academic-insurance-media complex.

This of course does not mean that we should not be involved in politics, only that **we must constantly be evaluating our every move for its long-term consequences to determine if those consequences in any way could compromise our integrity with the general public or with our principles.**

# Chapter 46
# THE EDUCATION OF THE HEALER

*"Gaining knowledge is one thing, and applying it
quite another. Wisdom is the correct application of
knowledge. . . to the development of a noble and
godlike character. A man may possess a profound
knowledge of history and of mathematics, he
may be an authority in psychology, biology, or
astronomy, he may know all about what has been
discovered, pertaining to general and natural
science; but if he has not with this knowledge
that nobility of soul which prompts him to deal
justly with his fellow man, to practice virtue
and holiness in his personal life, he is not
truly an educated man."*

— David O. McKay

## UNDER-ACHIEVEMENT

Quantum, expansionistic, vitalistic healing arts education has, in almost all cases, failed to achieve the lofty goals necessary to adequately train quantum healers. Most schools have bowed to pharmaceutical, academic, philosophical, insurance and political pressures and are trying to educate students of complementary healing according to the reductionistic, non-vitalistic mode. This approach is very much like trying to train airplane pilots in submarines. The pilots are completely out of their element and, therefore, the vast majority of them will probably never rise to their true potential.

G. Wilson, D.C., describes this reductionist attempt at education thus, **"Our schools are so concerned over the mental development of students that their emotional maturity is almost completely ignored. So they fail to give students the training that would completely balance their lives." Health is a dynamic balance of all aspects that constitute the total living being** and a student will never become a true healer until this most basic of principles is mastered.

Unfortunately, the faculty and staff of most of our educational institutions, being products themselves of this educational inadequacy, are not even aware of their individual and institutional shortcomings. This is one of the major reasons for writing this textbook. Without an accurate measuring device (the mastery of the laws of healing as outlined in this text) it is impossible to be able to determine the status of an individual, an institution or a profession.

Many of our professions currently lack clearly identified laws and well-defined goals which are the means of determining our present and future positions. **This lack of clearly defined goals is the unfortunate result of having lost our way, of abandoning our vitalistic, expansionistic, quantum philosophy, art and sci-**

ence. This is what is also so glaringly absent in allopathic medicine and is the reason that such chaos is found there. Allopathic, reductionistic, solid state medicine runs here and there and, lacking a clearly defined goal, it is susceptible to fads in surgery, medication and philosophical concept.

A. D. Speransky, himself an allopath, wrote, **"It must be frankly admitted that contemporary medicine does not owe its success in the sphere of treatment to science alone. Scores of its methods and procedures rest on empiricism and even on chance. Only in the sphere of infection, of mechanical therapy and of hygiene are its achievements connected with a really scientific analysis of the phenomena. For the rest, anarchy prevails, here and there corrected by separate facts and partial comparisons. We have an infinite number of medical theories, but we have not, and do not have, a theory of medicine, a theory capable of embracing all the data and directing them into channels where they can be actively utilized."**

# HISTORY

As our text has shown, numerous cultures throughout history have discovered these vitalistic, expansionistic, quantum principles. But the reality is that very frequently these same principles have been lost through neglect, political intrigue and indifference. For example, traditional Chinese Medicine was for many years outlawed by the communist government of the People's Republic of China and an entire generation was reared without its benefits. In America, naturopathy, homeopathy and chiropractic were and still are unmercifully and relentlessly pressured by the politico-allopathic-pharmaceutical-academic-insurance-media complex. Indigenous forms of quantum healing such as Native American and African healing have fared far worse, having been suppressed by the dominant cultural-politico-allopathic-pharmaceutical-academic-insurance-media complex for hundreds of years.

# PERSPECTIVE

All of this and much more must be remembered, understood and taught in a readily comprehensible manner to students of expansionistic, complementary, quantum healing in order for these professionals to grow and assume their proper places in society. **To do otherwise is to train nothing more than allopaths who treat with natural substances and procedures.**

# THE INSTRUCTOR

This leads us to the individuals charged with the training of the minds that will become the next generation of quantum, expansionistic, vitalistic healers. It is quite obvious that there have been great shortcomings in the past which have allowed so many quantum practitioners to graduate with such a lack of understanding of the true nature of health and dis-ease. **The unfortunate truth is that instructors cannot adequately teach healing if they have not themselves successfully mastered and internalized the quantum, expansionistic, vitalistic laws. A competent quantum healing arts instructor must be able to discuss, extemporaneously, the laws of healing because they have been assimilated and become an intricate part of his being.**

## THE LEARNING AND HEALING ENVIRONMENT

Any true healer who has endured the hospital experience knows the deplorable undercurrents of hospital politics and administrative attitudes - the stabbing your colleagues in the back and climbing over them to get to the top; the dollars-are-all that is important mind set that results in nurses being required to care for 12 or 15 patients at a time; the mentality that accepts the idea that people are expendable and you can work them until they drop and make their professional lives so miserable that they will burn out and quit and we won't have to pay them their retirement; the attitude that administrators should be paid a king's ransom but the floor workers should have their benefits cut.

**Such dis-harmony can never result in a healing environment.** Resentment, fatigue and intrigue are counter-productive to healing and yet we do much the same to our student healers. We frequently push them so hard and make their academic lives so demanding that we destroy their health, their families and their joy in healing. **A healthy academic and work environment should stimulate and enhance the students' health, their desire to learn and their ability to coordinate what they are learning into a useful, functional whole that will enhance their professional, community, personal and family lives. They must be acutely aware they are becoming a better human being because of their enlightened educational experience.** To give them less is to defraud them of what they are looking for and have a right to receive, a truly eclectic education.

## THE ADMINISTRATORS

But such dedication of faculty members and desire on the part of the students is very difficult, if not nearly impossible, to achieve if our college and university administrations have failed to master and internalize the same quantum, expansionistic, vitalistic laws and principles. Sadly, long and repeated experiences have documented that no **administrator who has not mastered and internalized the quantum, expansionistic, vitalistic concept of life and health is truly capable of leading a quantum, expansionistic, vitalistic institution of higher learning regardless of academic credentials and success in a reductionistic, non-vitalistic institution.** The disappointing track record of many of our schools indicates that they have become institutions that are clones of reductionist, non-vitalistic, allopathic medical schools. This has proven disastrous in every case where chiropractic, homeopathic, naturopathic, oriental, and ayurvedic education institutions have unwisely embraced the reductionist, non-vitalistic, limited, allopathic model of education.

## CONCLUSION

**We must avoid these suicidal mistakes at all costs or we may be in danger of destroying mankind's greatest hopes for a happy, healthy lifestyle. The sick and suffering of the world simply cannot afford to have inadequately educated, frustrated, pseudo-allopaths masquerading as quantum, expansionistic, vitalistic complementary healers.**

To make the necessary changes is a monumental task and will require exceptional individuals both as faculty and administrators, individuals who are willing to challenge the non-dynamic status quo of education, research protocols, our own professions, accrediting organizations, licensing boards, the media, and politics. **The paramount question for every complementary educator is, "Do I have the individual courage to become part of the answer or am I going to remain a part of the problem by simply doing nothing to change it?"**

# Chapter 47
# RESEARCH

*"Research is to see what everyone else has seen*
*and to think what nobody has thought."*
— Albert Szent-Gyorgyi

## THE CRITICAL FLAWS

**Researchers must not be seduced by the erroneous assumption that the standard reductionistic, non-vitalistic, double blind protocol is the only scientifically valid format for conducting research.** In fact, it has **major shortcomings,** the most glaring of which is the fact that modern quantum scientists are now acutely aware that the mere presence and observation of the researcher profoundly alters the results of experiments.

Secondly, conducting solid state Newtonian research to learn about quantum Einsteinian phenomena, which is the basis of life and health, is akin to studying apples in order to become the leading authority on oranges. Tiller's modifications of Einstein's Theories of Relativity show that researching quantum methods of healing in the incorrect reductionistic, solid state mode results in incorrect conclusions. This is precisely what limited reductionist science has done for years in its effort to discredit quantum healing.

The valid researcher must expand his/her protocol to circumvent these glaring deficiencies. You will note that the double blind protocol deletes all reference to the individuality of the test subjects while in properly conducted clinical trials, individuality of the test subjects becomes one of its cornerstones.

## PEER-REVIEWED AND CONTROLLED RESEARCH

An excellent example of these shortcomings in the currently accepted research protocol is that medical research has tested more than one million anti-cancer compounds but only about 50 of those substances have been approved by the FDA. None have significantly affected the continuing escalating cancer rate. In other words, literally millions of man-hours and tens of billions of dollars in cancer research have proven fruitless. Wouldn't it be logical to begin thinking that a chemical answer to cancer is not a logical approach to the problem? But conventional cancer research continues to lower its collective head like a bull in a china shop and make yet more plans to expend even more and more time and research dollars on what is literally a million-to-one long shot. Wouldn't it make far more scientific sense to begin looking at other aspects of the problem such as the quantum factors?

D. Black, Ph.D., speaking of Horrobin's writing, notes in his article in the *Journal of The American Medical Association,* "Between 1930 and 1960, before medical research became such a large industry, improvements in patient care were 'dramatic.' Since 1960, in contrast, despite major breakthroughs in science knowledge, improvements 'have been substantially smaller'."

Black supports this position with an example from his own field of psychiatry: "There are five major types of drugs used in psychiatry; the neuroleptics, the bensodiazepines, the tricyclic antidepressents and related compounds, the monoamine oxidase inhibitors and lithium. All five classes were discovered prior to 1960. Some new molecular variants have been introduced but all the original compounds are still extensively used and no major new therapeutic principles have been developed and shown to be effective clinically. This is in spite of the incomparably greater expenditure of funds on research into neurobiology and psychiatry since 1960." Thus, one fact becomes increasingly clear; **with peer-reviewed and peer-controlled research, we achieve mediocrity and minimal advancement of science. All become clones of the thinking of others. There is no longer any true independent genius at work and, as a result, humanity suffers as the advancement of science is stifled.**

## REVIEW OF BASIC LAWS

There are basic laws which govern all science.

1. Conservation - The sum of all matter, energy and anti-matter that ever has or ever will exist currently exists. Each is, however, under proper circumstances, interchangeable with the others.

2. Inertia - matter and anti-matter at rest tends to remain at rest unless acted upon by energy and once in motion they tend to remain in motion.

3. Gravity - all matter and anti-matter exert an influence on all other matter and anti-matter.

4. Definite Composition - Identical things have a single composition. For example, table salt is always NaCl, it is never SCl or PbCl.

5. 1st Law of Thermodynamics - Energy forms can change to other energy forms and to matter and anti-matter forms.

6. 2nd Law of Thermodynamics - Without a conceiving, organizing, guiding and sustaining intelligence all things are positively entropic (decompose to more basing forms).

7. Likes Make Likes - When an identical procedure is followed, the same results are always obtained; i.e., cows never conceive fish.

8. Intelligence - A conceiving, organizing, guiding, and sustaining intelligence is required in order to have negative entropy (more complex forms created).

## DOUBLE BLIND PROTOCOL

The double blind study is based upon the following supposedly indisputable laws:

1. Uni-dimensionality - all effects can be traced to a **single** cause.

2. Linearity - cause and effect are **always** of equal magnitude (small causes cannot produce large effects).

3. Uniformity of Class - cause and effect are always identical for all members of a class (mechanical causes can only produce mechanical effects, chemical causes can produce only chemical effects, etc.).

4. Generalization - data gathered from a simple, artificial laboratory experiment and or model (the classic double blind study) can be consistently applied to complex non-living and/or living systems.

5. Non-relation - the physical and/or energy presence of the researcher has no effect upon the outcome of the research.

6. Explainability - "scientific proof" is obtained only through the study of simple models that are units of complex systems, if they follow the one-dimensional, linear, class uniform, generalized theory (the double blind study) which includes the following:

   a. Uniform samples can be consistently formed of subjects who have identical dis-eases.

   b. All individuals with the same dis-ease may be treated in exactly the same manner.

   c. All variables may be eliminated by controls and thus all observations can be linked to a single cause.

   d. Statistically, even a small variation can be significant, even though the majority of test subjects may obtain no such results.

# QUANTUM PROTOCOL

The expansionistic, vitalistic Einsteinian concept of science is likewise based upon so-called indisputable laws.

1. Multi-dimensionality - The **ultimate effect depends upon the simultaneous action of many causes.**

2. Non-linearity - **Cause and effect may differ in magnitude, therefore, small causes may produce large effects and vice versa.**

3. Variance of Class - **When properly coupled, causes of one class may be registered as effects on another class** (mechanical causes may produce chemical effects, mental causes may produce physical effects, etc.).

4. Non-generalizability - **Data gathered from simple, artificial laboratory experiments and environments may not be reliably and consistently generalized to complex, real systems which must be studied in their undivided entities and fluctuating environments.**

5. Relationship - **The mere physical and/or energy presence of the researcher influences the outcome of the research.**

6. Reproducibility - **Natural phenomena that cannot be explained by current scientific understanding can nevertheless be reliably and consistently reproduced (clinical research) and therefore also constitutes valid scientific research because:**

   a. **No two patients have exactly the same dis-ease.**

   b. **Each patient must be cared for according to his/her unique needs.**

   c. **All variables must be considered in order to understand the totalities of the responses possible.**

   d. **The MOST MEANINGFUL outcome of research is the ability to consistently, and time- and cost-efficiently, restore and/or preserve the individual patient's health.**

# ENERGY VS. INFORMATION

To this point in the text, we have referred to the quantum or energy component of healing and this served very well at those levels of our development. Now that we are in the post-doctoral text, however, we must develop this concept still further in order to remain on the leading edge of technology. **Energy is capable of transmitting information, but energy itself is not necessarily information.** For example, a radio or television signal is pure energy but it need not be transmitting information; there may only be static instead of an intelligible program. Within biology, terms such as molecular recognition, genetic (DNA) code, receptors, transcription, translation, etc., are currently in daily use but life consists of far more than what these terms describe.

**A major difference between simple machines (even computers) and the living being is the number of critical internal interconnections and their degree of interrelation with the total environment.** Rubik, a Ph. D. in biophysics, states, "Living things have an immense network of internal and external interconnections, depending on habits and dispositions they have inherited or acquired. The continuous exchange of information in living systems to maintain their integrity is awesome." She continues, "For example, a living organism is much more than a collection of organs or tissues; it manifests a distinct wholeness, possessing a drive to exist, sustain itself, reproduce, constitute itself purposefully in response to its environment, and relate to other organisms and its ecological community."

# THE INFORMATION PARADIGM

Hence, a new paradigm is required when thinking in terms of subtle energies that relay or transmit information. Rubik has provided the basic beginnings of such a new thought process. To summarize:

1. The concept of information is already used successfully to explain various phenomena in the fields of molecular biology, computer science, thermodynamics and, more recently, quantum physics. Therefore, such a basis might be utilized as the launch pad for the more advanced concepts of the multidimensional living being.

2. Living systems are fundamentally different from non-living systems, in that they involve more levels of organization and more complex, dynamic interactions of their components and with their environment. Thus, higher levels of organization may involve additional principles that do not violate the laws of physics and chemistry but are not determined by and cannot be reduced to them. Examples of these higher principles are evolutionary design, consciousness, and the mind-body connection. As indicated earlier, the lowest levels of living organization (e.g., biomolecules) have already been described in mechanical molecular codes that convey information. Therefore, information is a unifying concept that spans the many levels of organization of living systems. Furthermore, information may also flow among levels of order in living systems. And when it does, it can produce different effects (e.g., a physical insult resulting in a psychological response, a biochemical shift resulting in structural derangement, or a frequency drift being manifest as a biological dysfunction).

3. Hence, local healing may be mediated by informational patterns of ultra-subtle, extremely low-frequency electro (and magnetoelectric) fields (in the range of 10-3 to 10-9 gauss range) emanating from the body of the healer(s) that are associated with altered states of consciousness such as hypnosis. This constitutes subtle, highly specific information that is distributed non-locally and has effects only for whom it is intended.

4. As stated previously, the concept of an informational paradigm goes beyond that of energy because it involves features of purposeful design, communication, communion and meaning, often on the part of both parties. Information is usually carried by energy or matter, but it transcends the conventional physical concept of both. Therefore, current solid state and in many cases, even our current crude methods of energy evaluation are inadequate to research the subtle energies involved and therefore provide inaccurate data when employed.

5. Information must be defined operationally at each level of order in living systems, and different working definitions are likely at each level. New ways of codification and utilization of qualitative or "soft" information

are needed. Recognition that and the acceptance of an extended science that encompasses higher levels of order such as the transpersonal domain will not be mechanical or quantitative. Such a perspective is **essential** in order to address all features that encompass life.

6. The observer participates in the quantum system by collapsing the wave function in the act of measurement. What we call data is more than a pile of numbers; it is information. **Scientific facts do not stand alone; they are theory-laden and content-dependent.** In other words, our interpretation of "science" always reflects our individual, educational, social, political, and cultural perspectives and prejudices in theory, execution, observation and measurement.

## THE CHALLENGE

This new paradigm of science must be driven by the following framework in order to generate appropriate answers.

1. To identify all the informational carriers. This text has identified energy, matter, anti-matter, physical touch, magnetic fields, prayer, hormones, mental telepathy, neurological, conscious, unconscious mind.

2. What does each specifically and, in concert, tell us?

3. What is the nature of each form of information?

4. What parameters are necessary to accurately monitor each form of information and its multiple interactions?

5. At what level(s) of the total being does each function?

6. How can each supersede or suspend other levels and produce healing in spite of apparent incurable conditions. For example, a person at a party in which many people are conversing in small groups can select and listen to a conversation nearby, despite the fact that the volume of this conversation may be much lower than the ambient background noise made up of all the chatter in the room. The volume, or sound energy intensity, of the voices is virtually irrelevant; it is the informational content of the conversation that is meaningful to the person who is able to "tune-in" specifically to low-level input based upon his interests.

7. Additional factors as they become evident.

Life, in order to fulfill its dynamic homeostasis, must receive, store, process and act upon the information for its own survival. Simple transmitters and receivers such as radios and televisions totally lack these abilities. For science to comprehend life's full potential, it must go far beyond reductionistic mechanical concepts that were developed for simple machines.

## LAWS OF QUANTUM RESEARCH

In testing the various forms of care it must be remembered that:

1. Strong heroic interventions, even in small amounts, bring about alterations in all people, even the robust and healthy; i.e., emergency cardiac drugs.

2. Milder forms of care must be given in larger volumes to cause change in all test subjects; i.e., chiropractic adjustments, acupuncture, phytotherapeutics, massage, etc.

3. Weak interventions reveal their therapeutic qualities only when tested on the hyper-sensitive who are dis-ease free.

**Because the scientific validity of the vitalistic healing arts and the well-being of all future generations depend upon this, no therapy should be administered except those that are thoroughly known to the practitioner. To do so is to be the potential cause of iatrogenic dis-ease.** For the purpose of learning, all therapies should be administered in their purest singular form otherwise prevent variants. For purposes of study, the tested individual's routine should be, for a considerable time, as consistent as possible and devoid of any other factors known or suspected to have therapeutic properties.

The tested individuals must be capable of accurately recording responses. But above all these individuals must guard against over-exertion of body and mind, against excess and disturbing passions, inactivity and any and all other variants that would invalidate the study. Additionally, the therapy must be proven on males and females, young and old, various constitutions, etc.

The full range of use cannot be known until the therapy's powers have been fully explored. Therefore, it may be necessary to test it from its weakest to its most powerful application. **When only weak effects are noted from a single administration, the therapy can be administered daily until effects become stronger, clearer and more constant.** This procedure gives excellent data regarding symptomatology but does not provide sequential data. If the correct strength (potency, force) is given at the beginning, there is the added advantage of the experiment establishing a chronological order to the symptoms. This provides a great deal more information about the character of the therapy such as its duration of action, contra-indications, types of patients best responding to it, primary and secondary actions, etc.

Once a particular symptom has been established, it is necessary to place the volunteers in varying circumstances in order to observe whether this increases, decreases or negates earlier data. Modalities such as eating, drinking, speaking, sleeping, exercise, inactivity, time of day, season, response to heat and cold, humidity and dryness, how many hours or days after the test therapy is administered do particular symptoms appear, etc., may prove significant.

It must also be kept in mind that the total dis-ease picture a particular therapy produces does not all come out in a single subject. For this reason, numerous observations are necessary before any degree of confidence can be achieved with respect to a given therapy. Of course, similar symptoms also reported by other investigators should also be considered.

If the previous requirements for a well-controlled experiment have been adhered to, all complaints, symptoms and changes in the physical, mental, emotional and spiritual health of the subjects under the influence of the therapy being investigated result from it and must be recorded as belonging to its therapeutic character. Even if the subject has experienced similar symptoms at some time in their past their appearance during the test indicates that the subject is especially predisposed to them by his/her constitution an/or miasmatic (diathic, doshic, phase) background.

# UNIQUE PROCEDURE

Not only must the researcher record data but the subjects also must have the capacity to record in the greatest possible accuracy and detail their experiences during the research. For this reason, some of the best research subjects have repeatedly proven to be students of the healing arts. **Such reports should as much as possible preserve the subject's own spontaneous terminology. Nothing recorded should be guesswork, interpretations, hunches, etc. However, the very best research data is always that which the researcher experiences her/himself. The researcher knows with the greatest certainty that which she/he has personally experienced.** A second benefit of this protocol of "self-testing" is that the healer develops a closer relationship with the patient who experiences the same symptoms.

## LAW OF SYMPTOMS OF THERAPY

Distinguishing symptoms produced by the therapy being tested from those of the dis-ease which it cures demands the highest discrimination. Hence the rule: **Symptoms that  were never before noticed, or that were noticed much earlier (before testing began), are new ones belonging to the tested therapy.**

## CLINICAL APPLICATION

This data  can now be used to monitor the healing process in a patient experiencing very similar symptoms. **When administering the tested therapy at just above threshold amounts, quick and permanent cures will be the results without secondary effects. Such an undertaking would seem to indicate trying a vast number of specific therapies in order to find an analogue for all dis-eases but such is not so. The vast majority of dis-eases can be indexed under a relatively small number of therapies. This is the reason that an accurate understanding  of the root cause, the constitution and miasma (diathesis, dosha, phase) is so critical to the successful clinical practitioner.**

## TRUE SCIENCE

Reductionists, such as allopaths, refuse to even consider the expansionistic aspects of science and many misguided expansionists refuse to consider the reductionist aspects. **The true scientist must, however, consider all aspects of science and apply each in its proper perspective and circumstances. To do less is to be unscientific.**

## SCIENTIFIC REALITY

**True healers and scientists accept the scientific reality that there never has been, is, or ever will be, enough reductionist, solid state facts, figures, or research projects to prove or disprove things of a quantum nature.**

## AN EXAMPLE

Solid state, reductionist, mechanistic science studies molecular mechanisms. Quantum, vitalistic, expansionistic science, on the other hand, studies far more. Take water, for example, two hydrogen atoms attached to a single oxygen atom in an unequal "V" formation with the oxygen atom at the base of the "V".

Structurally, water is one of the most basic of substances and solid state, reductionist, mechanistic science believes it functions according to well-understood laws causing it to act as a solvent and carrier. To them, water is water. There are no idiosyncrasies of water in living entities as compared to the non-living.

But modern quantum physics proves such an assumption to be totally incorrect. Black reports, "Water in living cells actively assists biological proteins, for example. Proteins have a bumpy surface with nooks and crannies that let them bind to other molecules. Antibodies bind to microbes; hemoglobin binds to oxygen;

hormones bind to 'receptors' on the surface of the cells; enzymes bind to chemical substances in order to juxtapose them so they react; and so on. Through binding, proteins direct the processes of life - and they rely on water to do it."

In 1992, quantum research documented that when four oxygen  atoms bind to hemoglobin, 60 water molecules are also bound! And when glucose binds to an enzyme, it releases about 100 water molecules at the same time. Again, Black comments, "Obviously, the role of water in biochemical reactions is not limited to its action as a mere solvent or carrier. On the contrary, water is directly involved in chemical exchanges, and may even play a key role."

What seems to be taking place is that within living cells, the protein molecules are bathed in water. Because the molecular valences of the water attract each other, they bind around the irregularly-shaped protein molecule capturing it. This, however, is a pulsating binding. It can push the protein to the surface or pull it inward and at the same time nudge it into the necessary shape to allow its chemical reaction(s) to take place.

This fact is, however, secondary to the following response. As the water binds the protein, it releases and reforms the bonds at a rate of 500 million  times a second. This is not a random activity, however, as water always return to the same configuration on the protein surface. At the same time this is taking place, the water molecules are also rotating in a direction oriented by their relation to the protein's surface. This is due to the unbalanced "V" formation mentioned earlier. As a result, they cannot form stable bonds and momentarily attempt to bond with every molecule they come into the vicinity of. This phenomenon is what causes water to be classified as "the universal solvent."

In the dynamics of the living entity, all this pulsation and rotation creates yet another phenomenon which literally allows water to form a communication medium in much the same manner that organized electrons conduct data in an electrical circuit, rhythmical patterns of light via a fiber optic circuit, or the dots and dashes in Morse Code. Black states, "Within a living cell, then, 'the entire region is filled with water fluctuating in a concerted way,' so that 'both  structure and energy are transmitted as waves'."

Thus, when a chiropractor adjusts a vertebra, a homeopath prescribes a similimum remedy, a Ch'i (Qi) Gong practitioner adjusts the energy, or an acupuncturist needles a point, the pattern and/or flow of biological energy is holographically generated and organized by the therapy administered.

If the behavior of simple water molecules is controlled by such intricate and rhythmic patterns of dynamic energy flow, it is even more likely, based upon the latest quantum research, that complex molecules such as enzymes, hormones, genes, vitamins, minerals and so on are too.

**The research that is being conducted by quantum, vitalistic, biodynamic sciences must be heavily involved with these complex and dynamic energy patterns which are proving, more and more, to be the underpinning of life and health. Our scientific research must more and more document these patterns of energy.**

## THE HOMEOPATHIC ANSWER

**This, then, is the scientific explanation of how homeopathic remedies in Microdoses can have such profound effects upon the psyche and physiology of the patient.**

# LAW OF MODE

No amount of money, time and/or solid state research can document why a cure takes place because **a therapy in and of itself does not cure.** This is proven by administering any form of care to a solid state cadaver with a clinically diagnosed dis-ease. **Nothing happens. This is because it is the quantum energy or life force, ch'i, innate, kundalini, and spirit, and likely the anti-matter modes that heal. The appropriate therapy only provides a template. To accurately understand the response we must study the mode in which it takes place. Research conducted in the incorrect mode only provides incorrect answers.**

# Chapter 48
# THE LEGALITIES OF HEALING

*"Let every man remember that to violate the law is
to trample on the blood of his father, and to tear the
charter of his own and his children's liberty. Let
reverence for the laws be breathed by every
American mother to her child; . . . let it be written in
primers, spelling books and almanacs; let it be
preached from pulpits, proclaimed in legislative
halls, and enforced in courts of justice. In short, let
reverence for laws. . . become the political
religion of the nation."*

— Abraham Lincoln

## THE ULTIMATE TRUTH

Obviously, Lincoln was referring to the constitutional and common laws of the United States of America in the above quoted statement. If such respect is due to manmade laws, how much more respect must be due to celestial law?

Our universe and the creatures that inhabit it function in accordance with universal laws. A dramatic number of these laws deal with the quantum or non-material components. To practice the healing arts only  by the reductionistic solid state laws is like trying to fly an airplane without navigational aids. True, in the good old days every pilot flew by the "seat of his pants", solid state tactics. But what these pilots couldn't do was to fly in rain, fog, snow, or at night, trans-continentally or trans-oceanically; nor did they fly at 30,000 feet or at 600 miles per hour, nor were they able to carry today's payloads. They could not re-fuel in mid-air or leave the earth's atmosphere and go into orbit. They were pilots but pilots of a very primitive standard compared to today's quantum pilots who use radio signals, radar, magnetic compasses, artificial horizons, altimeters, de-icers, etc.

The same is true of healing. **To remain a solid state reductionist-based practitioner and ignore the more advanced quantum vitalistic components of healing is to provide a very primitive form of health care.**

The challenge is that in western reductionist-oriented cultures, society at large has not been educated to think in quantum terms. This includes our reductionist-oriented legal system. Law is, to a great extent, based upon legal precedent. This means that whatever has been the established standard in past cases becomes the enshrined standard by which all such cases are evaluated in the future. The obvious shortcoming of this system is that **such a static standard becomes more and more archaic as time, research and understanding progress.**

Thus, the quantum vitalistic practitioner enters the legal arena with one strike against him already since he/she does not conform to the established legal precedent. The second strike is that almost no attorneys, being educated within the western, reductionistic, non-vitalistic educational system are capable of understanding the concepts of quantum expansionistic healing. Lacking such understanding, they prove incapable of adequately representing quantum health care in the courtroom and in the legal system. The third strike is that if a quantum vitalistic legal question goes to trial, the jury will be made up of members who are also products of the same reductionistic, non-vitalistic educational system and culture as that of the court officers and the attorneys. Number four is the fact that the judges are also products of this same reductionist educational system. Therefore, there is little hope of quantum, expansionistic, vitalistic science winning cases unless an attorney can re-educate the judge and jury within the established courtroom protocol and proceedings.

# ANSWERS

1. The first requirement necessary to resolve the above challenge is to create a post-graduate law school that specializes in teaching attorneys to understand and properly represent quantum healing within the confines of our current legal system.

2. A committee of such enlightened attorneys, quantum health  care professionals and vitalistically-oriented public relations individuals needs to be established to develop a battle plan of when and how issues of expansionistic, vitalistic, quantum health care are going to be addressed successfully and thereby change the basic thrust of health care issues within the legal system.

3. An independent war chest committee must be established to raise and  distribute funds and tightly monitor the recipients of the funds being dispersed. "Independent" means that no member of this committee can serve on any other committee simultaneously and no revolving door can allow members to move from one committee to another or to serve on any other committee within a period of five (5) years.

4. A committee or sub-committee needs to be established to constantly evaluate solid state medicine's response and to counter its plans to destroy these legal gains.

5. To the greatest extent possible, the quantum practitioner should document the progress of the patient being cared for by quantum means by conventional, legally acceptable, tests, examinations, etc.

6. Legally qualifying statements may need to be provided to and signed by the patient explaining to him/her in easily understood language what the proposed quantum procedures are designed to do, any risk factors associated with such procedures, cost involved, etc. Such a statement should also contain a legally qualifying release of legal liability whenever possible.

7. Second opinions from other quantum practitioners and, if possible supportive solid state practitioners, should be sought and documented in the patient chart whenever there is a question regarding the patient's progress.

8. Generous amounts of malpractice insurance from reputable long- standing companies should be carried by every quantum health care provider.

9. Personal assets, whenever possible, should be legally sheltered from access through legal actions against the provider. This likely would require another committee of appropriate professionals to make sure that assets protection is constantly being up-dated to conform with all current legal requirements and to advise appropriate modifications when such become necessary.

10. A committee is needed to advise practitioners of legal requirements of current governmental regulations regarding health and safety standard for in-office laboratories, X-ray facilities, rehabilitation facilities, etc.

11 Other committees should be established as deemed necessary and appropriate.

# Chapter 49
# THE QUANTUM HEALER

*"...But the student in his new-found enthusiasm
for pathology must not forget that it is the whole
patient who comes to consult the doctor, not just a
disordered liver, a cardiac lesion, a lump in the
breast, or a painful knee. In the words of an old
French proverb: 'There are no dis-eases,
but only sick people'."*

— William Boyd
Textbook Of Pathology, 7th Ed.

## LAW OF THE UNSYSTEM

Traditionally, anatomy, physiology, pathology, etc., have been taught and practiced by various systems; i.e., endocrinology, neurology, EENT, musculoskeletal, respiratory, and so on. Unfortunately, such artificial segregation creates an erroneous comprehension and compartmentalization that is perpetuated within education, practice, administration, professional organizations, insurance carriers, publishers, legislation and the legal system to the detriment of the sick and suffering and to society as a whole.

For example, the nervous system is not a distinct system from the hormonal. What affects one affects the other. In fact the pituitary and hypothalamus area of the brain appears to be the site of, the interchange between the two systems. The scientific reality is **all systems are members of a single inter-related and inter-dependent system - the living organism.** It's the old Three Musketeer motto: "All for one; one for all." **A healer, regardless of his or her specific discipline and/or procedures, affects the entire being!**

## SCOPE OF PRACTICE

Within the pages of this textbook we have covered the scope of practice of the quantum healer (QH). **The quantum practitioner's scope of practice is any and all things that affect the health for there is nothing that does not have an effect, great or small, upon the living being.**

This is an enormous responsibility. It dictates that every quantum physician be a true "Renaissance Man or Woman," that term meaning, "An individual who understands and does many or all thing well". Such a challenge requires far more of its practitioners than being a mere allopath, chiropractor, naturopath or oriental medical practitioner. In essence, it means mastering all knowledge and developing an understanding of how to employ it non-iatrogenically for the benefit of mankind. Obviously, such a trust encompasses a life totally dedicated to this ennobling goal.

Considering that our formal professional training only lasts eight to twelve years, it should be abundantly clear that we should be learning far more in the forty to sixty years of our practice than we did in the formal academic arena. This is especially true when we realize that during this forty to sixty  years, our learning should exponentially accelerate because we are constantly developing a greater data base with which we can evaluate, cross-reference and assimilate new concepts into our functional understanding.

It also requires being constantly on guard against the pernicious and irrational allopathic concept of treating the dis-ease that has the patient instead of the law of caring for the patient who has the dis-ease. This includes resisting the pressure that the patient brings to bear. Most of them have been repeatedly exposed to the sophisticated brainwashing of commercial "feel better fast, temporary relief" advertising and they mistakenly equate "temporary relief" with healing.

## THE TEACHER HEALER

As previously stated, the word "doctor" literally means "learned teacher". This is why we call individuals with advanced degrees in education "Doctor". **If a practitioner is not teaching his patients what true health is and how to maintain it, regardless of what else he is doing, he is not a teacher-healer.** This teaching aspect is one of the indispensable distinctions of the quantum physician.

## THE STUDENT HEALER

**The quantum healer is also humbled by his/her learning rather than made arrogant by it.** We realize that there is far more we do not know than what we do know about the living being. This is why a healthy respect for num, kundalini, innate, vital, ch'i, life force is so vital. If we learn how to **assist** the life force, master the Universal Laws of healing found in this text, and get out of the way and let the patient heal himself, then we are true healers. If, after studying this text, the practitioner is still caught up in the  misguided concept that he knows more than the innate intelligence that helped form and now runs the living organism, there is no hope of his becoming a great healer regardless of how many years of training he has, how many diplomas he earns, how many specialty qualifications he obtains, how big a practice he has or how financially successful he becomes.

# Chapter 50
# THE NEW PARADIGM

*"The only means of strengthening one's intellect is
to make up one's mind about nothing — to let the
mind be a thoroughfare for all thoughts."*
— George Keats, 1819

## THE FLUX OF THOUGHT

The human thought process is bound by numerous recognized and, as yet, unrecognized parameters. Alter our parameters and we alter our comprehension.

Since all knowledge is warped by the cultural norms to which we belong (in the case of healing allopathy, chiropractic, homeopathy, oriental medicine, ayurvedic, etc.), it is a major scientific mistake to accept as a fixed and ultimate truth one particular interpretation or philosophy. **Thus, there is no one scientific method as proposed by the reductionist solid state mind fix. Anything, anyone or any method can be a source of valid knowledge.**

As stated earlier in this text, science has documented that the entire universe and everything within it(including ourselves) are in constant flux or change. This fact leads to an inescapable reality. **We cannot create new paradigms if we are fixated on the old. Our philosophies and protocols, but not the Universal Laws that govern them, must change with the changing universe or we will become as extinct as the dinosaurs.**

Beyond the confines of our understanding, the universe is a vast ocean of uncharted knowledge and, more importantly, influences from past experiences much of which is likely to contradict our current finite knowledge and profoundly influences us. In the past, to speak of the cosmos was to speak of our limited world of knowledge. Figure 50.1 addresses this myopic perspective of western reductionistic, non-vitalistic "science".

As can readily be seen, there are vast amounts of knowledge and influences beyond any one culture and/or scientific discipline or method's ability to master. Thus, to reside in any one vortex (philosophy of healing, scientific approach, culture, etc.) is to miss far more than we are aware of and in the fullest sense of the word is unscientific.

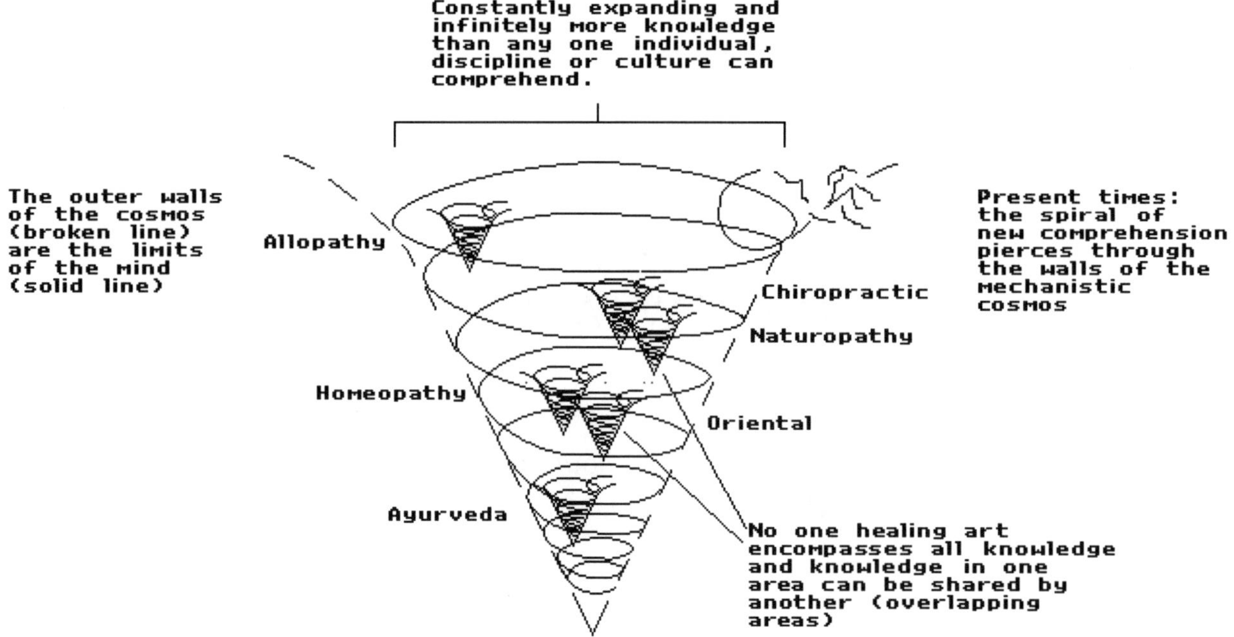


*Figure 50.1 — The Expanded Perspective Of Scientific*

## MORPHIC FIELDS

The quantum healing phenomenon must be characterized by specific patterns within the holographically regulated being rather than by mechanical and/or chemical effects exclusively. These quantum field dynamics are imprinted upon the being's organism and function with little or no distinction between the various levels of our total being (spirit, mind, emotion, thought, matter, anti-matter, etc.).

E. Whitmont, M.D., states, "What we are in the habit of separating into mind and matter appear rather like different levels of 'densification' or 'attenuation' of those transmaterial field-patterns or archetype fundamental 'essences' unrepresentable (*unanschaulich* in Einstein's terminology) as such, but underlying our dualistic experience of self and the world, mind and body."

This paradigm is in keeping with modern physics and brain research. Our material universe is increasingly seen as consisting of non-material entities, represented as eddies and whirlpools in an endless immaterial flow, or fields of information, forms, and structures or as Plato spoken of only in the language of mathematics. It is viewed as holographic in the sense that every part-aspect contains the patterns of the whole and that, conversely, the whole "knows" about and directs all of the part aspects. Our perceived hard reality rests upon our brain's interpretation of mathematical frequencies that originate in a space-time-transcending dimension. The unfolding of these archetypal information patterns in our brain translates into our illusion of concrete materiality.

## MORPHIC FIELD RESEARCH

Numerous research projects have documented the existence of "a priori" holographic fields of information and form, of "form prior to something that has form". Driesch uses Aristotle's term "Entelechy" which means "inherited goal directedness".

Seen in their entirety, these phenomena establish the fact that what we perceive with our five senses are space-time manifestations of experiences pertaining to a state in which the difference between spirit, body, mind, substance, space, and time are relatively insignificant. D. Bohm, Ph. D., termed this "enfolded order" the manifestations of which we experience as "explicate order". Yet, even though we perceive our universe in terms of innate or "a priori" representations, there exists a functional unity between our mental/emotional images and that which we call the "outer world of matter". The nature of this correlation rests on the principle of Simulium.

## SIMILIMUM PROGRAMMING

The similimum means expression of a similar basic programming in different languages or "codings". The different codes depend on what system(s) is/are responding to the basic program; i.e., the code may manifest as psoriasis on the skin but as a tic in the nervous system, as guilt in the mental, as asthma in the respiratory and as inability to reach orgasm in the reproductive system.

## CHANGE

It is impossible to remain constant. Just as our physical substance, our molecules and atoms, are in constant change, so also do our emotional, mental and vital energy constantly change. New impulses are generated, attitudes are modified and old programming is constantly and irrevocably modified by these new experiences and exposures. This change constantly conflicts with the status quo, both from without and from within. When any of these agents, be they thoughts, traumas, microbes, environmental changes, emotions, or new ideas, overpower the status quo, we experience dis-ease (lack of ease, balance, harmony, homeostasis). But when the new elements are successfully compensated for and/or assimilated with only minimal threat, we develop, grow, acquire immunity, develop heightened mental abilities, become more self-confident and experience a host of other desirable characteristics.

**Thus, we encounter difficulties and dis-ease in this life not only because of wrong living but also in order to evolve to higher planes which are a new, more refined and more efficient energy field pattern.** Hence, life is far more than Darwin ever envisioned,; it is not a mere struggle for survival. It is a perpetual process of creation, development and evolution on all levels of our total being. Its end result is the production of a being who has superseded all limitations on all of the levels of his total being, a being who has evolved to the point where dis-ease no longer has any effect.

## LESSONS OF HISTORY

History documents that static philosophies are always superseded by more expansionistic perspectives. For example, in the early Western context, myths, legends and poetry were the vehicles of conveying knowledge, to be supplanted by the Greco-Roman all-pervading logic. This was eclipsed by theology which was, in turn, was supplanted by the reductionist mechanistic concept that the cosmos and everything within it was a giant machine. Now that is, in turn, rapidly fading into obscurity before the quantum concept which will, in its turn, be replaced by yet more encompassing paradigms at some future date when our race has matured enough to begin to appreciate them.

Each cycle starts vigorously and lucidly and then becomes more and more complex until its very complexity becomes its greatest liability. Confidence in its precepts begins to wane as the philosophy becomes more and more incapable of answering the questions being asked and eventually collapses. A new and clearer paradigm unfolds that reinvigorates society and another upward spiral begins. This is nature's mechanism for reopening our minds to the bigger universal picture beyond our self-limiting philosophies.

## LAW OF DEPARTURE

**Departure from previous self/group limiting perceptions is inevitable.**

## LAW OF CHANGING LOGOS

**A change in perceptions goes hand-in-hand with a change in thought, words, speech, discourse, philosophy, actions, scientific findings, etc. In other words, it is a revolution/evolution of all aspects of our existence.**

## CURRENT STATUS

Currently (1980s to 2030s), we are in such a period of flux, whereby reductionistic mechanistic thought is rapidly giving way to the new more progressive quantum paradigm. With this metamorphosis, the objective attitude (reductionist, solid state scientific methodology and thought processes) and the unscientific attempts to limit science to the narrow perspective are collapsing. Objective assumptions that things exist in isolation, independent of the larger whole, is no longer valid in the scientific community.

We must learn to regain the deeper perspective and meaning of life. Versatility and depth depends on the individual context in which life is lived! Give it a shallow and trivial context and you end up with a trivial and unfulfilled life. But an understanding of its true deeper context provides the ultimate enthralling, challenging and enlightening spiritual experience.

Such a total experience provides a new perspective. We are no longer centered around the manipulation and domination of objects but rather around an innate reverence for our proper place in the cycle of life and the harmonious co-existence of all things.

## THE ULTIMATE GOAL

To settle for less is to accept a cheap counterfeit of what life is so desperately trying to offer us. Are we willing to continue to let our fears, our educational, scientific, political, professional, cultural, theological and racial prejudices, our false traditions, stand in our way? Or are we willing to open our minds and purge them of all that holds us back from achieving the ultimate purpose and goal of life? This is the grand question that each of us must struggle with and answer. It is the decisive issue that will determine if we truly become a great healer and a great human being. Are you willing to pay the price for such a prize? If so, then welcome to the ultimate struggle and thrill.

# Chapter 51
# CONCLUSIONS

*"When a man's knowledge is not in order, the more*
*of it he has, the greater will be his confusion."*
— Herbert Spencer

## THE GRAND OVERVIEW

We have been able to repeatedly document in this text that the universal laws of healing have been discovered by many cultures and groups throughout the world's history and geography. This is why we refer to them as "universal". While one group calls a law by one name and another by a different name, or one group applies its principles in one manner while  another takes a different tangent, **the basic concept of the law remains intact.**

Yet, with all of this universal wisdom, we have failed to appreciate the genius of each discipline's approach. Spencer's words have accurately described our situation in quantum medicine. This book has provided  data that is adequate to overcome that problem and allow all quantum health care disciplines to appropriate each other and work in close harmony for the benefit of the sick and suffering of the world. This **cooperation will allow us to leave the world a better place than we found it.** And that is the only reason that can justify the space and resources that we each utilize during our stay in mortality.

Together, we can accomplish what was merely each individual's dream. Now is the time to go out and **do it,** to become more educated in other quantum disciplines and work together. When we stop to think about it, an allopathic proctologist and an allopathic psychiatrist really have very little in common and yet in their minds they share an allopathic comradeship.

The comradeship of quantum healing arts makes far more sense than that of the psychiatrist and proctologist. And the sick and suffering of the world will benefit far more from it than any of us can envision. Let us put aside our ignorance and preconceived prejudices and move healing forward to this worthwhile goal at a vastly accelerated rate.

## THE HUNDREDTH MONKEY PRINCIPLE

Scientists have repeatedly observed a very interesting phenomenon, which they have dubbed the "Hundredth Monkey Principle" because it was first observed among the behavior of such primates. This law states, **"When a critical mass of individuals achieve an academic understanding and working knowledge of a particular concept, a spontaneous spreading or ideological breakthrough occurs across individuals of** the group irrespective of the fact that they have or have not studied the principle(s) involved or are in physical proximity of others who have and all members of the group begin to think and respond in a manner congruent with the new knowledge."

In order to preserve expansionistic, vitalistic, quantum healing, a critical mass of healers educated in the true principles of healing must be achieved. To fail to achieve this goal is to abandon the sick and suffering of the world to a future of ever-increasing suffering and woe. The laws set forth in this text are the principles necessary to move healing to this higher level but only if healers are willing to internalize them into their practice and personal life. Only you can make that commitment. The quality of the future depends you. Are you willing to pay the price to be that quality of a leader?

## WHAT IS SCIENTIFIC?

Some will read this text and make brash statements such as, "There is no scientific support for such and such a statement." We need only think of Columbus. Many of the so-called "scientists" of his day told him, "You can't sail west to reach the Orient." Fortunately, he knew otherwise from his own scientific studies.

Currently, our most brilliant electrical engineers freely admit that they do not completely comprehend electricity. Does this mean that the use of electrical appliances such as toasters, radios, TVs, microwaves and even computers are unscientific because we don't completely understand electricity? Of course not!

So-called "science" states, "The bumblebee cannot fly." Such "scientific" inconsistencies bring us to the realization that **science is what is true not what is currently the thinking in vogue.** To quote Shakespeare's Hamlet, "There are more things in heaven and earth, Horatio, than are dream't of in your philosophy." And Einstein wrote, "Science is the attempt to make the chaotic diversity of our sense experience correspond to the logically uniform system of thought."

Time is the great determiner of truth; therefore, I commit this text to the acid test of time. It is my firm conviction that time will prove the controversial issues contained herein to be scientifically (universally) correct.

## FINAL ANALYSIS

In conclusion, we must again remember what Einstein taught, **that we can neither create nor destroy anything only change its state of being. If it is not matter it must be energy or anti-matter.** Therefore, from a scientific, as well as a theological perspective, we have always existed and will always continue to exist. This leads to the inescapable conclusion that **we are not solid state (mortal) beings who only exist temporarily having quantum (spiritual) experiences, but rather we are quantum (spiritual) beings who exist infinitely, in the past and in the future, having a solid state (mortal) experience. Therefore, all healing must focus on the true eternal nature of the being we are attempting to heal.**

Second; ALL healing proceeds according to laws and if we understand and apply these laws, we can be consistent healers. **If we don't properly understand and apply the laws, we will be hit-and-miss healers.**

If you have mastered these grand truths, which are the basic principles taught throughout this text, then you are well on your way to being a true healer. If not, then you are, sadly and in reality, the major threat to the life, health and welfare of your patients.

We must constantly keep in mind and evaluate ourselves in light of the old adage, **"Forever learning but never coming to an understanding of the truth."** Many potentially great healers search for it throughout their entire lifetimes but are unable to identify, comprehend and apply truth in their personal and professional lives. They are their own roadblock. The ultimate question each of us must answer is, **"Am I willing to pay the price?"** If not, then why become a practitioner? Let each of us accept the goal of becoming part of the answer and not part of the problem.

## THE ULTIMATE GOAL

Remember, **the ultimate goal of all quantum complementary healers is to work ourselves out of a job. To assist the human race, through personal, social, scientific and professional responsibility, in arriving at a point where we are living in harmony with the universal laws and, therefore, there is no dis-ease at any level of any of our total beings.**

## THE BEGINNING OR THE END

This book is not the ultimate end but rather it is the beginning. In time, the text will have to be revised in order to remain current, not because the universal laws have changed but because we have discovered more laws and our understanding and ability to more effectively utilize them has increased. This is the natural result of being more and more in tune with the Universal Intelligence.

# REFERENCES

## SELECTED REFERENCES FOR BOOK I: FRESHMAN TEXT


Barnett, L., The Universe And Dr. Einstein, W. Sloane Associates, 1948

Black, Inner Wisdom: The Challenge Of Contextual Healing, Tapestry Press, 1990

Carrel, A., Man, The Unknown, Harper Brothers, 1935

Crile, G., A Bipolar Theory Of Living Processes, Macmillan Co., 1926

Crile, G., The Phenomenon Of Life, W. W. Norton & Co., 1936

Cerasoli, P., The Science And Logic Of Chiropractic, 8th Ed., 1956

Floyd, E., Hinze, J., Liu, R., Wilcher, C., 21st Century Chiropractic: The Neuropathophysiological And Quantum Physics Components Of Homeopathy, Acupuncture And Endocrinology, Digest Of Chiropractic Economics, Vol. 33, 6, May/June, 1991

Hahnemann, S., Organon Of Medicine, 6th Ed., J. P. Tarcher, Inc., 1982

Inlander, C., Take This Book To The Hospital With You, Pantheon Books, 1991

Kaptchuk, T., The Web That Has No Weaver; Understanding Chinese Medicine, Congdon & Weed, 1983

Kent, J. T., Lectures On Homeopathic Philosophy: Fundamental Doctrines In Healing, North American Books, 1981

Kent, J. T., New Remedies, Clinical Cases, Lesser Writings, Aphorisms And Precepts, B. Jain Publishers Pvt. Ltd., 1994

Manning, C., Vanrenen, L., Bioenergetic Medicines, East And West; Acupuncture And Homeopathy, North Atlantic Books, 1988

Ouspensky, P., A New Model of the Universe: Principles of the Psychological Method in the Application To Problems Of Science, Religion And Art, Vintage Books, 1971

Ouspensky, P., The Fourth Way, Vintage Books, 1971

Palmer, B. J., Chiropractic Clinical Controlled Research, W. B. Conkey Co., 1951

Palmer, D. D., The Science, Art And Philosophy of Chiropractic, Portland Publishing House Co., 1910

Peat, F., Briggs, J., Turbulent Mirror: An Illustrated Guide To Chaos Theory And The Science Of Wholeness, 1989

Peat, F., Einstein's Moon: Bell's Theorem And The Curious Quest For Quantum Reality, 1990

Peat, F., Philosopher's Stone: Chaos, Synchronicity, And The Hidden Order Of The World, 1991

Peat, F., Lighting The Seventh Fire: The Spiritual Ways, Healing And Science Of The Native American, Birch Lane Press Book, 1994

Sakar, B., Hahnemann's Organon With Commentary, Battacharyya & Co., 1987

Speransky, A. D., A Theory For The Basis Of Medicine, International Publishers, 1943

Stephenson, R., Chiropractic Textbook, Vol. XIV, Palmer School Of Chiropractic, 1927

Tole, D., Chiropractic And Homeopathy, The Prover: The Journal Of The Academies Of Homeopathy, Vol. 7, No. 2, Summer, 1996

Vithoulkas, G., The Science Of Homeopathy, Grove Press, 1980

Wilcher, C., Heritage Of Naturopathy Medicine, Journal Of Naturopathic Medicine, Vol. 2, No. 4, October, 1984

Wilcher, C., Liu, R., Floyd, E., Plant, R., Roder, C., Beyond The mechanical Subluxation: The Science, Art and Philosophy Of Comprehensive Chiropractic, Digest of Chiropractic Economics, Parts I - VI, Vol. 35, No. 6, May/June, 1993 to Vol. 36, No. 7, September/October, 1994

Wilcher, C., The Chronic Subluxation Complex, 2nd National Subluxation Conference, 1994

Wilson, G., The 2nd Factor In Chiropractic, 2nd Ed., Standard Research Laboratories, 1959

# SELECTED REFERENCES FOR BOOK II: SOPHOMORE TEXT

Choudhuey, H., Indications Of Miasmas, Jain Publishers Pvt. Ltd., 1991

Hahnemann, S., Organon Of Medicine, 6th Ed., J. P. Tarcher, 1982

Hahnemann S., Dudgeon, R., Organon Of Medicine, 5th & 6th Ed., B. Jain Publishers Pvt. Ltd., 1990

Health Returns In Cycles, Parker Chiropractic Research Foundation, 1994

Kent, J. T., Lectures On Homeopathic Philosophy: Fundamental Doctrines In Healing, North Atlantic Books, 1991

Kent, J. T., New Remedies, Clinical Cases, Lesser Writings, Aphorisms And Precepts, B. Jain Publishers Pvt. Ltd,. 1991

Lindlahr, H., Philosophy Of Natural Therapeutics, Vol. I, Maidstone Osteopathic Clinic, 1975

Palmer, D. D., The Science, Art And Philosophy Of Chiropractic, Portland Publishing House Co., 1910

Palmer, B. J., Chiropractic Clinical Controlled Research, Vol. XXV, Conkey Co., 1951

Sarkar, B., Organon Of Medicine With Commentary, M. Battacharyya & Co., 1984

Speransky, A. D., A Basis For The Theory Of Medicine, International Publishers, 1943

Stephenson, R., Chiropractic Textbook, Vol. XIV, Palmer School Of Chiropractic, 1927

Vithoulkas, G., The Science Of Homeopathy, Grove Press, 1980

Wilcher, C., Liu, R., Floyd, E., Plant. R, Roder, C., Beyond The Mechanical Subluxation: The Science, Art And Philosophy Of Comprehensive Chiropractic, Digest Of Chiropractic Economics, Part 5, Vol. 36, No. 6, May/June, 1994

# SELECTED REFERENCES FOR BOOK III: JUNIOR TEXT


Acupuncture: A Comprehensive Text, Shanghai College Of Traditional Medicine, Eastland Press, 1988

Airola, P., How To get Well, Health Plus Publications, 1974

Aliviastos, A., Semiconductor Clusters, Nanocrystals And Quantum Dots,Science, 1996

Arnold, E., Rational Fasting, Beneficial Books, 1971

Ball, K., Berry, R., Kunz, E., Li F. et al., From Topographics To Dynamics On Multidimensional Potential Energy Surges Of Atomic Clusters, Science, 1996

Beck, M., Milady's Theory And Practice Of Therapeutic Massage, 2nd Ed., Milady Publishing Co., 1994

Beinfield, H., Korngold, E., Between Heaven And Earth: A guide To Chinese Medicine, Ballantine Books, 1992

Bash Bhagwan, Basic Principles Of Ayurveda, B. Jain Publishers

Becker, R., Sledon, G., The Body Electric: Electromagnetism And The Foundation of Life, W. Morrow Co., 1985

Becker, R., Cross Currents; The Perils Of Electropollution, The Promise Of Electromagnetic Medicine, J. P. Tracher, 1990

Bieler, H., Food Is Your Best Medicine, Vintage Books, 1973

Black, D., Vital Controversy: Why Educated People Are Turning To Chiropractic, Tapestry Press, 1989

Black, D., Inner Wisdom: The Challenge Of Contextual Healing, Tapestry Press, 1990

Bohm, D., Wholeness And The Impicate Order

Boyd, Sheldon, Introduction To The Study Of Disease, 8th Ed., Lea & Febrifer, 1980

Brewster, R., McEwwn, W., Organic Chemistry, 2nd Ed., Prentice-Hall, 1963

Channana Dev Raj, The Classic Doctrines Of Indian Medicine, B. Jain Publishers

Chappell, P., Emotional Healing With Homeopathy: A Self-Help Manual, Element, 1994

Chavuduka, G., Traditional Healers And The Shona Patient, Gwelo Mambo Press, 1978

Chinese Acupuncture And Moxibustion, Foreign Language Press, 1990

Choudhary, H., Indications Of Miasmas, Jain Publishers (P) Ltd., 1991

Coulter, H., Homeopathic Science And Modern Medicine: the Physics Of Healing With Microdoses, North Atlantic Books, 1981

Coulter, H., Divided Legacy: The Conflict Between Homeopathy  And The American Medical Association, North Atlantic Books, 1982

Brown, J., Among The Bantu Nomads, 1926

Dachs, A., Livingstone: Missionary Explorer, Salisbury Central African Association, 1973

DeCava, J., The Real Truth About Vitamins And Antioxidants

Dennis, C., The Role Of Dinagka Tsa Setswana From The 19th Century To The Present, Botswana Notes And Records, Vol. 10, 1978

Diamond, H., Diamond, M., Fit For Life II: Living Health, Warner Books, 1987

Du Toit, B., Abdalla, I., African Healing Strategies, Trado-Medic Books, 1985

Fabrega, H., Toder, P., African Health And Healing Systems, University Of California Press, 1982

Gelfand, M., Livingstone The Doctor: His Life And Travels, A Study In Medical History, Oxford, 1957

Gerber, R., Vibrational Medicine, Bear & Co., 1988

Hahnemann, S., Dodgeon, R., Organon Of Medicine, 5th & 6th Ed., B. Jain Publishers (P) Ltd., 1990

Harner, M., The Way Of The Shaman, Bantam Books, 1982

Hinkson, D., Don't Mortgage Your Life For Your Health III, New Ideas For Nutritional Healing

History And Culture Of The Incas, 1960

Homewood, A. E., The Neurodynamics Of The Vertebral Subluxation, 1962

Hulbert, R., The Sun Is Always Shining, Arrow Graphics, 1996

I-Lok, C., Macon, N., Acupuncture And Moxibustion: A Handbook For The Barefoot Doctors Of China, 1975

Illich, I., Medical Nemesis, Modern Medical Mistakes, Indiana University Press, 1978

Inglis, B., The Case For Unorthodox Medicine, Berkley Medallion Book, 1969

Irons, V. E., There Is A Difference Between Man's And Nature's Handiwork, Whether It Be In Soil, Foods, Vitamins Or Food Supplements: The Chromatograms Show The Difference, 1960

Juhan, D., Job's Body: A Handbook For Bodywork, Station Hill Press, 1987

Kamal, H., Encyclopedia Of Islamic Medicine, General Egyptian Book Organization, 1975

Kapchuk, T., The Web That Has No Weaver: Understanding Chinese Medicine, Condon & Weed, 1983

Kent., J. T., Lectures On Homeopathic Philosophy, North Atlantic Books, 1981

Kent, J. T., New Remedies, Clinical Cases, lesser Writings, Aphorisms And Precepts, B. Jain Publishers (P) Ltd., 1996

Kervran, C., Biological Transmutation, Beekman Publishers, Inc., 1980

Knapp, D., Gesundheit: Erkntnis des Ledens, Jarl F. Verlag, 1983

Kraines, S., Thetford, E., Managing Your Mind, Macmillan Co., 1943

Kuntz, D., Boiling Energy: Community Healing Among The Kalahari 'Kung

Lappe, M. When Antibiotics Fail, North Atlantic Books, 1986

Lee, R., Hanson, W., Protomorphology: The Principles Of Cell Auto-Regulation, Lee Foundation For Nutritional Research, 1947

Lesmore, F., The Shaman And Modern Medicines, El Palacio XLII Nos. 45-46

Feb. 10, 1937

Lewis, A., Hormesis And Homeopathy, Professional Health Products, Ltd., 1995

Liu, K., Cruzan, J., Saykally, R., Water Clusters, Science, 1996

Lindlar, H., Philosophy Of Natural Therapeutics, Vol. I, Maidstone Osteopathic Clinic, 1975

Lindlar, H., Natural Therapeutics, Vol. II, C. W. Daniel Co., Ltd.

Livingston, C., Cancer: A New Breakthrough, Publishing House Publishers, 1972

Manning, C., Vanrenen, L., Bio-Energetic Medicine: East And West: Acupuncture And Homeopathy, North Atlantic Books, 1988

Means, P., Ancient Civilizations Of The Andes, 1931

Mendelson, R., Confessions Of A Medical Heretic, Contemporary Books, Inc., 1979

Mincin, J., The Whole Truth About Vitamin Supplements, 1993

Moinuddin, H., The Book Of Sufi Healing, Inner Traditions International, 1991

Murry, R., Natural vs Synthetic, Life vs death, Truth vs Lies, Selene River Press, 1995

Murry, R., Doctor's Seminar On Nutrition

Pauling, L., New Dynamics Of Preventive Medicine, 1974

Ott, J., Health And Light, Pocket Books, 1976

Peat, F., Lighting The Seventh Fire: The Spiritual Ways, Healing And Science Of The Native American, Birch Lane Press Book, 1994

Peterson, A. R., Segmental Neuropathy: The First Evidence Of Developing Pathology, Canadian Memorial Chiropractic College

Pottenger, F., Pottenger's Cats: A Study In Nutrition, 1938

Pottenger, F., Symptoms Of Visceral Disease, C. V. Mosby Co., 1944

Pribram, K., Quantum Information Processing In Brain Systems And The Spiritual Nature Of Mankind, Frontier Perspectives, Vol. 6, No. 1, Fall/Winter, Temple University, 1997

Reckeweg, H., Homotoxicology: Illness And Healing By Antihomotoxic Therapy, Menaco Publishing Co., 1980

Reid, B., Aspects Of Intangible Energy Functions In Biosystems, Frontier Perspectives, Vol. 5, No. 1, Fall/Winter, Temple University, 1995

Rubik, B., Energy Medicine And The Unifying Concept Of Information, Hemi-Sync Journal, Vol. XV, No. 1, Winter, 1997

Sarkar, B. K., Hahnemann's Organon With Commentary, M. Battacharyya & Co., (P) Ltd., 1984

Sankaran, R., The Spirit Of Homeopathy, Homeopathic Medical Publishers, 1991

Sankaran, R., The Science Of Homeopathy, Homeopathic Medical Publications, 1994

Schapere, I., Livingstone's Private Journals, 1851 - 1853, 1960

Schmid, F., Profile: Water Clusters, Biological Therapy, Vol. XIV, No. 3, 1996

Sharma, P., Ayurvedic Medicine: Past And Present, Krishnadas Academy, 1987

Sharma Shiva, The System Of Ayurveda, B. Jain Publishers

Sheldrake, R., The New Science Of Life, J. P. Tarcher, 1981

Shepard, D., Homeopathy In Epidemic Diseases, Health Science Press, 1981

Speransky, A. D., The Basis For The Theory Of Medicine, International Publishers, 1943

Steiger, B., Medicine Power: The American Indian's Revival Of His Spiritual Heritage And Its Relevance For Modern Man, Doubleday & Co., 1974

Stephenson, R. W., Chiropractic Textbook, Vol. XIV, Palmer School Of Chiropractic, 1948

Stone, E., Medicine Among The American Indians, Paul B. Hoeber, 1932

Tadlock, D., Tadlock, B., Teachings From The American Earth: Indian Religion And Philosophy, Liveright, 1975

Taggart, L., Medical Madness: How To Prevent The Leading Cause Of Poor Health, LLC, 1995

Talbot, M., The Holographic Universe, Harper Perennial, 1992

Tilden, J., Toxemia: The Basic Cause Of Disease, Natural Hygiene Press, 1974

Tipler, F., The Physics Of Immortality, Doubleday, 1994

Tole, D., Miasmas: A Theoretical Review Of An Antiquated Concept, The Prover: The Journal Of the Academies Of Homeopathy, Vol. 7, No. 1, Spring, 1996

Tole, D., Chiropractic And Homeopathy, The Prover: The Journal Of The Academies Of Homeopathy, Vol. 7, No. 2, Summer, 1996

Tushnet, L., The Medicine Man, St, Martin's Press, 1971

Turnbull, C., The Forest People

Udupa, K., Science And Philosophy Of Indian Medicine, B. Jain Publishers

Ullman, D., Homeopathy: Medicine For The 21st Century, North Atlantic Books, 1988

Vathoulkas, G., The Science Of Homeopathy, Grove Press, 1980

Verner, J., The Science And Logic Of Chiropractic, P. J. Cerasoli, 1956

Watkins, R., All Or None, Digest Of Chiropractic Economics, March/April, 1975

*The Universal Laws of Healing*

Wendal, P., Standardized Naturopathy: The Science And Art Of Natural Healing, P. Wendal, 1951

Wilson, G., The 2nd Factor In Chiropractic, Standard Research Laboratories, 1959

Williams, R., Kalita, D., A Physician's Handbook On Orthomolecular Medicine, Pergamon Press, 1977

Wilson, G., Emotions In Sickness, Standard Research Laboratories, 1963

Wilson, G., A New Slant On Diet, Standard Research Laboratories

Wolfe, F., Space - Time And Beyond: Towards An Explanation Of The Unexplainable, Bantam Books, 1982

Wolfe, F., The Body Quantum: The New Physics Of Body, Mind And Health, Macmillan Publishing Co., 1986

Wolfe, F., Parallel Universes; The Search For Other Worlds, Touchstone, 1988

Wolfe, F., Taking The Quantum Leap: The New Physics For Non-Scientists, Perennial Library, 1989

Wolfson, E., From The Earth To Beyond The Sky: Native American Medicine, Houghton Mifflin Co., 1993

Wysong, R.L., Wysong Catalogue, 1998

Yang Jwing-Ming, Chinese Qigong Massage, YMAA Publication Center, 1992

Zimmerman, M., Phytochemicals And Disease Prevention, Alternative & Complementary Therapies, April/May, 1995


# SELECTED REFERENCES FOR BOOK IV: SENIOR TEXT

Barton, A., Communities In Disaster: A Social Analysis Of Collective Stress Situations, Doubleday & Co., 1969

Bascom, R., Wiles, S., Nasal Inhalation Challenges Studies: An Approach To The Study Of Health Effects Of Indoor Air Pollutants, Indoor Air 90, 5th International Conference On Indoor Air Quality And Climate, 1990

Bell, I., Environmental Illness And Health: The Controversy And Challenge Of Clinical Ecology For Mind-Body Health, Advances, 1987

Bares, P, et al., Ten-Year Mortality Study Of the Population Involved In The Seveso Incident In 1976, American Journal Of Epidemiology, 1989

Bechuana, A., Investigation Of The mechanism Of Action Of Atmospheric Pollutants On The Central Nervous System And Comparative Evaluation Of Methods Of Study, Environmental Health Perspectives, 1976

Boil, T., Vaccinations Don't Work, Health Consciousness, Vol. 13, No. 5, 1992

Buttram, G., Live Vaccines and Genetic Mutation, Health Consciousness, April, 1990

Colubris, E, Pollutants And High Risk Groups: The Biological Basis Of Increased Human Susceptibility To Environmental And Occupational Pollutants, John Wiley & Sons, 1978

Campbell, D., The Riddle of the Mozart Effect, Natural Health, January-February 1998

Cartwright, F., Bibb, M., Disease and History, Dorset Press, 1972

Chaitow, L., Vaccination and Immunization: Dangers, Delusions and Alternatives, C. W. Daniel Co., 1987

Chaltin, L., Vaccination Damages, A Surprising and Frightening Reality, The Prover: The Journal of the Academies of Homeopathy, Vol. 7, No. 3, Fall, 1996

Chishti, S., The Book of Sufi Healing, Inner Traditions International, 1991

Cone, J., Hodgson, M., Problem Buildings: Buildings Associated Illness And The Sick Building Syndrome, Occupational Medicine: State Of The Art Reviews, 1989

Coulter, H., Vaccination, Social Violence and Criminality: The Medical Assault on the American Brain

Coulter, H., Fisher, B., A Shot In the Dark, Abery Publishing Group, Inc., 1982

Crump, K., et al., Cancer Incidence Patterns in the Denver Metropolitan Area in Relation to the Rocky Flats Plant, American Journal of Epidemiology, Vol. 126, No. 1, 1987

Dettman, G., Viral Vaccines: Vital Or Vulnerable, Health Consciousness, Vol. 14, No. 3, August, 1998

Eizayaga, F., Treatise on Homeopathic Medicine, Edicones Maracel, 1991

Fisher, J., The Plague Makers: How We Are Creating Catastrophic New Epidemics - And What We Must Do To Avert Them, Simon & Schuster, 1994

Gaublomme, K., Vaccinations, A Bad Case of Scientific, Homeopathic Link, 1994

Garrett, L., The Coming Plague, Penquin Books, 1994

Gershon, S., Shaw, F., Psychiatric Sequelae Of Chronic Exposure To Organophosphorus Insecticides, Lancet, 1961

McNeill, W., Plagues and People, Doubleday Books, 1989

Golden, I., Vaccination: A Review of Risk and Alternatives, Blessington Word Service, 1989

Hagidikian, B., Media Monopoly, 3rd Ed., Beacon Press, 1990

Hanford Thyroid Disease Study, Fred Hutchinson Cancer Research Center, August, 1994

Howard, A., An Agricultural Testament, Oxford Press

Hoye, R., Parasites: Are They Misdiagnosed In The U.S.?, Part I, The Prover: The Journal of the Academies of Homeopathy, Vol. 7, No. 3, Fall, 1996

Hoye, R., Parasites: Are They Misdiagnosed In The U.S.?, Part II, The Prover: The Journal of the Academies of Homeopathy, Vol. 7, No. 4, Winter, 1996

Hume, D., Decamp or Pasteur, Essence of Health, 1989

Jensen, B., Anderson, M., Empty Harvest

Kratz, A., Vaccinations and Their Toxic Effects, The Prover: The Journal of The Academies of Homeopathy, Vol. 7, No. 3, Fall, 1996

Lappe, Germs That Won't Die

Liebig, V., The Natural Laws Of Husbandry

Lise-Gotzsche, A., The Fluoride Question: Panacea Or Poison? Stein & Day, 1975

Mangano, J., Cancer Mortality Near Oak Ridge, Tennessee, International Journal Of Health Sciences, Vol. 24, No. 3, 1994

Maniquet, X., Survival: How To Prevail In Hostile Environments, Barnes and Noble, 1996

Mendelsohn, R., Confessions of a Medical Heretic, Contemporary Books, Inc., 1979

Merisgaard, M., Black Water, Poisoned Lives, The Independent, 1991

Miller, Z., Vaccines: Are They Really Safe and Effective?, New Atlantean Press, 1993

Molhave, L., et al., Human Reactions To Low Concentrations Of Volatile  Organic Compounds, Environmental International, 1986 1967

Neustaefter, R., The Immunization Decision, North Atlantic Books, 1990

Neustaefter, R., The Vaccine Guide: Making An Informed Choice, North Atlantic Books, 1996

Nussbaum, R., Kohnlein, W., Inconsistencies and Open Questions Regarding Low Dose Health Effects of Ionizing Radiation, Environmental Health Perspectives, Journal of the National Institute of Environmental Health Sciences, Vol. 102, No. 8, August, 1994

Preston, R., The Hot Zone, Doubleday Books, 1994

Radiation Health Effects: An Overview, Hanford Health Information Network, Vol. 1, Winter, 1993-94

Radiation Health  Effects and Hanford, Hanford Health Information Network, 1995

Radionuclides in the Columbia River: Possible Health Problems in Humans and Effects on Fish, Hanford Health Information Network, 1995

Russia's Secret Cities, The Economist, 1994

Scheibner, V., Vaccination, Australia Print Group, 1993

Scheibner, V., One Hundred Years of Orthodox Research Shows That Vaccines Represent the Medical Assault on the Immune System

Schmidt, M., Smith, L., Sehnert, K., Beyond Antibiotics, North Atlantic Books, 1994

Sheppard, D., Homeopathy in Epidemic Diseases, Health Science Press, 1981

Skousen, W. C., The Miracle Of America, The Freeman Institute, 1980

Skousen, W. C., The American Heritage and Constitutional Study Course, The Freeman Institute

Steele, K., Making Warheads, Hanford's Bitter Legacy, Bulletin of Atomic Scientists, 1988

Scheibner, V., Vaccination: One Hundred Years of Orthodox Research Shows That Vaccines Represent the Medical Assault on the Immune System

Stevens, W., Leukemia in Utah and Radioactive Fallout From The Nevada Test Site, Journal of the American Medical Association, Vol. 264, No. 5, 1990

Technical Steering Panel, Hanford Environmental Dose Reconstruction Project, Fact Sheet No. 2, No. 16, 20 May, 1989, revised February, 1992

Technical Steering Panel, Hanford Environmental Dose Reconstruction Project, Fact Sheet No. 12, The Green Run, March, 1992

The Release of Radioactive Materials from Hanford: 1944-1972, Hanford Health Information Network, Winter, 1994

The Vaccine Reaction, Vol. 1 , No. 3, July, 1995

Tilden, J., Toxemia: The Basic Cause Of Disease, Health Hygiene Press, 1974

Tole, D., Vaccination Has Nothing to do With Immunization, The Prover: The Journal of the Academies of Homeopathy, Vol. 7, No. 3, Fall, 1996

Tole, D., The Microbial Wars: Homeopathy Versus the Micropredator, The Prover: The Journal of the Academies of Homeopathy, Vol., 7, No. 4, Winter, 1996

Waldbott, G., Health Effects Of Environmental Pollutants, C. V. Mosby Co., 1973

Walene, J., Immunization: The Reality Behind the Myth, Bergin & Garvey, 1995

Weisenberger, S., Parasites: An Epidemic In Disguise, Healing Within Products, 1993

Whooping Cough: The DPT Vaccine and Reducing Vaccine Reactions, National Vaccine Information Center, 1989

Wilcher, C., Philosophy 303, What Does the Future Hold?, The Prover: The Journal of the Chiropractic Academies of Homeopathy, Vol. 6, No. 2, Summer, 1995

Wollan, M., Controlling The Potential Hazards Of Government Sponsored Technology, George Washington Law Review, Vol. 36, No. 5, July, 1968

Wysong, R. L., Wysong Catalogue, 1998

Zimmerman, B., Zimmerman, D., Killer Germs: Microbes and Disease That Threaten Humanity, Henry Holt & Co., 1994

# SELECTED REFERENCES FOR BOOK V: POST-DOCTORAL TEXT

Amato, I., A New Blueprint for Water's Architecture, Science, 22 June, 1992

Asimov, I., The Gods Themselves, Doubleday, 1972

Bass, L., A Quantum Mechanical Mind-Body Interaction, Foundation of Physics, Vol. 5, No. 1, 1975

Becker, R., Seldon, G., The Body Electric: Electromagnetism And The Foundation of Life, William McMorrow & Co., 1985

Black, D., The Need to Broaden the Law, Share International, 1995

Black, D., Choreographing the Dance of Life, Share International, Vol. XXXVI, No. 439, September, 1996

Black, D., Mutually Helpful Relationships, Share International, No. 5259, 1997   Bryant, R., Water at the Protein Surface, Frank, F., Biophysics of Water, John Wiley & Sons, 1982

Bohm, D., Wholeness and the Implicate Order, Bantam Books, 1974

Bohr, N., Light and Life, Atomic Physics and Human Knowledge, Wiley, 1958

Caro, P., Water, McGraw-Hill, 1993

Clegg, J., Alternative Views on the Role of Water in Cell Functions Frank, F., Biophysics of Water, Wiley & Sons, 1982

Davis, K., Day, J., Water: The Mirror of Science, Anchor Books, 1961

Davis, P., God and New Physics, Simon & Schuster, 1983

DeWitt, B., Quantum Mechanics and Reality, Physics Today, September, 1970

DeWitt, B., Grahm, N., The Many Worlds Interpretation of Quantum Physics, Princeton University press, 1973

Doolittle, F., Proteins, In the Molecules of Life, W. H. Freeman, 1985

Driesch, H., Science and Philosophy of Organisms, 1908

Epstein, L., Relativity Visualized, Insight Press, 1983

Gurber, R., Vibrational Medicine, Bear & Co., 1988

Homewood, A., The Chiropractor and the Law, Chiropractic Publications of Canada, 1961

Horrobin, D., The Philosophical Basis of Peer Review - And the Suppression of Innovation, Journal of the American Medical Association, 9 March, 1990

Hoyle, F., The Intelligent Universe, Holt, Rinehart & Winston, 1983

Kent, J., Lectures on Homeopathic Philosophy: Fundamental Doctrines in Healing, North Atlantic Books, 1981

Pannisi, E., Water, Water Everywhere, Science News, 20 February, 1993

Pierre Teilhard de Chardin, The Phenomenon of Man, 1959

Platt, R., Water: The Wonder of Life, Prentice-Hall, 1971

Rubik, B., Energy Medicine and the Unified Concept of Information, Hemi-Sync Journal, Vol. XV, No. 1, Winter, 1997

Sarkar, B., Hahnemann's Organon with Commentary Bhattacharya & Co., 1984

Schmid, F., Profile: Water Clusters, Biological Therapy, Vol. XIV, No. 3, 1996

Scholten, J., Homeopathy and the Elements, Stiching Alonnissos, 1996

Sharma, P., Ayurvedic Medicine: Past and Present, Karishnadas Academy, 1987

Sheldrade, R., The Presence of the Past, Random House, 1988

Skolimoweski, H., The Participatory Mind, 1994

Skolimoweski, H., The Participatory Universe And Its New Methodology, Frontier Perspectives, The Center for Frontier Sciences at Temple University, Vol. 5, No. 2 Spring/Summer, 1996

Stillinger, F., Water, Learner, R., Trigg, G., Encyclopedia of Physics, VCH Publishers, 1991

Toben, B., Wolf, F., Space-Time and Beyond: Toward an Explanation of the Unexplainable, Bantam Books, 1987

Talbot, M., Beyond the Quantum, Bantam, Macmillan Publishing Co., 1968

Tailbot, M., The Holistic Universe, Harper Collins, 1991

Wendel, P., Standardized Naturopathy: The Science and Art of Natural Healing, 1951

Wheeler, J., The Universe as Home for Man, The American Scientist, November/December, 1974

Whitmont, E., Psyche and Substance: Essays on Homeopathy in Light of Jungian Psychology, North Atlantic Books, 1980

Whitmont, E., The Role of Mind in Health, Disease and the Practice of Homeopathy, Frontier Perspectives, The Center for Frontier Sciences at Temple University, Vol. 5, No. 2, Spring/Summer, 1996

Wolf, F., The Body Quantum: The New Physics of Body, Mind and Health, Macmillan Publishing Co., 1966

Wolf, F., Taking the Quantum Leap: The New Physics for Non-Scientists, Perennial Library, 1989

Wolf, F., Parallel Universes: The Search for Other Worlds, Touchstone Books, 1990

# INDEX

## CCC





## DDD

## EEE



## FFF

Microwaves 268–269

Military 269

Minerals 122

Mission 25

Mohammed 191, 192, 193

Morphic fields 354

Mortimer 243

Moses 151

Mozart 272–273

   Mozart Effect 273

Multidimensional 6, 90, 98, 342

Multiple Being 13

Muranaka 260

Murray 64, 161

Muses 271

Music 272–273

Mutations 156, 246–247, 299

Myelin sheath 106, 248

## NNN

NASA flu 260

Native American Medicine 7, 198. *See* Medicine: Native American and Oceanic

Natural dis-ease 37, 74

Natural disaster 41, 255

Naturopathic Medicine 141, 184, 212. *See also* Medicine: Naturopathic

Navajo 133

Nazi 260, 290

Neafsey 116

Neuro-endrocrine

   behavioral disorders 261

Newtonian 7, 10, 139, 212, 339

Ngaka 70

Niebuhr 201

Non-corporal 3, 7, 9, 13, 19, 35, 82, 99, 103, 143, 148, 207, 209, 329

Num 70, 169

Nutriceuticals 160

Nutrition 144, 153. *See also* Medicine: Nutrition

## OOO

Obstetricians 252

Oceanic Medicine. *See* Medicine: Native American and Oceanic

Organophosphates 260

Oriental Medicine 7, 169, 198, 324. *See also* Medicine: Oriental

Ostrander 273, 274

Ott 275

Oxidizers 167–168

## PPP

Pain 13–14, 74, 99, 104, 147, 149

Palliative vs. healing 40, 229, 288

Palmer, B.J. 16, 23, 59, 95, 107, 311

Palmer, D.D. 16, 81, 84, 87, 91, 92–93, 95, 99, 101, 102, 104, 105, 106, 203, 208, 212, 275

Paracelsus 41, 95, 116

Paradigm 5–6, 353

   change of 355

   departure, law of 356

   energy 9–10

   flux of thought 353–354

   goal 356

   information 342–343

   lessons of history 355–356

   logos 356

   morphic fields 354

     research 354–355

   similimum programming 355

   status 356

Parasite 251

Passion 13–14

Pasteur 49, 62, 64

Patient 47, 49, 53

   closed 45, 231, 232

   open 45, 230, 233

Pauling 161

Peat 135, 138

Pediatricians 244, 252

Peterson 90

Petrochemical 257, 260, 311, 312

## QQQ



## RRR

## UUU



## VVV



## WWW



## YYY

# ABOUT THE AUTHOR

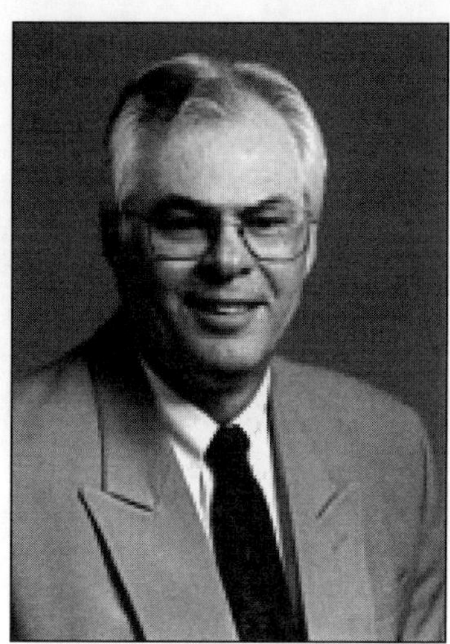

**Dr. C. C. Wilcher** practices acupuncture, chiropractic and naturopathy in Boise, Idaho. He has studied in Europe, Latin America and the Orient, as well as with Indian, Native American and Western healers.

Dr. Wilcher teaches patho-physiology, philosophy, homeopathy and the quantum physics of healing at several colleges. He has authored numerous professional and lay articles, written a newspaper column, and hosted a weekly health care radio talk show.

He has held many professional and academic offices and is a past president of the Board of Homeopathic Examiners, Inc., the inter-professional examining board for homeopathy. He was involved in the successful passage of acupuncture licenser in the State of Idaho, and is currently involved in similar efforts for naturopathic physicians and masseuses.

**Dr. Wilcher is available for the presentation of lectures and workshops.** For more information, contact him by phone at (208) 286-9654 (evenings), or by e-mail at cwilcher@cyberhighway.net

DO YOU HAVE A FRIEND, RELATIVE OR STUDENT
WHO IS INTERESTED IN HEALTH?

THE UNIVERSAL LAWS OF HEALING
MAKES A WONDERFUL GIFT!

Yes, I want to have a personal copy of this book.
Send me _______ copies of **The Universal Laws of
Healing,** by C.C. Wilcher.

Please add $5.00 per book for postage and handling. Idaho residents include 5% state sales tax ($2.25) per book. Make checks payable to :

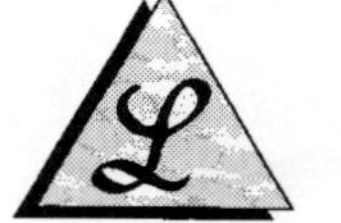

**Legendary Publishing Company
Lorry Roberts, Publisher
P.O. Box 7706
Boise, Idaho 83707-1706
1-800-358-1929**

VISA and MasterCard accepted

Print Name _______________________________

Address _______________________________

City _______________ State _______ Zip _______

**The Universal Laws of Healing**   $45.00  x ___ # books = _______

Postage and Handling            $5.00  x ___ # books = _______

Idaho Sales Tax (ID residents only)   $2.25  x ___ # books = _______

**Enclosed is my check/money order**
                    **for the total amount of  $ _______**

Quantity Orders Invited
For bulk discount prices, please call: (208) 342-7929
Please photo copy this page if additional forms are needed.


DO YOU HAVE A FRIEND, RELATIVE OR STUDENT
WHO IS INTERESTED IN HEALTH?

THE UNIVERSAL LAWS OF HEALING
MAKES A WONDERFUL GIFT!

Yes, I want to have a personal copy of this book.
Send me _______ copies of **The Universal Laws of
Healing,** by C.C. Wilcher.

Please add $5.00 per book for postage and handling. Idaho residents include 5% state sales tax ($2.25) per book. Make checks payable to :

**Legendary Publishing Company
Lorry Roberts, Publisher
P.O. Box 7706
Boise, Idaho 83707-1706
1-800-358-1929**

VISA and MasterCard accepted

Print Name _______________________________

Address _______________________________

City _______________ State _______ Zip _______

**The Universal Laws of Healing**   $45.00  x ___ # books = _______

Postage and Handling            $5.00  x ___ # books = _______

Idaho Sales Tax (ID residents only)   $2.25  x ___ # books = _______

**Enclosed is my check/money order**
                    **for the total amount of  $ _______**

Quantity Orders Invited
For bulk discount prices, please call: (208) 342-7929
Please photo copy this page if additional forms are needed.

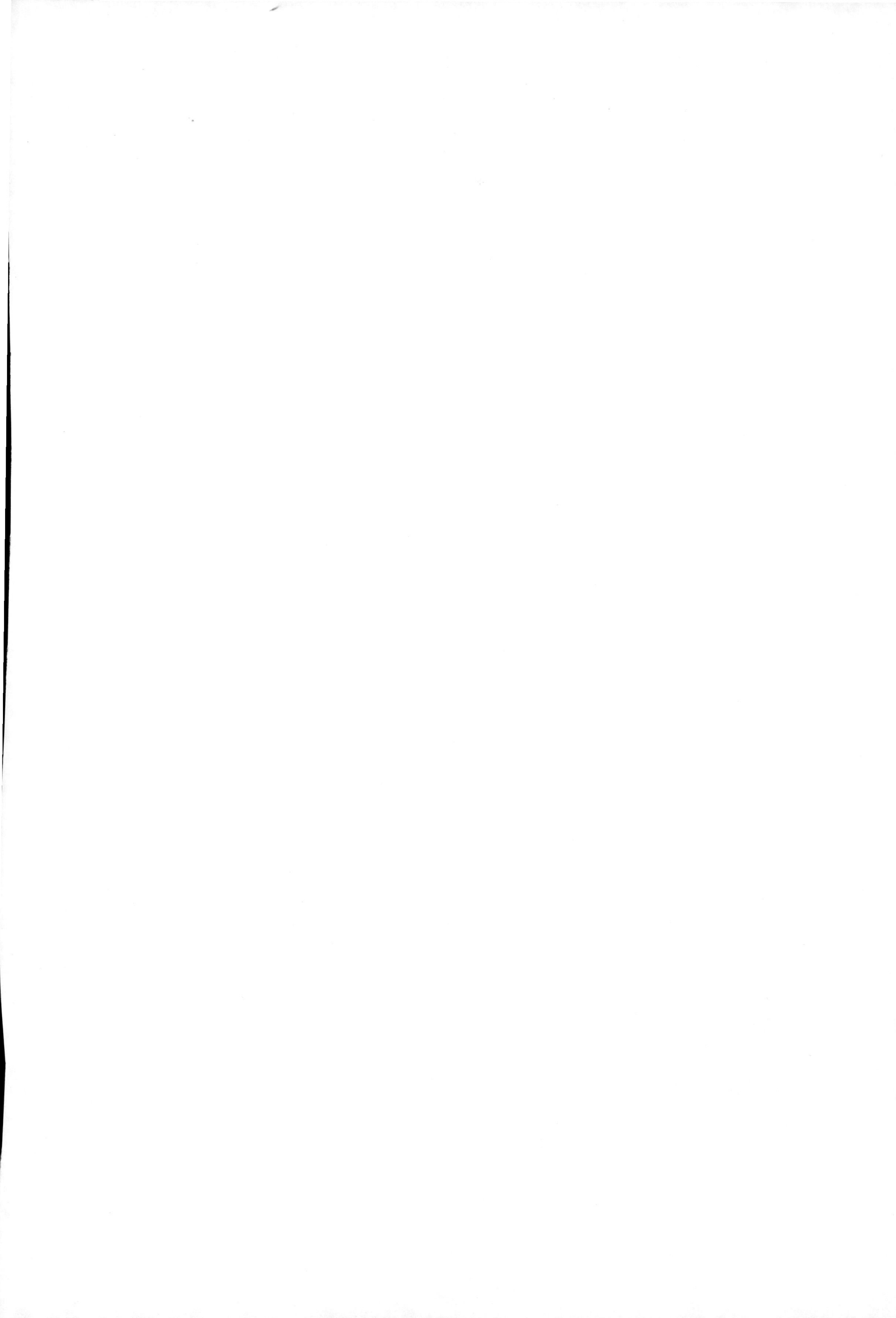